EXPECTING INEQUITY

The MIT Press's publishing mission benefits from the generosity of our donors, including Diana Chapman Walsh.

EXPECTING INEQUITY

How the Maternal Health Crisis Affects Even the Wealthiest Black Americans

KHIARA M. BRIDGES

The MIT Press
Cambridge, Massachusetts
London, England

The MIT Press
Massachusetts Institute of Technology
77 Massachusetts Avenue
Cambridge, MA 02139
mitpress.mit.edu

© 2026 Khiara M. Bridges

All rights reserved. No part of this book may be used to train artificial intelligence systems or reproduced in any form by any electronic or mechanical means (including photocopying, recording, or information storage and retrieval) without permission in writing from the publisher.

The MIT Press would like to thank the anonymous peer reviewers who provided comments on drafts of this book. The generous work of academic experts is essential for establishing the authority and quality of our publications. We acknowledge with gratitude the contributions of these otherwise uncredited readers.

This book was set in Adobe Garamond Pro by New Best-set Typesetters Ltd. Printed and bound in the United States of America.

Library of Congress Cataloging-in-Publication Data is available.

ISBN: 978-0-262-05155-2

10 9 8 7 6 5 4 3 2 1

EU Authorised Representative: Easy Access System Europe, Mustamäe tee 50, 10621 Tallinn, Estonia | Email: gpsr.requests@easproject.com

Contents

Introduction: "I Think I'm Dying"—Class Privilege and the Persistence of Racial Disadvantage *1*

1. **How We Got Here: The Peculiar (But Not Uncommon) Racial History of San Francisco** *19*
2. **Healthcare Segregation in the City by the Bay** *45*
3. **The Many Contributors to Racial Disparities in Maternal Mortality** *87*
4. **Covering the Black Maternal Health Crisis** *117*
5. **Going to the Doctor in Yale Sweatpants: Techniques for Avoiding Racial Disadvantage During the Clinical Encounter** *143*
6. **The Racially Concordant Care Intervention (and Its Discontents)** *181*

Conclusion: If We Really Cared—How to Solve the Black Maternal Health Crisis *223*

Acknowledgments *227*
Notes *231*
Bibliography *269*
Index *295*

Introduction: "I Think I'm Dying"— Class Privilege and the Persistence of Racial Disadvantage

In February 2022, I began my research in the obstetrics department at Golden Health,[1] a world-renowned academic medical center offering state-of-the-art healthcare to the San Francisco Bay Area community. However, my investigations into maternal health had begun more than a decade prior, when I was conducting research at Alpha Hospital, a public hospital in New York City that cares for the city's most marginalized.[2] It was there that I first encountered what is now a well-known, often-heard statistic: Black people die from pregnancy-related causes at three to four times the rate at which white people die.[3] As appalling as that is, it isn't the entire story. A fuller picture of black maternal health in the United States reveals that *racial disparities in maternal mortality persist across income levels and socioeconomic statuses*.[4] Poor black people die from pregnancy-related causes more frequently than poor white people do, middle-class black people die from pregnancy-related causes more frequently than middle-class white people do, and upper-middle-class black people die from pregnancy-related causes more frequently than upper-middle-class white people do.[5] In other words, the higher rates of black maternal deaths in the United States are not because black people disproportionately bear the burdens of poverty, which we know compromises the health of those forced to live in it. Rather, black people have higher rates of maternal deaths than white people *across all income levels*. This devastating fact reveals that racial disparities in maternal mortality are not a problem of class. They are a problem of race—of racism, to be precise.

Further, the fact that wealthier black people die more frequently from pregnancy-related causes than wealthier white people do means that *class privilege is not protecting black people from racism.* That is what led me to Golden Health. I wanted to investigate how racism showed up in the lives of wealthier pregnant black people and, most of all, what wealthier black people were doing to survive pregnancy and childbirth in a country that allows so many black people to fall victim to preventable deaths from pregnancy-related causes. This book details what I've learned.

From my first day at Golden Health, I saw clear differences between it and Alpha Hospital. Yet perhaps the most striking difference was how orderly and efficiently Golden's obstetrics department was run. Indeed, I felt the need to document—to pull out my iPhone and take a picture of—a whiteboard that hung behind the check-in desk to the immediate left of the intake workers' heads. The whiteboard reported when individual providers were running behind schedule, and it gave patients estimated wait times for those providers. While I never witnessed a wait time that was greater than thirty minutes—and while the whiteboard was smugly blank on most days because there were no delays to share—this was not the most remarkable aspect of the whiteboard to me. Instead, I was simply blown away that Golden announced patient wait times. The whiteboard signaled that Golden patients expected to be seen by their provider at their scheduled appointment time and that the clinic understood that not meeting that expectation was an exceptional circumstance, not business as usual. In this way, the whiteboard signaled that Golden Health was light-years away from Alpha Hospital. The pregnant, indigent patients who turned to Alpha for prenatal care could expect to wait *hours* for their scheduled appointments, sometimes spending their entire morning or afternoon waiting to see their provider. This partially explains the confrontations between patients and staff—the smart-alecky exchanges, the hurled curse words, the raised voices—that regularly erupted in Alpha's waiting room. Golden's waiting area was not the site of these types of showdowns.

This is not to say that there were no confrontations in Golden's waiting area. Rather, the confrontations that I observed at Golden were just different. For example, a patient who had recently given birth arrived at her postpartum appointment with her newborn, her husband, and her nanny. Despite the clinic's COVID-19 precautions, which allowed only one guest in the exam room, the patient insisted on bringing all three members of her party into the exam room with her, and she argued her case with Pamela, a medical assistant. The disagreement was resolved when Pamela told Tammy, the midwife who was scheduled to see the patient that day, that the patient refused to be seen if her newborn, husband, and nanny could not accompany her during her exam, and Tammy relented. Tammy later told me, "The policy is there for everyone's safety—mine and theirs. But I'm not going to argue with these entitled patients all day. They don't pay me enough for that." When I later asked Pamela about it, she closed her eyes, squeezed the bridge of her nose, and said, "I. Do. Not. Understand. Why couldn't the nanny wait in the waiting room with the baby? What's the point of bringing your nanny if she's not actually going to look after your kid?"

Over time, the journal in which I recorded the notes that I took at Golden Health was filled with minor observations that collectively described the gulf that existed between Alpha Hospital and Golden. I kept a tally of the number of patients wearing Patagonia jackets, the $240 piece of outerwear that is so ubiquitous among the middle- and upper-middle-classes in the Bay Area that outsiders may mistakenly believe that it is a regional uniform. I jotted down the names of the companies (Apple, Google, Meta, Salesforce, Uber) whose logos were embossed on the backpacks, messenger bags, tote bags, and laptop bags that patients carried—bags that probably had been gifted to them as swag at a company event. I recorded the brand names of the strollers that recently postpartum patients pushed into the clinic (Bugaboo, Nuna, UPPAbaby), and I would be stunned when I looked up the strollers' sticker prices ($1,299.99, $825, and $999.99, respectively). I overheard patients on work calls where they discussed market contractions, growth opportunities, client relationships, change management, and, of course, artificial intelligence. Fifteen years prior, when I sat in the waiting room of Alpha Hospital's obstetrics clinic observing its patients as they came and went, the conversations that I overheard never touched on such things. I was reminded again and again of the enormous gulf that separated Golden and Alpha.

When I began conducting in-depth interviews with the Golden Health patients who generously agreed to talk to me for this book, I discovered that the interviews were invariably as interesting (and fun!) as the ones that I had

had with Alpha Hospital patients. Orchestrating the conversations was a bit of a challenge, however. At Alpha, I could interview patients in the clinic while they waited for their appointments. But things were more complicated at Golden due to the efficiency of its obstetrics clinic, since patients never had to wait very long for their appointments. So to recruit Golden patients for this study, I began by pitching my research project to the patient. If patients expressed an interest in participating, I asked for their contact information, followed up via text message or email, scheduled a time for a Zoom or in-person interview, and then met to conduct the interview. This process was so prolonged that many patients who initially were willing to be interviewed eventually disappeared. (Indeed, I was ghosted by Golden patients more times than I care to admit.) Nevertheless, I managed to interview over two hundred pregnant or recently postpartum people for this book. All of the patients I interviewed were cisgender women, with the exception of one transgender man.

When it was finally time to transcribe my interviews with Golden patients, I noticed that I had spent a good deal of time during the conversations connecting with patients about things that we had in common. One patient and I discovered that we both attended Columbia University at the same time; she was in the business school when I was in the law school. Another patient and I bonded over our love of the Madeira wine made at the V. Sattui Winery in Napa Valley, a vineyard that we both visited whenever we found ourselves in the wine-making area, about an hour's drive north of the city. Another patient and I connected over the highs and lows of book writing. When I saw her in the clinic for her postpartum appointment, she signed a copy of her first book for me, and I signed a copy of my first book for her. These were the types of shared experiences that I never had with the Medicaid-insured, low-income folks who comprised Alpha's patient population.

Nevertheless, there were many things that were common to both Alpha Hospital and Golden Health. The most significant commonality is that they both were places where the United States' failure to protect the health of the nation's pregnant people comes to a head. However, that failure looks different depending on whether it unfolds in sites where poor people receive their healthcare or in sites where the more affluent are cared for.

COMPARING HARMS: MEDICAID VERSUS COMMERCIAL INSURANCE

My fieldwork in Alpha Hospital's obstetrics clinic led me to have a deep and nuanced understanding of New York State's problematic efforts to provide healthcare to the most dispossessed and vulnerable pregnant people living within its borders. I describe these efforts as problematic even though they certainly have prevented many miscarriages, stillbirths, and neonatal deaths and have reduced the incidence of death and severe injury among pregnant and recently postpartum people. However, the government sometimes harms as it helps. There are three harms inflicted by New York State's prenatal care program for Medicaid beneficiaries worth mentioning here. First, because Medicaid insists on addressing the far-ranging and far-reaching injuries that poverty inflicts with an abundance of technology, the pregnant poor cannot opt out of the medicalization of their pregnancies. Their ability to direct their own medical care is denied as they are forced to receive prenatal care from a system that assumes that pregnancy is not a healthy state of the body but rather a medical event that invariably kills if not properly managed. Second, Medicaid denies the wide range of needs, experiences, and capacities of the poor in this country, creating a fictional uniform population on which the government acts. The unique wishes and desires of individual pregnant patients within that larger patient population get lost in the process. Third, the entire system of public healthcare is made politically possible by the idea that it would be bad for *everyone else* if poor people did not receive medical care during their pregnancies. The fear is that without prenatal care, poor folks would give birth to sick children who would require expensive, government-funded healthcare for the rest of their lives and would burden the nation's public schools and social safety net programs. Of course, these narratives unduly and unfairly pathologize the poor.

When I was conducting research at Alpha, I thought about the government a lot. But anyone who is examining healthcare for low-income pregnant people in the United States will find it impossible to avoid thinking about the government, since it is the entity that provides health insurance to the poor in this country. However, the government disappears almost entirely when one examines healthcare for pregnant people who are not poor. This is because in the United States, large portions of the population disparage proposals that would guarantee citizens access to healthcare at all times—although these proposals, if implemented, would make the country more like the other high-income nations that it considers its peers. Naysayers call such schemes "socialist" and deride them as "un-American." They say that America is exceptional and that universal healthcare has no place in the land of the free and the home of the brave. It is because of this commitment to American exceptionalism that the government falls out of view when a study focuses on healthcare for those with some degree of class privilege. For those who are pregnant and not poor in the United States, society does not expect that the government will provide healthcare and guarantee health. Instead, society expects that the *market* will do that work.

When individuals in the United States are class-privileged (and are not serving or have not served in the military), they do not rely on the prenatal care programs that the government furnishes through Medicaid (or to service members and eligible veterans). Instead, they rely either on the health insurance that an employer (theirs, their spouse's, or their parent's) provides or on an individual or family insurance plan that they have purchased from a health insurance exchange. Employer-based health insurance and individual or family health insurance plans are what people who are younger than age sixty-five and who earn above a certain income threshold use to access healthcare in the United States. Importantly, when people under the age of sixty-five attempt to access healthcare after surpassing that income threshold, they have entered a place where the market reigns and the profit motive rules. While the government definitely regulates this side of the healthcare industry, our healthcare system is based on the foundational principle that the private market—and not the government—will generate the highest-quality healthcare at the lowest cost.

Unfortunately, the United States has fallen far short of expectations on both counts. The country has the highest healthcare costs among high-income nations,[6] and the quality of the healthcare provided in the United States is uneven, at best.[7] This is undeniably true in the context of maternal health. The rates of maternal morbidity and mortality in the United States are much higher than those in other high-income nations. As a point of comparison, in the United Kingdom and Canada, nations where the government administers a system of universal healthcare, the maternal mortality rates are close to half the rates in the United States.[8] Notably, while other industrialized nations' maternal mortality rates have been falling, the United States' rates have been steadily increasing. In fact, the United States is one of just thirteen countries that have experienced upticks in their maternal mortality rates over the past twenty-five years.[9] The United States is the only developed country among the thirteen: "Bahamas, Georgia, Guyana, Jamaica, North Korea, St. Lucia, Serbia, South Africa, Suriname, Tonga, United States, Venezuela, and Zimbabwe."[10]

While my focus in this book is on the fact that maternal mortality rates are particularly bad for black people in the United States, it is important to understand that the maternal mortality rates for white people in the country should also be the stuff of national shame. People in twenty-four other industrialized nations have better chances of avoiding a pregnancy-related death than white people in the United States.[11] Yet the state of black maternal health in the United States is even more dire than the terrible state of white maternal health in the country. And this is why I was first drawn to study pregnancy and childbirth in the United States: The tragedy of maternal mortality does not befall racial groups equally.[12] And I was drawn to Golden Health specifically because *even wealthier black people are dying more frequently than wealthier white people during pregnancy, childbirth, and the postpartum period.* Indeed, the most privileged black people have maternal health outcomes that are more dismal than the least privileged white people. As obstetrician and activist Joia Crear-Perry explained in congressional testimony, "A White woman with less than a high school education has a better chance to live in childbirth than a Black woman with a college degree. . . . [A] Black woman who initiates prenatal care in the first trimester has a worse outcome in birth than a white woman with late or no prenatal care."[13] In the compelling words of Crear-Perry, "As a Black mother, I cannot buy or educate my way out of dying at three to four times the rate of a white mother in the United States."[14] Anthropologist Dána-Ain Davis puts it even more bluntly: "To believe that one's educational attainment and insurance coverage will serve as a protective mechanism against adverse birth outcomes in an anti-Black society is ideological pablum and offers a false sense of security."[15]

Startingly, statistics show that racial disparities in maternal mortality actually *increase* as one moves up the socioeconomic ladder. A report released by the Centers for Disease Control and Prevention reveals that black people with less than a high school education are 1.8 times as likely as white people with less than a high school education to die from a pregnancy-related cause.[16] However, black people with a college education or more were 5.2 times as likely as white people with a college education or more to die from a pregnancy-related cause.[17] In other words, the rates at which uneducated black people and uneducated white people die are closer than the rates at which highly educated black people and highly educated white people die. In this way, class privilege leaves black people exposed to a racial inequity that their low-income counterparts manage to avoid.

The same is true in the context of infant mortality.[18] One study relying on data out of California shows that if you are black and poor, your baby is almost twice as likely to die as the baby born to your poor, white counterpart.[19] However, if you are black and wealthy, your baby is 2.5 times more likely to die as the baby born to your wealthy, white counterpart.[20] Again, the rates at which low-income black babies and low-income white babies die are closer than the rates at which wealthier black babies and wealthier white babies die. Thus, class privilege, when enjoyed by black people, produces a distinct type of vulnerability.

What this means is that while the notion that the United States has achieved racial equality is, in most cases, enthusiastically untrue, the country has managed to achieve some degree of racial *equalization* with respect to low-income people's infant and maternal mortality rates. When it comes to the likelihood that a newborn or a pregnant or recently postpartum person will die, race matters less when one is poor than when one is wealthy.

This is a striking fact that must be explained in terms of the Medicaid programs designed to ensure that low-income pregnant people can access prenatal care—the ones that I studied during my research at Alpha Hospital. Moreover, it is likely that Medicaid narrows racial disparities in infant and maternal mortality through the three harms described above—through its denial of poor people's ability to direct their medical care and its insistence on medicalizing pregnancy, its erasure of the vast differences among those who are low income, and its construction of the pregnant poor as a danger to the rest of the nation. That is, Medicaid delivers a uniform program of prenatal care to the poor. By standardizing care, it denies pregnant patients the freedom to direct the course of their care and removes opportunities for providers to exercise discretion. While this standardization problematically limits patient and provider autonomy, *it also reduces racial disparities in infant and maternal mortality*. In so doing, Medicaid serves antiracist goals. In a country where race matters so very much, Medicaid, in the context of infant and maternal mortality, has managed to make race matter just a little less.

Pregnant, class-privileged black people are holders of insurance cards that typically are provided through an employer. These cards allow them an escape from the lower tier of the United States' two-tiered healthcare system. They are free from the standardization, regularization, and forced conformity that Medicaid demands. Yet that freedom from standardization, regularization, and forced conformity comes at a cost: It also frees pregnant, class-privileged black people from a government oversight that, in this context, shields patients from some of the market-driven, profit-maximizing, discretion-packed processes found in the profit-generating side of the healthcare industry. The result is that black people with higher incomes and higher levels of education die more frequently than white people with higher incomes and higher levels of education; their babies suffer the same fate. Class privilege leaves these socioeconomically fortunate black people susceptible to a race-based harm. That irony pulled me to Golden Health, determined to investigate it.

THE FRAGILITY OF THE PROTECTION THAT CLASS PRIVILEGE OFFERS

It is common in the United States to collapse racial disadvantage and class disadvantage, resulting in a misperception that all black people are poor (and, conversely, that all white people are *not* poor). The collapse does more than make class-privileged black people invisible. It also suggests that class-privileged black people, when they are visible, are not racially disadvantaged. According to this logic, graduate degrees from elite universities and high-paying jobs ensure that the black people who obtain them can enjoy freedom from negative experiences due to their race. In the context of healthcare, this logic suggests that wealthier black people never have the demeaning, degrading, demoralizing encounters inside of healthcare institutions that low-income black people frequently report. However, this is a fallacy. Dozens and dozens of black people who spoke with me as I was conducting research for this book shared disturbing experiences that they had once had with healthcare providers. These encounters made vivid for me the fragility of class privilege's ability to shelter wealthier black people from race-based disadvantage. Consider Rita's and Annette's stories.[21]

At the time of our conversation, Rita, who identified as "a black Jew," was forty-five years old and pregnant with her second child. Rita's father, who was a white Jewish man, was a physician until his retirement; her mother, who was black and not Jewish, was a schoolteacher before her death. Rita grew up in Washington, DC, and attended elite private primary and secondary schools. When she was fifteen years old, she traveled to Italy on a trip organized by her high school. While there, she experienced the trauma of what she called "unwanted sex." It was her first sexual experience. Soon after, she developed painful ulcers on her vulva. She was able to return to the United States and seek medical care shortly after the onset of her symptoms. Not ready to tell her parents what had happened to her in Italy, Rita went to the doctor's appointment by herself. The gynecologist that she saw was unaware that Rita was a high-achieving student at a competitive high school, had enjoyed a solidly middle-class upbringing, and had a Jewish father—an aspect of her background that she, in retrospect, believed would have shielded her from what ultimately happened to her during the appointment. (Although she has her father's last name, it is not recognizably Jewish.) The doctor saw only a fifteen-year-old black girl with a sexually transmitted infection. In Rita's recounting, he permitted antiblackness to fill in the details.

Rita said, "The way he treated me.... It was just so extreme. I lost speech because it was so extreme—how awful he was to me." Rita remembered that he said to her, "You're promiscuous. You've brought this on yourself. You're the type of person who would have sex with anyone on the street. You would probably eat garbage out of a trash can." Rita also described her sense during the appointment that if she somehow could have gotten the doctor to understand who she was, he would treat her differently: "I was thinking to myself the whole time, 'Oh, he doesn't know that my father is Jewish.' The doctor was Jewish as well. And I kept thinking, 'If only he knew that my father is Jewish—that he's a Jewish doctor like him. . . .'" Rita told me that the experience was memorable not simply because of the outrageousness of the physician's conduct but because a part of her believed him:

> I already felt stupid that [the sexual assault] had happened to me. I already felt like an idiot and every negative thing. I already felt dirty, disgusting because I had these sores on my vagina. But the cruelest part about the way he treated me was not what he said but that it made sense to me. It didn't roll off my back. It *did* make me feel bad. I now have the wisdom of age. I now have tens of thousands of dollars of therapy under my belt. [laughs] I know that [the sexual assault and the sexually transmitted infection] do not define me. But the gynecologist, that day, he was like, "No. This *does* define you." It took me so long—decades—to learn that he was wrong.

When Rita explained her present-day decision to receive her prenatal care from a black obstetrician, she pointed to her first gynecology appointment.

Consider Annette as well, who was in her mid-thirties when she became pregnant with her first and only child—her now five-year-old daughter. Annette earned her law degree from an elite university and worked as a lawyer for a nonprofit in the Bay Area. She described herself as multiracial; however, "if I have to check one box, I check 'black.'" I talked to Annette about her pregnancy over Zoom during the worst of the pandemic in 2020 as her little girl popped in and out of frame throughout the conversation.

Annette told me that when she was in her sixth month of pregnancy, her heart sometimes beat irregularly. The irregularity would last for hours at a time. Occasionally, her heart raced for so long and with such unevenness that she went to an emergency room for help, but the irregularity always went away when she was being observed. Annette always reported her symptoms to her midwives at the prenatal care appointments that followed her emergency room visits, and her midwives always dismissed the possibility that the symptoms were a sign of a more serious condition: "They all said, 'Your body does weird things when you're pregnant. Or maybe it's stress.' But no tests, no nothing."

When Annette finally went into labor—after several more trips to the emergency room—the heartbeat irregularity returned. Because she was already in the hospital, her providers decided to perform an electrocardiogram, which revealed a pregnancy-triggered heart condition. Because of the condition, Annette had to deliver her baby in the cardiac intensive care unit (ICU). Her labor and childbirth were nightmarish.

Nearly everything went wrong. The physician who attempted the Foley bulb induction[22] was a fairly unskilled resident, and the procedure was "excruciating" as a result: "They had a resident doing all of these things. It felt to me that they were saying, 'Resident, this is a great way for you to get practice. This is a great opportunity for you to get your hands on a really once-in-a-lifetime thing.' They made that choice instead of saying to themselves, 'Wow, this is probably the most physically traumatic day of this woman's life. Let's just have the actual [attending physician] insert the Foley bulb.' No. They didn't consider my experience of the whole thing. Instead, they had this fucking resident who's like, 'Ahhhh, I can't . . .'"

Then when it was time to push, Annette suffered a third-degree vaginal tear,[23] which her providers, again, allowed a resident to suture: "They had the resident do it! And he was doing it wrong! And so, [the attending physician] had to come in and be like, 'Oh, no, no, no, no!'"

Finally, when Annette was in the recovery room, resting after the birth of her daughter, her heart began to beat irregularly again, making it necessary for her to go back to the cardiac ICU—without her daughter: "And it's seared off in the most awful way in my brain—the sound of her crying when they took her out of my arms."

Five years later, Annette still became visibly angry when she talked about her experiences during her pregnancy. By the end of our conversation, her face was flush and her voice quivering:

It's upsetting. I mean, I didn't die. My daughter didn't die. I'm well aware that it could have been so much worse. But for me, it comes back to this question. . . . I don't know. . . . If I was some pretty, rich, thin, white lady having my heart race, would my midwives have been like, "Oh, we've got to get you into the—. . . ."? You know what I mean? As opposed to, "Oh, I think it's just stress," when it was a fucking heart condition that could kill me or cause my daughter to die if it's not managed. No one paid attention the whole time that I was paging the doctor quite *literally* saying, "I think I'm dying."

Annette's class privilege—her juris doctor degree from a top law school, her status as a civil rights attorney—did not guarantee her a positive experience with reproductive healthcare. During her routine prenatal care appointments, her midwives did not insist on figuring out why a racing heart had sent her to the emergency room on multiple occasions. During her labor and delivery, Annette's doctors did not think about what it must have felt like to her to be diagnosed with a potentially fatal cardiac condition on the day that she was to give birth to her first child.

Now, of course, it is not clear that Rita's and Annette's black race explains why they had such traumatic experiences. People of all races in the United States have terrible encounters with healthcare institutions. Further, scores of women of all races report disempowering experiences with obstetricians and gynecologists.[24] Black people do not have a monopoly on receiving poor healthcare in this country. But we would be naïve if we did not ask the question: What role did Rita's race play in her physician's decision to treat her with such contempt? What role did Annette's race play in causing her providers to dismiss her symptoms of a serious heart condition? If Annette had, in fact, been a "pretty, rich, thin, white lady," would she have managed to avoid a hellish childbirth experience?

We do not know. We cannot prove that *but for* Rita's and Annette's black race, their providers would have given them excellent healthcare. But this lack of proof is always true. Although we may have damning statistics describing the higher rates of injury and death that black people suffer in hospitals and healthcare facilities, we do not know in any individual case whether the person's black race caused them, in particular, to suffer an injury or death. This is a reality that makes racism both deniable to racism skeptics and elusive to many who are confident that racism persists in countless ways in the post–civil rights era. (As Annette said, "You'll never know, right? Unless they show up in white hoods to the appointment, you don't entirely know—which is one of the mind-fucks about it.") Nevertheless, many of the class-privileged black women who spoke with me for this book were confident that even though they enjoyed some degree of affluence, their black race mattered—or had the potential to matter—as they navigated healthcare systems in the pursuit of a healthy pregnancy, childbirth, and newborn. Many of the class-privileged black women that I interviewed were confident that their race placed them at a distinct disadvantage—despite their advanced degrees from competitive universities, high-status jobs, and amassed wealth. As a result, they adopted strategies for diminishing the effects of that felt disadvantage and for avoiding what Dána-Ain Davis calls "obstetric racism"—the fact that racism "materialize[s] during Black women's medical encounters" involving reproductive healthcare and "threat[ens] maternal life and neonatal outcomes."[25]

THE EXPLORATION TO COME

It is not surprising that the wealthier black San Francisco residents interviewed for this book experienced disadvantages on account of their race, as San Francisco has a long history of imposing race-based burdens on nonwhite people. In this way, the racial burdens faced by the black women who spoke with me began long before they set foot in a provider's office for prenatal care: As black San Franciscans, their lives are set within a historical context of race-based disadvantage. Chapter 1 provides a racial history of the City by the Bay—a history of genocide, exclusionary zoning, banishment to internment camps, racial covenants, redlining, urban renewal, and gentrification. This chapter explains how San Francisco's current racial and socioeconomic demographics—black people comprise only 5 percent of the city's population, and close to half of them live in poverty—are not random or arbitrary but are the product of policy decisions made over generations. These policy choices have led the people who are the focus of this book—affluent black

San Francisco residents—to be rarities. Unicorns, in fact. But a caveat is in order. Although there is a distinctiveness to San Francisco's history and to black people's absence from the city, there is nothing unique about the techniques that San Francisco used to manage nonwhite people's place in the city. Genocide, exclusionary zoning, racial covenants, redlining, urban renewal, and gentrification have been features of every major city in the United States. As a result, San Francisco's story is every city's story. Consequently, this book both is and is not about San Francisco. It is a book about race, class, and reproduction in the United States that simply is set in San Francisco.

With this in mind, chapter 2 analyzes how the efficient, orderly operation of Golden Health's obstetrics clinic is made possible by the existence of "the General," the public hospital in San Francisco that cares for the city's indigent residents. This type of healthcare segregation—in which wealthier, commercially insured people and poor, Medicaid-insured or uninsured people receive their healthcare from different institutions—is not unique to San Francisco. It is a phenomenon that exists in most cities in the United States. Beyond simply noting the existence of healthcare segregation in San Francisco and in the country at large, chapter 2 argues that the "nice" hospitals and healthcare facilities where wealthier people receive their care can possess features that make them nice because there are other "not nice" hospitals— "poor people's hospitals"—that care for the publicly insured and uninsured. In this way, the comfort that wealthier people enjoy is made possible by the discomfort that poor people endure. Further, chapter 2 allows us to begin to see how Golden and other hospitals that cater to the "haves" benefit from the nation's failure to protect the health of black pregnant people. Racial disparities in maternal mortality mean that these hospitals will be virtually guaranteed a customer base that includes commercially insured black patients who will understand the creature comforts and small luxuries that these hospitals offer as evidence of a superior healthcare that is also on offer. The sad state of black maternal health in the United States means that these commercially insured black people can be expected to take their commercial insurance (and its higher reimbursement rates) to these institutions as a strategy to survive the nation's black maternal health crisis—a strategy that pours money into these institutions' coffers.

Racial disparities in maternal mortality and morbidity—and racial disparities in health, more generally—are the product of many different contributors, which chapter 3 explores. It begins by discussing genes and culture—two factors that defenders of the racial status quo propose to explain why people of color are sicker and die earlier than their white counterparts. Genes and culture are particularly problematic explanations of racial disparities in health. Not only is there scant evidence showing that they cause people of color to have shorter, sicker lives, but genes and culture absolve society of any responsibility for addressing racial disparities in health. Essentially, if black people's genes or culture is killing them, what can society possibly do to save them? After exploring why it is troubling to explain the higher rates of sickness and death among black people in terms of genes or culture, the chapter then investigates more likely contributors to racial disparities in health—differing access to healthcare across racial lines, epigenetics, stress and weathering, inferior quality of care provided to people of color on both individual and systems levels, and patient mistrust. In keeping with the critical orientation of this book, chapter 3 subjects even these more likely contributors to racial disparities in health to critical examination.

Chapter 4 analyzes the abundance of recent media attention to what has been called the "black maternal health crisis." While there are many positive aspects of this media attention, it has problematic facets. As chapter 4 observes, coverage of black maternal deaths can be profitable for media companies and other third parties. It asks whether some individuals who engage with this coverage may be consuming it as entertainment—because many have found it pleasurable to read, watch, or listen to accounts of black suffering and death. Additionally, the chapter questions the effect that these journalistic accounts of black people who die or come close to dying during pregnancy, childbirth, or the postpartum period have on black people who are pregnant or desire pregnancy. Interviews with study participants provide some insights into how pregnant black people are experiencing the steady stream of coverage of "the black maternal health crisis."

Chapter 5 continues this inquiry, investigating the various strategies that the class-privileged black patients interviewed for this book adopted to avoid becoming part of the statistics that reflect the nation's failure to care for the lives of pregnant and recently postpartum black people. While wealthier black people deployed many techniques to survive—and to thrive during—their pregnancies, this chapter sits with patients' choice to receive their care from black providers. It delves deep into this choice, seeking to identify precisely what black patients hope a provider's black race will give them. Chapter 5 explains that there is no single answer to this question. The answer depends on the patient. Some patients believe that a provider's black race will protect them from the medicalization of their pregnancies, while others believe that a provider's black race will *perfect* the medicalization of their pregnancies. This chapter also explores a phenomenon that I call "racial renunciation"—when a black patient refuses to believe that race and racism have impacted their healthcare experiences despite all evidence to the contrary. It probes racial renunciation, wondering why it may be disquieting to those (like myself) who are convinced that because race structures society in the United States, race invariably impacts individuals' experiences.

Chapter 6 conducts an even deeper exploration into black people's choice to receive their prenatal care from black providers as a technique to survive pregnancy and childbirth. This chapter considers Golden Health's response to pregnant black patients' desire to be cared for by black obstetricians, midwives, and nurses. Golden's Black Wellbeing Clinic allows black-identifying people to receive their obstetric and gynecological care from black-identifying providers. Racially concordant care—where patients and providers share racial identities—has been offered as the latest, most effective tool in the struggle against racial disparities in health. This chapter probes the racial concordance innovation alongside the approaches to addressing racial health disparities that came before it. Implicit bias trainings within medical education, while popular, have been revealed to be insufficient (and protective of the status quo). Cultural competence trainings have been subjected to extensive (and justified) critiques and may produce more problems than they solve. Diversity, equity, and inclusion (DEI) initiatives frequently are performative and, for that reason, ineffective; moreover, the Trump administration and conservative activist organizations have waged an extensive war against them, making it difficult for institutions to continue to implement them. Structural competence trainings allow for a more critical understanding of racial disparities in health—which may explain why they have not been taken up more widely within medical education. Many have looked to racially concordant care to protect black lives and health when the other tools at our disposal have failed. Chapter 6 examines Golden's race concordance clinic, and it considers critiques of such race-conscious efforts to address racial disparities in health that have come from a relatively unexpected place—the political left. A brief conclusion follows.

1 How We Got Here: The Peculiar (But Not Uncommon) Racial History of San Francisco

When I was in the early planning stages for this book, I identified five characteristics for the people I most wanted to interview. They would be residents of San Francisco, over the age of eighteen, pregnant or recently postpartum, in possession of commercial health insurance, and black. Years later, when I finally began conducting research at Golden Health, I always felt a rush of adrenaline whenever I recruited someone with these five qualities. It was as though I had met a living, breathing unicorn, and the unicorn had agreed to sit down and chat with me. (Over two years of research, I eventually interviewed seventy-five unicorns and 125 nonblack people who otherwise met the study's inclusion criteria.)

Whenever I encountered a San Francisco resident who was over the age of eighteen, pregnant or recently postpartum, commercially insured, and black, my heart raced and I felt giddy. And this was simply because the class-privileged black San Francisco resident is a rarity. It deserves emphasis that the scarcity of high-income black people in San Francisco is not a fluke, but rather is a product of a series of racially discriminatory processes—including government-funded urban renewal and government-approved gentrification—that have pushed virtually all but the poorest black people out of the city. Importantly, the processes that have worked to exclude all but the most indigent black people from San Francisco are not unique to the city. San Francisco is merely an amplified version of Every City, USA.

This chapter discusses the racial history of San Francisco, explaining why the high-income black people who are the focus of this study are in short supply in the City by the Bay. It begins by describing the general invisibility of class-privileged black people as a result of the common cognitive practice of conflating racial disadvantage with class disadvantage—that is, blackness and poverty. It then describes the racial and class demographics of San Francisco, emphasizing the dramatic absence of black people from the city and the even more dramatic absence of wealthier black people from the city. The chapter then provides a short version of San Francisco's long history of racial exclusion—a history that has sequentially marked Native people, then people of Chinese descent, then people of Japanese descent, and then black people as targets for expulsion. The chapter ends by describing my pursuit of unicorns.

THE CONFLATION OF BLACKNESS AND POVERTY

Researchers learn how to describe their research projects in a couple of words (or less). Although we construct dense prospectuses that are filled with theory so abstract that it borders on the impenetrable, we learn to give a concise version of our research to anyone who asks. So when I began fieldwork at Golden Health and curious nurses, doctors, front desk workers, ultrasound technicians, administrators, and other hospital employees asked me why I was at the obstetrics clinic every day with a pen and notebook in hand, I learned to avoid mentioning the scholars whose work I aimed to build on, the racial disparities in infant and maternal mortality that increase as people move up the socioeconomic ladder, and my desire to investigate the unexpected vulnerability of being black and class-privileged during the event of pregnancy. Instead, I learned to say, "My study is about how race and class affect experiences of pregnancy and prenatal care." Over time, I noticed a pattern in how people at Golden responded to this description.

Many of these folks regretfully informed me that I probably was not going to find what I was looking for at Golden and that I would be more successful if I conducted my study at Zuckerberg San Francisco General Hospital and Trauma Center ("the General," for short). The General, which is the focus of chapter 2, is a "poor people's hospital" that provides healthcare to the proverbial tired, poor, huddled masses yearning to breathe free. (In fiscal year 2021–2022, the overwhelming majority of patients who received care from the hospital were uninsured or had publicly funded health insurance [Medicare or Medicaid]. Only 5 percent of the patients cared for at the General that year had commercial health insurance.)[1] Some folks at Golden Health suggested that Tuesdays were the best days to try to recruit patients for my study, as Tuesdays were when Dr. Sitara Davani conducted her clinic on the East Hills campus, and Dr. Davani saw more Medicaid-insured patients than any other provider in the obstetrics practice. Others said that I should go to the obstetrics department on the Yerba Buena campus on Thursday afternoons, which was when the department held a clinic for young people that also tended to see Medicaid-insured patients of all ages.

Essentially, my declaration that I was interested in "race and class" prompted people to respond with "Medicaid patients." It did not take long for me to unpack why this call-and-response happened so frequently.

First, people understood my interest in "race" to be about nonwhite people. This is consistent with what critical scholars of race have long proposed about the denial of whiteness as a racial identity.[2] While people of color in the United States typically think of themselves as having a race—out of necessity, people of color may have to remain aware of their race as they move through society—white people do not experience their race similarly. Scholars have proposed that this is because society is organized in a way that allows *white people to be unconscious of their racial identities and ascriptions.* The result is that whiteness becomes invisible, leaving nonwhite people to be the only people imagined as having a race. My status as a black woman probably played a role in people's assumptions that my stated interest in race was not just about nonwhite people generally, but about black people, specifically. It may have been contrary to most people's intuitions that a black woman researching race would be interested in Latine, Asian, or Native people—let alone white people.

Second, once people connected my interest in race with an interest in black people, they assumed that my interest in "class" was about poverty or low income. To be clear, they associated black race and poverty. Hence, they pointed me toward sites where Medicaid-insured—that is, impoverished—black people could be found, such as the General, Dr. Davani's clinic, and the Thursday clinic for young people.

Black people do disproportionately bear the burdens of poverty in the United States. While black people were only 13.5 percent of the country's total population in 2022, they comprised close to 20 percent of those living below the poverty line that year.[3] However, disproportionate indigence is not total indigence. Nevertheless, the conflation of black race and poverty is common.[4] Consider Donald Trump's campaign for the presidency in 2016. In one well-reported instance from the campaign trail, Trump spoke directly to black people in an effort to secure their votes, declaring, "You're living in poverty. . . . Your schools are no good. You have no jobs. Fifty-eight percent of your youth is unemployed."[5] He later promised that, if elected, he would be a president for everyone, "African Americans, the inner cities[.]"[6] Here, Trump made plain his assumption that to speak about black people is to speak about poor people. Perhaps this helps to explain why during his first presidency, Trump appointed a black retired neurosurgeon with no obvious experience with housing policy, Dr. Ben Carson, to head the US Department of Housing and Urban Development[7]—the federal agency whose primary charge is to address the housing needs of low-income people in the country. If black race and poverty are one and the same, as Trump apparently believed them to be, then Carson, a black man with no expertise in matters pertaining to poverty, would be perfectly suited to run an agency that concerns itself with matters pertaining to poverty.

The correlation of black race and poverty is interesting for a number of reasons, the most relevant of which is that it obscures the fact that many black people are not, in fact, poor.[8] Scores of black people are class-privileged—a fact that may alter their experiences with racial disadvantage. Indeed, the hope that drove my investigation into wealthier black people's experiences with pregnancy and prenatal care was that I would be able to study how their relative affluence transformed their experiences of racism and racial inequality. When we presuppose that impoverished black people's experiences of racism represent the entirety of racism, then it seems to me that we miss essential aspects of the phenomenon of racism. In other words, antiblack racism is not manifested solely when poor black people have to attend racially segregated, underfunded public schools; live in substandard public housing; or receive inferior, Medicaid-subsidized healthcare from public hospitals. Antiblack racism also may be manifested when wealthier black people are among only a handful of other nonwhite people attending racially segregated, well-funded public and private schools; live in expensive housing that nevertheless is of poorer quality and lower value than the housing that their wealthier white counterparts call home;[9] or think it necessary to hire a doula to survive childbirth even while receiving healthcare in the best hospitals that money can buy. By focusing on black people who were not poor, this book seeks to expand our understanding of the forms that racism takes in the United States.

RACE AND CLASS IN SAN FRANCISCO

Eventually, I smiled to myself when I said "race and class" and the people I was speaking with revealed that they had heard "blackness and poverty." However, about a year into my fieldwork, I was struck with a disconcerting thought: What if people at Golden Health were not entirely wrong when they conflated black race and poverty? What if something about San Francisco made thinking about poverty when thinking about black race more reasonable than it is in other parts of the country—in Los Angeles, New York City, Chicago, Atlanta, or Washington, DC?

As it turns out, San Francisco's numbers with respect to black race and poverty are an extreme version of those that can be found in other parts of the nation. Some 43 percent of black San Francisco residents—close to half—is in poverty.[10] Meanwhile, only 13 percent, 22 percent, and 23 percent of white, Asian, and Latine San Francisco residents, respectively, are impoverished.[11] Further, while close to half of the black population in San Francisco lives in poverty, only 20 percent is upper middle class.[12] Of white San Francisco residents, 53 percent are upper middle class.[13] That is, almost half of the black population in San Francisco is at the bottom of the socioeconomic ladder, and over half of the white population in the city is at the top.

While these numbers do not suggest that it is appropriate to collapse white race and wealth or black race and poverty in San Francisco, they do suggest that when one encounters a white San Franciscan, there is a good chance that person enjoys class privilege, and when one encounters a black

San Franciscan, there is a good chance that person is living in poverty. That said, the likelihood of simply encountering a black San Franciscan is low. This is because only 5 percent of San Francisco residents are black.[14]

The percentage of black people living in San Francisco has not always been so small. In 1970, black people comprised 13 percent of the population in the city.[15] In the intervening years, other racial groups have moved into the city while black people increasingly have abandoned it. Further, the black people who have sought greener pastures outside of the city have tended to be from the working class, middle class, and upper middle class, while the black people who have elected to tough it out in the City by the Bay have tended to be poor. Between 2000 and 2015, San Francisco's black population dwindled in all income categories—except for extremely low-income households.[16]

The combination of wealthier black people leaving San Francisco and poor black San Francisco residents remaining has resulted in the fact that close to half of black San Franciscans today live in poverty. It is important to understand that the exodus of black people from the city—with greater proportions of working class, middle class, and upper middle class black people deserting the city—is not an accident of history. Nor can it be attributed to black people's "preferences." As one set of researchers has written, "The rampant displacement seen today in the San Francisco Bay Area is built upon a history of exclusion and dispossession, centered on race, and driven by the logic of capitalism. This history established massive inequities in who owned land, who had access to financing, and who held political power, all of which determined—and still remain at the root of deciding—who can call the Bay Area home."[17]

It is ironic, perhaps, that the racial expulsion recounted in the next section occurred in a city with a reputation of being decidedly left of center. As anthropologist Savannah Shange writes, "San Francisco is mythologized as a land of liberal tolerance, progressive politics, and picturesque cosmopolitanism."[18] Surely, San Francisco deserves some of that mythologizing. It was the home of Harvey Milk, the prescient civil rights leader who was one of the first openly gay elected officials in the country.[19] It is the origin of many forward-thinking environmental approaches and was one of the first cities to ban plastic straws and single-use plastic bags.[20] It was the site of Bloody

Thursday, the deadly culmination of the 1934 West Coast longshoreman's strike.[21] After the strike and Bloody Thursday, all of the West Coast ports in the United States were unionized, thus cementing San Francisco's reputation as a city with progressive labor policies.

Despite being a place with a rich progressive past when it comes to sexual, environmental, and labor politics, it is also a place with a vile racial history. Indeed, a place known for being a bright blue city in a bright blue state actually invented many of the techniques for excluding and segregating unwanted nonwhite Others that have been deployed in communities across the nation.

San Francisco has come to be associated with liberals, and liberals are imagined to be more concerned than the other side with equality. But San Francisco is a city with dramatic inequality. In fact, the inequality found in San Francisco is so severe that it seems unsustainable. Many of its residents are employed in the tech industry and enjoy high salaries and generous benefits, like no-cost egg freezing and in vitro fertilization. They live in million-dollar homes that they own, or they pay amounts in rent that would incite laughter from folks living in other parts of the country. They do weekend getaways in Napa Valley, Big Sur, or Monterey Bay. They pay $9 for a cup of coffee without hesitation. Meanwhile, other San Francisco residents experience vividly different realities. If they are poor and lucky, they are crowded into dilapidated housing projects in polluted neighborhoods where residents tell me that even the cats get leukemia.[22] If they are poor and unlucky, their "home" is a tent beneath an expressway or in an abandoned storefront.

These almost criminally different worlds exist within city blocks of one another. On one typically lovely northern California day, I walked from Golden Health's East Hills campus, where I had ended a day of fieldwork, to a yoga studio where I had hoped to sweat, stretch, and unwind before heading to my home on the other side of the Bay. As the walk began, I passed beautiful parks with views of the sparkling, glittering waters of the San Francisco Bay where dog parents let their fur babies run free. I eyed $100 yoga pants in the window of a Lululemon store. I saw Tesla after Tesla after Tesla drive past me. But the neighborhood soon changed, and I found myself hopping over piles of human excrement on the sidewalk. I witnessed at least a half a dozen people inserting needles into the crooks of their elbows. I saw my first crack pipe. I observed a woman ambling down the sidewalk wearing only a dirty T-shirt, the lower half of her body exposed. I eventually walked by the soiled pants that she had just discarded. I saw all of this in the warm light of the northern California sun. In San Francisco, people do not have to wait for night to witness the suffering of fellow human beings.

A LONG HISTORY OF RACIAL EXCLUSION

The story of San Francisco as a site of racial exclusion begins with the genocide of the Native people who inhabited the lands that would come to be California—a beginning shared by every major city in the United States. Fifteen thousand Muwekma Ohlone people once populated the region that is now the San Francisco Bay Area.[23] Their numbers began to dwindle in 1769, when Spanish troops and missionaries arrived and began to dispossess the Indigenous people of their ancestral land, oftentimes through violent means.[24] The decimation of Ohlone people continued over the next decades, as the land they inhabited was claimed first by Spain and then by Mexico. By 1830, there were only two thousand Ohlone people living in the Bay Area, less than a seventh of the population that had existed just sixty years prior.[25] The number of Native people in the region, and in the state more broadly, plummeted after the California Gold Rush of 1848 to 1855 brought tens of thousands of fortune seekers to the state, which by that time had come to belong to the United States as spoils of the Mexican-American War. During the Gold Rush, private militias composed of white aspiring settlers slaughtered over 100,000 Indigenous people—more than two-thirds of the Native population in the state—in order to claim the lands that these peoples had lived on for thousands of years.[26]

Once Native people had been sufficiently decimated and San Francisco had developed into a city of opportunity for white people hailing from other parts of the nation and the world, people of Asian descent became the objects of racial exclusion. Public and private actors in the city adopted a variety of mechanisms to contain the threat that Chinese immigrants were imagined to pose. Some of these efforts proudly bore race on their face, like the Bingham

Ordinance of 1890, which required all people of Chinese descent to move to a small area of the city that had been set aside for them. The Democratic County Committee passed a resolution in support of the law that made clear the rank racism that drove the ordinance:

> Whereas we have in our midst hordes of Chinese who have located in the heart of our city and there erected one of the most pernicious plague spots ever known in the history of civilization, where in utter disregard of the laws of our State are maintained gambling hells, houses of prostitution and opium dens, to which are allowed not only people of their own race, but where white men and women are dragged down to ruin, and where have been erected arsenals so strong that our police consider it a vain task to attempt the suppression of the constant violations of law there occurring; and
>
> Whereas experience has shown that the filth, offal and refuse existing in Chinatown is a consistent menace to the health of the people of our city, and that it is impossible to secure obedience to the sanitary ordinances adopted for our protection.[27]

The Democratic County Committee considered the Bingham Ordinance a necessary measure to protect "our citizens, their wives and children" from the menace of walking through the neighborhoods where Chinese people lived, worked, and played and "see[ing] all the scenes and dens of vice there openly exposed to their gaze."[28] Notably, the Bingham Ordinance allows San Francisco to hold the ignominious title of the first city to use a zoning law to explicitly segregate on the basis of race.[29] In other parts of the country, officials looking for ways to contain unwanted nonwhite people within their municipalities later took up the useful device of racial exclusionary zoning and adapted it to their own local circumstances.

Other techniques of racial exclusion forged in San Francisco were facially race neutral, like the 1880 laundry ordinance, which most law students become familiar with at some point in their legal education. The ordinance required all laundries in wooden buildings to have a city-issued permit.[30] Although people of Chinese descent operated most of the laundries in San Francisco, the city did not grant a single permit to a Chinese-owned laundry.[31] The result was that over 150 Chinese owners of laundromats were prosecuted for operating a laundry without a permit. Notably, not a single non-Chinese laundromat owner was prosecuted under the law.³² The United States Supreme Court ultimately struck down the ordinance in an 1886 decision, holding for the first time that a facially race-neutral law administered in a racially discriminatory manner violated the guarantees contained in the equal protection clause of the Fourteenth Amendment to the United States Constitution.³³ As the Court pronounced, "Though the law itself be fair on its face and impartial in appearance, yet, if it is applied and administered by public authority with an evil eye and an unequal hand, . . . the denial of equal justice is still within the prohibition of the Constitution."³⁴

People of Chinese descent living in San Francisco were not the only nonwhite targets of white ire in California. The entire state has a history of anti-Japanese sentiment. In 1913 and 1920, the state adopted laws that prevented "aliens ineligible to citizenship" from owning, selling, leasing, and inheriting land. Because federal law prohibited Japanese nationals from naturalizing as United States citizens, the state law made it impossible for Japanese people to participate fully in the agricultural economy in California, thus "undermining the economic foundation of Japanese immigrant society."³⁵

Anti-Japanese sentiment tragically peaked during World War II, when military officials claimed that people of Japanese descent were likely to participate in acts of espionage and treason to help bring about the triumph of Germany, Italy, and Japan in the global conflict. Impelled by the racist certainty that people of Japanese descent were more predisposed than people of German or Italian descent to retain a devotion to their ancestral homelands, the federal government ordered the confinement of both Japanese Americans and Japanese nationals living on the West Coast for the duration of the war. The effects of Japanese internment were deeply felt in San Francisco. As the *San Francisco Chronicle* reported in May 1942:

> For the first time in 81 years, not a single Japanese [person] is walking the streets of San Francisco. The last group, 274 of them, were moved yesterday to the Tanforan assembly center. Only a scant half dozen are left, all seriously ill in San Francisco hospitals. Last night Japanese town was empty. Its stores were vacant, its windows plastered with "To Lease" signs.³⁶

Most historians agree that in the mid-nineteenth through mid-twentieth centuries, when anti-Chinese and anti-Japanese racism animated San Francisco and the surrounding Bay Area, few black people lived in the region, and there was little antiblack racism. The 1930 Census documented that 3,803 black people lived in San Francisco, constituting a little over one half of one percent of the city's total population.[37] However, during World War II, the United States' entrance into the global conflict led to a demand for labor, as the country had to produce the materials necessary to fight a war. California became the site of shipbuilding efforts. Initially, California shipyards attempted to satisfy the demand for labor solely with white workers, as nonwhite workers were largely considered "untrainable and unemployable[.]"[38] Yet, as scholar of segregation Richard Rothstein writes of the shipyards, "[A]s the war dragged on, unable to find the sufficient number to meet their military orders, they were forced to hire white women, then black men, and eventually black women as well."[39]

Many of the black people who flocked to California during World War II were fleeing the *de jure* brutality of the South, where white people used both banal and spectacular forms of racist violence to maintain the racial hierarchy. Black émigrés from the South were also fleeing unemployment brought about by the contraction of the demand for agricultural labor. The recruitment strategies that employers used to lure black people out West are storied:

> Tales abound about how Kaiser advertised nationwide and even sent trains through the southwest and South to recruit workers for shipyards. According to some stories, trains stopped at each crossroad and recruiters called farmers and sharecroppers from the fields to pack up and get on board for California—good jobs, more cash than they'd ever seen, and decent places to live.[40]

This siren song proved irresistible for many black southerners, and the number of black people living in California increased by an astounding 272 percent between 1940 and 1950.[41]

Many black workers who migrated to San Francisco during the war found employment in the shipyard in the Bayview–Hunters Point neighborhood.

However, this does not explain why so many black families also lived in that neighborhood. Instead, *racial discrimination* explains why large portions of the black workers who came to San Francisco to participate in the war effort ended up living in Bayview–Hunters Point. The racist ire that once focused on Chinese and Japanese persons quickly shifted to black people, whose rapidly expanding presence in the city had become impossible to ignore. With Japanese people "confined in distant relocation centers and with Chinese Americans now allied in the anti-Japanese campaign, black migrants became the prime target of local bigotry."[42] Unsurprisingly, this new antiblack racism took the form of restrictions on where the despised racial group could live—the same form that racism took when it had been directed against people of Chinese descent just half a century earlier. Black workers and their families were prohibited from living in many neighborhoods, but they were permitted to live in temporary war housing that had been constructed close to the shipyards in Bayview–Hunters Point. White lawmakers felt that it was unacceptable for white workers to live alongside black workers, so this temporary war housing was racially segregated, and many white workers were housed in all-white residences in other parts of the city. After lawmakers designated Bayview–Hunters Point as a corner of the city where black people could live, there was a mass exodus of the white people who had once resided there. Hunters Point had been 98 percent white in 1940 but became 87 percent black by 1970.[43]

In addition to Bayview–Hunters Point, black migrants were permitted to live in segregated temporary war housing that had been built in the Fillmore neighborhood, which abutted Japantown. The tragedy of internment for Japanese people during World War II became an opportunity for black people, who had been crowded into the Fillmore and Bayview–Hunters Point. Once the Japanese were compelled to report to concentration camps or risk criminal punishment—a black boy who lived near Japantown "reported that one day all of his Japanese schoolmates and neighbors disappeared" and "[n]o one said where they had gone or what happened to them"[44]—the tenements that people of Japanese descent had been forced to abandon in Japantown "were filled virtually overnight with black migrants seeking the warmth of other suns."[45]

As large numbers of black newcomers arrived in the Fillmore, many of the neighborhood's white residents fled to the suburbs, purchasing homes with the assistance of the GI Bill and loans subsidized by the Federal Housing Administration.[46] However, many white residents resisted the allure of white flight and stayed put. The result was that although the Fillmore neighborhood had the highest density of black people in San Francisco during and immediately following World War II, the community was racially mixed. In 1947, two years after the end of the war, the Fillmore was 65 percent white, 26 percent black, 5 percent Chinese American, and 4 percent Japanese American.[47]

Although white segregationists had created the Fillmore as a dumping ground for black people—a place that would save white people from the indignity of having to call a black person "neighbor"—black people built the Fillmore district into a space of black excellence. The streets became filled with black-owned businesses—restaurants, nightclubs, clothing stores, groceries, hair salons, and funeral parlors. It also became a center of black religious life, with churches that cared for the spiritual needs of the black community. The jazz scene in the Fillmore was rivaled only by the one found in New York City, earning the neighborhood the moniker of "the Harlem of the West."[48] The Fillmore became the obvious destination for those seeking out good food, good drinks, good music, and good times among incandescent black folk.

The end of the war meant the end of the demand for labor in the industries that had drawn black people to San Francisco and had sustained their well-being. Moreover, the return of soldiers from battlefields abroad meant an increase in competition for the unskilled and low-skilled jobs that remained. The result was massive unemployment—some estimates put black unemployment during the postwar years at 30 percent—and massive poverty in Bayview–Hunter's Point and the Fillmore, where black people had been corralled.[49] Further, the temporary war housing that had been constructed for black workers was turned over to public housing authorities and began to function as "projects." As sites of concentrated poverty, Bayview–Hunters Point and the Fillmore deteriorated. These neighborhoods, "which had been vibrant with hope and economic vitality 15 to 20 years before," became "low income ghettoes."[50]

The decline of Bayview–Hunters Point and the Fillmore is the result not just of the disappearance of jobs associated with the war effort in San Francisco but also of racist housing policies designed and implemented by the federal government. With its redlining practices, the federal government, through an agency called the Home Owners' Lending Corporation (HOLC), identified neighborhoods that were deemed deserving of federal monies for investment and development and neighborhoods that were deemed underserving. The government was willing to pour federal money in the form of loans and mortgages into neighborhoods that did not have old buildings and did not face the "threat of infiltration of foreign-born, negro or lower grade population[s.]"[51] In other words, the neighborhoods that benefited from federal investment were white. These neighborhoods were traced in green or blue lines on official maps that HOLC created. Meanwhile, the neighborhoods where black and other nonwhite people lived were traced in red on these maps, marking these communities as "bad" investments and cutting them off from federal money.[52] As a consequence of this redlining, black and other nonwhite people were denied mortgages to purchase homes in the neighborhoods where they lived. Additionally, both black and nonblack people who already owned property in these neighborhoods were unable to obtain loans to rehabilitate buildings that were in need of repair. These buildings fell further into dilapidation.

The "social experiment" of urban renewal began during this period of formal disinvestment in neighborhoods of color.[53] After World War II, the nation faced both a housing shortage and the exodus of the white middle class from cities (and their crumbling infrastructure). Elites, many of whom were politically liberal, were taken by the idea that these problems could be solved if they could clear "slums" in cities across the nation and construct adequate housing—alongside educational, commercial, and recreational facilities—in their place. In 1949, President Harry Truman declared in his State of the Union Address that "slum clearance" was the solution to the imminent demise of cities across the country.[54] The goal was to "remak[e] the industrial cities of America into rational and car-friendly metropolises."[55] To facilitate this project, Congress passed the Housing Acts of 1949 and 1954, allocating federal monies to revitalize urban areas and construct housing for those who would be displaced from sites of revitalization. Title I of the Housing Act of 1949, aptly titled "Slum Clearance and Community Development and Redevelopment," empowered local governments to acquire "slums" through eminent domain and to hand over these blighted lands to private developers, investors, and builders for redevelopment. (It is worth noting that although the US Constitution requires that persons whose property is seized through eminent domain must receive "just compensation," those whose property was taken in the neighborhoods that were subject to urban renewal rarely were paid the market value of their property.[56])

In cities across the nation, local lawmakers identified neighborhoods—usually those where nonwhite people lived[57]—as either hopelessly blighted and desperately in need of regeneration or hopelessly blighted and ideal sites for the construction of a highway that would make it easier for suburbanites to travel to the heart of the city. (It often seems as though neighborhoods that had a significant number of people of color—and not simply deteriorated buildings—were the neighborhoods that were deemed to be "blighted." As one professor of urban planning explains, "[I]n the discourse of urban planning in the mid-20th century in the United States, blight was often synonymous with people of color and with African Americans, in particular."[58]) Local governments then began acquiring large parcels of land in these communities through purchase, condemnation, or eminent domain. Once the existing structures in the neighborhood were razed, they were replaced by "gleaming office towers, highways, stadiums, and high-rise apartment buildings."[59] San Francisco was not spared the upheaval of urban renewal, which swept through the country in the 1950s and 1960s.

When James Baldwin visited the Fillmore neighborhood in 1963, he said that urban renewal was, in fact, "Negro removal"[60]—a term that became widely affixed to these projects of revitalization, which commonly destroyed black neighborhoods. Local lawmakers had declared that the Fillmore was blighted beyond redemption and an embarrassment to the city. (Of course, they did not acknowledge the role that HOLC and federal housing policy had played in producing the blight that they found in the neighborhood.) Shortly thereafter, the City Planning Commission, which was responsible for designing the renewal of the Fillmore, issued a report that described the neighborhood in ways that were not altogether different from the way that the Democratic County Commission had described San Francisco's Chinatown sixty years earlier. Similar to how the Democratic County Commission's resolution depicted Chinatown as a location rife with "gambling hells, houses of prostitution and opium dens," the City Planning Commission described the Fillmore as a site with "71 bars, 45 liquor stores, numerous smoke shops and magazine stands suspected of gambling joints and bookies in disguise," and "'hotels' that accommodate members of the 'world's oldest profession.'"[61]

Decision-makers at the time saw no value in the Fillmore in its current state. They said the area was ugly and consisted of "architecture [that] was a hodgepodge of styles."[62] They maintained that the homes in the neighborhood, which had been built in the late nineteenth century through the early twentieth century, were not worth saving, as they were not "'old enough to have historical interest' and had 'little salvage value.'"[63] And yet, as noted by one journalist writing a half a century after city elites concluded that the buildings in the Fillmore were worthless, "[t]oday, one floor of a Japantown Victorian can be yours for $1 million."[64]

Decision-makers also declared that Geary Boulevard, which cut through the Fillmore, should be widened to make it easier for those who had abandoned San Francisco for the suburbs to travel downtown. Thus, lawmakers, realtors, and commercial interests all agreed that the Fillmore should be dramatically transformed. Meanwhile, the actual residents of the Fillmore had no say in what happened to the neighborhood where they had grown up, raised their children, worshipped, and eked out a life worth living. These residents had no political clout. They sat on no commissions or committees. They had no friends in high places. There was not much that they could do to stop their homes and their community from being sacrificed on the altar of "progress."

Most estimates put the number of people exiled by the urban renewal of the Fillmore at ten thousand.[65] These displacements were permanent in large part because no one thought it was important to ensure that the residents whose homes were destroyed would be able to afford the newly constructed housing in the neighborhood—even though federal funding for urban renewal efforts had been made contingent on local authorities making affordable replacement housing available to uprooted families. Prior to the commencement of the urban renewal project in the Fillmore district, a planning committee released a proposal that estimated that the new housing that would be built after the "slums" were cleared would be affordable for those who earned the region's average income. However, this committee also acknowledged that those who currently resided in the neighborhood earned less than this amount: "In view of the characteristically low incomes of colored and foreign-born families, only a small proportion of them may be expected to be in a position to occupy quarters in the new development."[66] Thus, the inability of the families who had lost their homes to return to the neighborhood after it had been "renewed" was entirely predictable. In some cases, though, the permanent expulsion of the families who had resided in the Fillmore prior to its "renewal" was not only predictable but entirely intentional. One official who worked with the San Francisco Redevelopment Agency confessed (after his retirement), "One of the purposes of slum clearance was not only to get rid of the people and the structures but to make sure those blighting influences didn't come back. And so there was no intent to rebuild for the kind of people who were being displaced."[67]

Many displaced residents ended up in high-density public housing—some of which was constructed in the Fillmore district but most of which was built in the Bayview–Hunters Point neighborhood. Many more of these residents left the city altogether, joining the scores of other low- and middle-income families who found the increasing cost of living in San Francisco untenable. Remaining in the city in a home that was not public housing was not an option for many black people who had been exiled from the Fillmore, as housing discrimination in San Francisco made these units unavailable to them. One survey of the housing landscape during the time of this mass displacement reported that "34 out of every 35 apartments in the city prohibited African Americans."[68] Black Fillmore expatriates had nowhere to go. So they moved into the projects in Bayview–Hunters Point, or they deserted San Francisco altogether.

There is nothing unique about this history of the Fillmore. What happened to the Fillmore happened in cities across the nation.

In New York City, the San Juan Hill neighborhood on the Upper West Side of Manhattan was the home of thousands of black and brown people. The black people who lived there had fled the South during the Great Migration, and the brown people who lived there had migrated from Puerto Rico to the mainland in search of industrial jobs. The neighborhood was declared to be "blighted," "crime-ridden," "inefficient," "substandard," and "unsanitary"—that is, a "slum."[69] The city used federal funds, made available under Title I of the Housing Act, to acquire eighteen city blocks through eminent domain. Lincoln Center—the exquisite, twinkling landmark of the performing arts—now sits where the San Juan Hill neighborhood once did. Over seven thousand poor families of color and eight hundred businesses were expelled in the pursuit of "urban renewal."[70]

In Chicago, the Near West Side abuts the downtown of the city and its attractions. In the 1940s, during the Great Migration, the neighborhood became the destination of over 40,000 black people fleeing the South. By the 1950s, the Near West Side had also become the home to close to 28,000 Latine migrants. Predictably, HOLC redlined the neighborhood, declaring that "[t]he entire area is just as bad, if not worse, than the large colored blighted area where Chicago's three hundred odd thousand colored people live [the Black Belt].... [It] is becoming, increasingly, a serious problem and a menace."[71] Thus, the neighborhood suffered formal disinvestment. Crime, poverty, and unemployment followed. Elites in the city became worried that the neighborhood would continue to expand and imperil the downtown—which was already being "eclipsed by new suburban markets."[72] Urban planners declared the area "blighted," and Democratic mayor Richard J. Daley spearheaded a project of urban renewal.[73] With the help of Title I federal funds, the "slums" in the Near West Side were cleared, and housing projects were erected that would more efficiently contain the poor black and brown families who lived there.[74] So contained, the city's downtown was saved from the encroaching threat of color.

In Washington, DC, low-income people of color were concentrated in a corner of the city—Southwest DC. By the mid-twentieth century, some 70 percent of the 23,000 people who lived in the neighborhood were black, and close to 90 percent were poor.[75] Most of their homes lacked "basic amenities, such as electricity, central heating, an indoor toilet, and interior running water."[76] City planners declared the area blighted. With the assistance of Title I federal funds, the city began acquiring large parcels of land through eminent domain, razing the existing structures, and handing over the cleared land to private developers for redevelopment. Although these private investors had initially promised that a third of the newly constructed housing would be affordable—thereby ensuring that the neighborhood's residents would not be permanently displaced—investors eventually "determined that it would not be feasible to offer one-third of the units at an affordable rent, arguing that cost increases had made the rent limit impractical and that affordable housing was available in other parts of the city."[77] In the end, the area's rents, which had been half of the city's average, became double the city's average[78]—transforming the neighborhood from a community that was 70 percent black to one that was 70 percent white:[79] "[M]ost residents never had the chance to move back to their old neighborhood, even though early promises by the [project's planners] had suggested that possibility."[80] Ultimately, some 1,500 businesses and 23,000 residents were expelled.[81]

In Miami, the neighborhood of Overtown had been the center of black life in South Florida, earning it the name "the Harlem of the South."[82] Jim Crow laws, which mandated racial segregation, led the community to be self-contained and self-reliant. Black doctors, restaurants, grocers, barbers, and beauticians thrived, and an "'all Negro' municipal court" heard cases in the neighborhood.[83] In the 1950s, elites concluded that Miami would benefit if a highway were built that connected the suburbs to downtown, and another highway were built that connected the beach to the airport. Federal funding was available for construction: President Eisenhower signed the Federal-Aid Highway Act of 1956, allocating funds for the sort of project being proposed for Miami.[84] Decision-makers eventually concluded that the highways—eventually called I-95 and I-395—should cut through Overtown.[85] They used eminent domain to acquire the necessary land, compensating owners for their property at amounts that were far less than market value.[86] Some estimate that 30,000 black residents of Overtown were displaced.[87] And Overtown itself was destroyed: "[T]he combination of land purchases and evictions decimated the all-black enclave economy that had sustained the multi-cultural and multi-classed spaces of black Miami over the previous sixty years"[88]

In Los Angeles, the Sugar Hill neighborhood became the home of the black elite after the white families who once lived there sought larger homes in more fashionable neighborhoods, like Beverley Hills.[89] Indeed, the first black Oscar winner, Hattie McDaniel, had a mansion in Sugar Hill where she hosted parties attended by Duke Ellington and Ethel Waters.[90] Even after McDaniel sold her home and moved away from the neighborhood, Sugar Hill remained a site of black affluence. Despite this, city planners declared the area "blighted." In the 1950s, without input from residents, the California Highway Commission approved the construction of a highway through Sugar Hill that would make it easier for people living in the suburbs to travel to the city center.[91] (The California Division of Highways also proposed another highway that would run through Beverley Hills, but "when that wealthy white community protested, officials cancelled construction.")[92] The government used eminent domain to acquire parcels in Sugar Hill for what would be called the Santa Monica Freeway.[93] Most of the black residents of Sugar Hill were permanently exiled, and those who remained were left with the pollution and noise generated by the thousands of cars that drove past them daily.

* * *

Today, like many center-city neighborhoods from which white people fled after nonwhite people moved in, the Fillmore is a "highly gentrified space" where young, monied, overwhelmingly white and Asian professionals live in expensive condominiums.[94] In this respect, urban renewal as "Negro removal" was a resounding success. Restaurants and ateliers and furniture stores and clothing boutiques and wine shops and art galleries—all with price points that are high enough to keep out the residents of the public housing that stubbornly sits on Fillmore Street—currently dot the sidewalks. The Fillmore of yesteryear—"the once-thriving district studded with minority-owned businesses, nightclubs and hotels"—is gone, existing solely "in faded photos and oral histories."[95]

IN SEARCH OF UNICORNS

Today, the words "San Francisco" and "expensive" are often spoken in the same breath. As Savannah Shange has written, "The rise of the tech economy over the past twenty-five years and the role of San Francisco as one of its command centers now positions it as a global city. . . . [T]hese dynamics combined with a dearth of manufacturing jobs and skyrocketing costs has made San Francisco one of the most unaffordable places to raise a family in the nation."[96] Of course, the city is easily affordable if one is rich, and many San Franciscans are just that, resulting in a place with one of the highest per-capita incomes of the largest cities in the country.[97] Even so, many people living in San Francisco are *not* rich, making continued residence in the city increasingly unachievable. Large numbers of black people, who disproportionately populate the ranks of the "not rich," have left the city for more affordable areas. The black people who have stayed behind in San Francisco tend to be those who are so poor that they qualify for housing benefits, which explains why one journalist could write in 2016 that "most of the city's 46,000 blacks liv[e] in public housing."[98]

The short version of the long history of racial exclusion in San Francisco is that working-class and middle-class black people were pushed out of the city after their neighborhoods were destroyed and, due to housing discrimination, were unable to relocate to homes in other parts of the city. The black people who have remained in San Francisco are either wealthy enough to afford the high cost of living in the City by the Bay or poor enough to live in public housing. Because black people are underrepresented at the higher end of the socioeconomic ladder and in the tech industry,[99] which employs many high-income San Franciscans, there are disproportionately fewer high-income black people in San Francisco relative to other racial groups. This confluence of factors has made class-privileged black San Francisco residents into unicorns.

Many of the unicorns who spoke with me for this study—doctors, lawyers, executives, engineers, and tech industry employees—were aware of their uniqueness. Their singularity was a source of pride, joy, and comfort. But it was also a source of exhaustion. Indeed, that was the word that many of my interviewees used to describe their experience of being black and class-privileged in San Francisco—exhaustion.

Evelyn, a pretty, petite, thirty-four-year-old black woman, was twenty-two weeks pregnant with her first child when I met her at her obstetrics appointment at Golden Health. On the day of our Zoom meeting, she was cradling a mug of tea and wearing a fluffy, off-white sweater. Her "hello" echoed against what sounded to me like walls in an empty room, and she apologized in advance for any possible interruptions to our conversation: "We're getting some work done to our house, and the construction workers are downstairs. I might need to pop out if they need me for something." Evelyn explained that she and her husband had bought their Cole Valley home four months earlier. Cole Valley is a charming enclave next to Golden Gate Park where the median home price was $1.8 million in 2024[100] (down from a median price of $2.4 million in 2017).[101] She gushed, "This is my dream neighborhood to get into because I really liked the walking areas around it. I'm still so shocked that we managed to find housing here." She was talking to me in what eventually would become the nursery, and the project of decorating the room was far from complete: "I've been dealing with analysis paralysis on fucking nursery wallpaper for, like, ages—which is absolutely unhinged in the grand scheme of things."

Evelyn was born and raised in the Bay Area and was the daughter of two physicians. She grew up in a suburb thirty minutes south of San Francisco that she described as "some fancy town on the peninsula." She had left California for college and returned after earning a doctorate in biostatistics from an East Coast Ivy League university. She currently worked as a researcher at a biotechnology firm. She and her husband, a white man who was also a researcher, had married two years before our interview. She told me with a laugh, "I'm a data girl. He's a data boy. We are both data lovers. It's a match made in nerd heaven."

Our conversation—which was filled with lots of laughter, loads of curse words, and occasional interruptions by construction workers—eventually turned to the question of Evelyn's singularity as a self-described "rich" black woman who called San Francisco home. Because I felt like we were comfortable with one another, I asked her pointedly, "What has it been like for you to *not* be poor and to be black in San Francisco?" She responded with a sigh, a pause, and then this:

> That is such an intense question. It almost makes me emotional. Ahh. . . . [long pause] I think the black population in San Francisco right now is like 5 percent or something really low, right? My dad's family is from San Francisco. But they've all since either passed away or moved out. I think there's three people who are left in the city. But all of them—every single one of them—would be considered low income.

Her eyes looked toward a corner of the room, seeming to seek the words that would form an adequate response to my question: What is it like to be a unicorn? The words came to her:

> The phrase I would use to describe it—being black and high-income in San Francisco—is "jarring for other people." I mean, I grew up in a wealthy suburb. So I'm very used to being the only black person in a room of hundreds of people or thousands of people. Like, that's fine. But it feels different here—in a city where most black people are poor or living in the projects or, worse still, are drug addicts on the street. I do not fit that mold in San Francisco, and it throws people off. And they don't really know how to deal with it. It's not easy for them. But it's not easy for me either. It's not pleasant.

Like all of the class-privileged black people who spoke with me for this study, Evelyn was very well educated. What might have made Evelyn unusual was that, as a Bay Area native whose father also was from San Francisco, she was well-educated about the history of San Francisco. This informed her race- and class-informed attachment to the city:

> I love San Francisco because I like what it actually means to live here. But I also feel very strongly—like, a bit militantly—that I *deserve* San Francisco. They drove out all the black people—fucked us over in every single fucking which way. . . . Me and my family of kids—who are going to be black and *not poor*—are going to be in San Francisco. And they can take it from my cold dead hands. San Francisco is my fucking birthright.

Evelyn described the purchase of her multimillion-dollar home in Cole Valley as "putting the flag down for one black family. It feels a little bit like a clawing back."

Evelyn's statement suggests the complexity of the position that high-income black San Franciscans occupy. In many respects, black people are a subordinated racial group in San Francisco. They largely have been driven out of a city that they helped to build, and close to half of those who remain are subjected to the violence that is poverty. However, when Evelyn says that buying a home in San Francisco felt "a little like clawing back" a piece of the city, we have to ask: Whose land is she clawing back? Evelyn probably would answer that she was clawing back the land of her black forebearers, who were denied the opportunity to purchase property in San Francisco. But Evelyn's black forebearers were denied the opportunity to purchase property on land that white settlers had brutally expropriated from Muwekma Ohlone people. Thus, Evelyn, rightfully, was claiming property for her black family, but the property that she was claiming sits on land that belonged to Native people who have been asking for their #LandBack.[102] This is the complex position in which wealthier black San Franciscans find themselves. The truth of their victimization does not erase the reality that they participate in a system that victimizes.

Moreover, affluent black San Franciscans are not simply participating in a system that victimizes; they are *thriving* in a system that victimizes. Wealthier black San Franciscans are on the winning side of the stunning income inequality that describes contemporary life in the United States. They are amassing wealth. They are enjoying privileges. And to the extent that great wealth can be accumulated only by denying laborers the full value of their labor—and to the extent that privileges are produced only by refusing universal access to the thing that we call a privilege—then affluent black San Franciscans are members of the class that exploits and refuses. Again, this is the complex position that high-income black San Franciscans occupy.

And yet we cannot forget that although wealthier black San Franciscans—like wealthier black people across the United States—are succeeding in a system in which success often depends on the subordination of others, their success is tinged with their own marginalization. They die more frequently than their white counterparts from pregnancy-related causes.[103] Their babies die during their first years of life more frequently than the babies born to their white counterparts.[104] Their children are much more likely than the children of their nonblack peers to slip out of the middle class and to fall into the working class or the impoverished class. In other words, there is a higher frequency of intergenerational downward mobility among black people than among nonblack people.[105] This is the complex position that high-income black San Franciscans occupy.

Evelyn was defiant in her insistence that San Francisco is hers, and she described the "exhaustion" of living in a city where few black people live and where most of the few black people who live there are poor: "The exhaustion is real. It is something that like—it just all kind of sucks. It just feels very unfair. Black people here—we do a lot of heavy lifting for a place that hasn't valued us. I love San Francisco. But it doesn't love us back."

The exhaustion that many of my class-privileged black interviewees reported experiencing is not inconsequential. As chapter 3 explores, there are many possible explanations for the racial disparities in health that exist even at the top of the socioeconomic ladder. But one explanation that has captured the attention of researchers is the likelihood that racism-related stress may contribute to the poorer health of wealthier people of color. According to one research study, "Racial discrimination is a unique source of stress reported by African Americans and has been associated with hypertension, weight gain, adverse birth outcomes and persistent inflammation."[106] Class-privileged black people have frequent contact with nonblack people—in college and university classrooms, at high-paying jobs, and in affluent neighborhoods. Class privilege allows them to exit sites of concentrated black poverty and to enter predominately white spaces. While entrance into these spaces comes with great benefits—college degrees that make accessible the halls of power, jobs that pay higher salaries, and personal connections that constitute invaluable social capital—it also comes with some costs. One cost may be the exhaustion that is a consequence of navigating overwhelmingly white spaces as a racial Other.[107] This exhaustion may help to explain why "high socioeconomic position 'does not buy the same level of health for African Americans relative to Whites.'"[108]

Nevertheless, high-income black people try their damnedest to buy the level of health enjoyed by their white counterparts. In the United States' two-tiered healthcare system, this typically means that black people who can afford to do so seek and receive their healthcare from institutions that cater to commercially insured patients, carefully avoiding hospitals and clinics that care for large numbers of the uninsured or Medicaid-insured. In the context of a black maternal health crisis, receiving healthcare from institutions that care for the class-privileged can be the difference between life and death. In this way, there seems to be a parallel between yesterday's urban renewal and gentrification and today's failure to protect the health of black pregnant people. Just as urban renewal and gentrification harmed black people but benefitted developers, contractors, and those who could afford to remain in the city, racial disparities in maternal mortality harm black people but benefit places like Golden Health, where class-privileged black people attempt to purchase an escape from the nation's black maternal health crisis. Distilled to its essence, it appears that black vulnerability can be profitable. The next chapter examines Zuckerberg San Francisco General Hospital and Trauma Center, which has helped to make Golden Health the site where unicorns like Evelyn—and high income San Franciscans of all races—receive their healthcare.

2 Healthcare Segregation in the City by the Bay

One afternoon during my second summer conducting research at Golden Health, I wandered around the obstetrics clinic on the Yerba Buena campus, willing myself to see things that I had not yet seen. A corkboard in one of the clinic's employee-only hallways eventually caught my eye. Among the various papers it displayed was a chart created by Golden's administration that presented various metrics of how well the obstetrics and gynecology (OB/GYN) department was performing. Columns on the chart included "Patient safety," "Patient security," and "Financial security." However, I was struck by the final column on the chart: "Patient satisfaction." The administration had evaluated the OB/GYN department's performance with respect to patient safety, patient security, and financial security as "Excellent," "Excellent," and "Very good," but with respect to patient satisfaction, it had evaluated the department only as "Good." A footnote at the bottom of the document explained how the administration planned to improve performance in the area: "Emphasize patient experience and a concierge-like approach."

About five miles away from Golden's Yerba Buena campus sits Zuckerberg San Francisco General Hospital and Trauma Center, or "the General," for short.[1] The General is San Francisco's "poor people's hospital"—the place where the city's indigent, dispossessed, and marginalized can receive healthcare. While Golden's administration might aspire to "emphasize patient experience and a concierge-like approach" when caring for its mostly commercially insured pregnant patients—aspirations that some Golden patients would say the health system has achieved, while other patients would say it has not—the General's administrators cannot afford to worry about its patients' experience and offering them a "concierge-like approach." Instead, the General's administrators know that the hospital succeeds wildly when it provides healthcare to every impoverished person who enters its doors—even if there is nothing pretty, efficient, or concierge-like about the healthcare experience that is delivered.

I came to understand that Golden Health and the other private San Francisco hospitals and health systems that are Golden's competitors can hope to provide "concierge-like" care to their overwhelmingly commercially insured patients *because* the General cares for large numbers of the city's uninsured and publicly insured patients. In other words, the General's designation as the place for poor people enables other hospitals in San Francisco to offer class-privileged people the care that middle-class and upper-middle-class people expect from their healthcare institutions.

The General informs the healthcare choices of all San Franciscans—especially those whose relative affluence permits them to receive their care from other institutions. Indeed, wealthier San Franciscans see the General as a place that they should avoid at all costs. This fact was made crystal clear to me in spring 2022, when I attended a Zoom webinar that Golden hosted for its patients who were in their third trimester of pregnancy. The webinar provided patients with information about the hospital's labor and delivery (L&D) department so that they could finalize plans for the births of their babies. The presenters shared information on COVID-19 restrictions (for example, patients were allowed no more than two visitors, both of whom were required to wear face masks) and described the amenities that would be available in the recovery rooms (for example, patients could schedule a photoshoot with their newborns and specify in advance whether they had any dietary restrictions). Things got a little less tame, however, when the L&D director mentioned that if all of the beds in Golden's birth center were filled with patients in labor, then the center would be put "on divert," and newly arriving patients in labor would be sent to deliver their babies in another San Francisco hospital. This piece of information clearly rankled the webinar's attendees, as shown by the questions they posed in the chat:

How often does divert happen?

Has the birth center been on divert frequently in the past few months?

If you are already scheduled for an induction, does that guarantee you will not be diverted?

Are high-risk patients commonly diverted?

Are we able to request a specific location or express a preference for [an] alternate birthing location if on divert?

Is SF General one of the hospitals where patients are sent if you're on divert?

If Golden is on divert, can we ask not to be sent to the General?

Is there a way for a patient to guarantee that they won't have to deliver at the General if Golden is diverting patients?

For the patients posing these questions, it seemed as though that the General was the last place they wanted to deliver their baby. It was a worst-case scenario.

Like many safety-net hospitals, the General has been mythologized in San Francisco. In the minds of most San Franciscans, the General is the place for poor people, the place that will not provide the healthcare experience that you desire, the place that delivers inferior care. The fact that the General is the negative example against which all other San Francisco hospitals are compared becomes particularly interesting in light of racial disparities in maternal mortality. When class-privileged pregnant black people—in their efforts to avoid becoming another tragic case in the ongoing black maternal health crisis—choose to receive their prenatal care from Golden, they are, in many important respects, choosing *not* to go to the General. These commercially insured black patients are deploying their class privilege to achieve an exit from the institutions where their impoverished counterparts go and where they think they are more likely to become yet another black maternal death.

While high-income people of all races in San Francisco steer clear of the General in order to dodge the second-rate experience and substandard healthcare they imagine that the hospital will deliver, high-income black people steer clear of the General for those reasons *and* because they are seeking to dodge a race-based harm. More affluent black people in San Francisco suppose that if the black maternal health crisis is happening somewhere in the city, it probably is unfolding at the General. By staying away from the General and receiving their prenatal care from hospitals with wealthier patient populations, affluent black people are attempting to achieve the superior maternal health outcomes that their white counterparts enjoy. Avoiding "poor people's hospitals," then, is a strategy for avoiding the burdens of nonwhiteness. Importantly, in the United States' profit-generating healthcare system, this particular strategy for avoiding the burdens of nonwhiteness is lucrative for Golden and its competitors. These institutions can count on receiving the business of high-income black patients who are trying to survive pregnancy. In this way, the black maternal health crisis accrues to the benefit of hospitals that cater to wealthier clienteles.

This chapter begins by describing healthcare segregation in San Francisco—where Golden Health and its competitors provide attentive, responsive, courteous care to their largely commercially insured patients, and the General provides care that likely will win no awards for patient experience to its largely uninsured and publicly insured patients. The chapter then examines the common assumption that the poor patient experience that one can expect at the General correlates with poor-quality healthcare. Then, after a discussion of how hospitals that cater to commercially insured patients seek to maximize their profits by minimizing the number of Medicaid-insured patients they care for, this chapter explores how the General's existence enables hospitals like Golden to provide its commercially insured patients with the patient experience that they seek from healthcare institutions. The chapter ends by showing that there is nothing particularly distinctive about healthcare segregation in San Francisco, briefly sketching what healthcare segregation looks like in New York City.

Before diving into this exploration, it might be helpful to clarify a few things. First, Medicaid is the government program that provides health insurance to low-income individuals in the United States.[2] Individual states administer their own Medicaid programs, funding the state's version of Medicaid through a mix of federal and state monies.[3] California has dubbed its Medicaid program "Medi-Cal."[4] Second, Medicare, which is different from Medicaid, is the government program that provides health insurance to individuals over age sixty-five in the United States.[5] Medicare is largely irrelevant to an analysis of insurance coverage of prenatal care and other pregnancy-related expenses because most people are unable to become pregnant after age sixty-five. Third, in this chapter, "commercial insurance" refers to health insurance that is administered by private corporations, not the government. Individuals typically access commercial insurance through their employer (or the employer of their spouse or parent) or through an individual or family health insurance plan they have purchased directly from a private insurer.

SAN FRANCISCO-STYLE HEALTHCARE SEGREGATION

In the imaginations of San Franciscans, the General is the place where the dispossessed—poor people, unhoused persons, sex workers, drug users, people struggling with substance use disorders, mentally ill individuals—receive their healthcare. For the most part, this perception aligns with reality. The hospital's 2022–2023 annual report reveals that over half of its patients—almost 59 percent of its inpatients and 58 percent of its outpatients—were Medi-Cal insured.[6] Additionally, 1 percent of its inpatients and 8 percent of its outpatients were uninsured.[7] Thus, close to two-thirds of the General's patients were poor enough to qualify for Medi-Cal or were so disenfranchised that they lacked health insurance altogether.[8] Meanwhile, commercially insured individuals comprised only a small percentage of the General's patient population—4 percent of inpatients and 3 percent of outpatients.[9] So people with enough class privilege to exit the constraint-riddled world of public insurance rarely visit the General for healthcare, but poor people turn to the institution in droves. Because of the enduring relationship in the United States between class privilege and race privilege—with racially unprivileged people disproportionately bearing the burdens of poverty—the General's status as San Francisco's "poor people's hospital" also means that it is San Francisco's black and brown people's hospital. While black and Latine people comprise, respectively, 5 percent and 15 percent of the city's population, they comprised 13 percent and 41 percent of the General's patient population in 2022–2023.[10] Compare the overrepresentation of black and Latine people at the General with the underrepresentation of white and Asian people: While white and Asian people constitute, respectively, 43 percent and 34 percent of the city's population, they constituted only 16 percent and 21 percent of the General's patient population in 2022–2023.[11]

Comparing the General's demographics with those of Golden Health is illuminating. While commercially insured patients comprised less than 4 percent of the General's patient population in 2021–2022, 33 percent of Golden's inpatients and 48 percent of its outpatients were commercially insured.[12] Moreover, while Medi-Cal-insured patients comprised almost two-thirds of the General's patient population, they comprised only 29 percent and 16 percent of Golden's inpatients and outpatients, respectively.[13] In essence, while class-privileged, commercially insured people avoided the General like the plague, they frequently elected to receive their healthcare from Golden. In contrast, while poor people made up the overwhelming majority of those who received their healthcare from the General, they were much less likely to be found among the thousands of people that Golden Health cared for every year. And so we may begin telling a story about more affluent people receiving their medical care from institutions from which the poor are absent.

Scholars recently have begun to call this pattern "healthcare segregation."[14] And as one set of researchers notes, "[S]egregated care can take many forms."[15] Healthcare segregation sometimes results from the common practice of departments in academic medical centers assigning Medicaid-insured patients to the care of residents while assigning commercially insured patients to the care of faculty.[16] At other times, healthcare segregation occurs when Medicaid-insured patients are scheduled at different times of the day than commercially insured patients.[17] Healthcare segregation may also result when Medicaid-insured patients are seen in different parts of a single hospital or facility than commercially insured patients.[18] Indeed, when I was conducting research for my first book, a patient, Annalise, told me about receiving prenatal care from a New York City hospital that physically separated patients along the lines of insurance status in this way. As she told me:

> They had an area for high-risk patients with Medicaid. And then there was the pretty lounge over there [for commercially insured patients]. You know? And they were—they call them perinatologists. They had the Perinatology Suite [for commercially insured patients]. And sitting over there were . . . white

ladies, upscale black ladies. . . . All up in there. And I'm like, "Well, damn! Let me go get on my mama insurance or my daddy insurance." I'm like, damn! They were looking good. They had beautiful, comfy chairs. The lighting was nice. It was beautiful. It was a *suite*. After I had my son, for some reason, I don't know why, I went back on my job's insurance. I don't know if the hospital messed up, but I used it. I was a private patient then. I was in the pretty area. I was in the suite. Over here. All the Medicaid patients were in the crazy area over there—yelling and screaming and carrying on. I was on this side.

The healthcare segregation that I witnessed in San Francisco while conducting research for this book primarily took the form of physical separation between institutions, with the obstetrics clinics at Golden Health and its competitors operating as places for more affluent people and the obstetrics clinic at the General operating as the place for the poor. But as I studied the city's healthcare landscape in greater depth, I found that the story was more complex. The numbers showing that 29 percent and 16 percent of Golden's inpatients and outpatients are Medi-Cal-insured hides healthcare segregation *within* the health system and *between* departments.

Healthcare Segregation within Health Systems

Golden Health has three campuses—Yerba Buena, East Hills, and John Muir. I conducted fieldwork only on the Yerba Buena and East Hills campuses, as the John Muir campus does not have an obstetrics clinic. The buildings on the Yerba Buena campus are older and less appealing than those on the East Hills campus, which tend to have a lot of glass, shiny metal, vaulted ceilings, and art on the walls. The East Hills campus is located in a neighborhood that I will pseudonymously call Morristown Flats—one of the many communities in San Francisco that the well-heeled call home. In Morristown Flats, condos of twelve hundred square feet are sold for $1.3 million.[19] Meanwhile, the Yerba Buena campus is located in a neighborhood that I will pseudonymously call Valerio—a community that while still unaffordable to most buyers and renters in the United States, might be *slightly* more accessible than Morristown Flats due to its proximity to housing projects and other low-income housing. When low-income people find their way to a Golden Health hospital, they are more likely to end up on the Yerba Buena campus than the East Hills campus. The statistics describing Medi-Cal-insured patients as composing 29 percent and 16 percent of Golden Health's inpatient and outpatient population do not reveal the distribution of Medi-Cal-insured people within the hospital system. It is likely that Golden's Yerba Buena campus cares for many more low-income patients than Golden's East Hills campus. In this way, Golden achieves healthcare segregation *within* its individual health system.

Statistics describing Golden Health's primary competitors—which I will pseudonymously call Synoptic Health and Mercy Medical Center—make this plain. Medi-Cal-insured patients comprise 42 percent of the outpatient population at one of Synoptic Health's two hospitals, Synoptic East, and only 15 percent at its other hospital, Synoptic West.[20] In this way, Synoptic East becomes a quasi poor people's hospital, while Synoptic West becomes a hospital for wealthier people. Similarly, Medi-Cal-insured patients comprise 22 percent of the patient population at one of Mercy Medical Center's two hospitals, and they comprise only 12 percent at the other. (Golden Health's other competitor is a managed-care conglomerate that I will pseudonymously call the Brighton Leary Foundation, which integrates its health insurance, providers, and medical facilities. Medi-Cal-insured patients comprise just 6 percent of the inpatient population and 10 percent of the outpatient population at Brighton Leary's San Francisco medical center.)[21]

Healthcare segregation within an individual health system might not be simply a function of location, as when the system locates some of its hospitals in economically depressed areas of a city or region and some of its hospitals in more affluent areas. The health system might also do things—intentionally or unintentionally—that direct low-income patients toward the system's quasi poor people's hospitals and away from the system's hospitals for wealthier clientele. For example, Golden Health operates a Young Women's Clinic that, at least initially, was designed to provide reproductive healthcare to minors. A former director of the clinic once described it as a place that "offered an evidence-based caring and safe space for birthing adolescents to learn about the experience of pregnancy and delivery through empowerment and trust."[22] Because poverty is a predictor of adolescent pregnancy, many of the pregnant patients who received their prenatal care at the Young Women's Clinic were poor. Over time, however, the clinic transformed from a place that cares for young pregnant patients to one that cares for low-income pregnant patients. Significantly, this clinic is located on Golden's Yerba Buena campus. In this way, Golden directs some of its already small low-income patient population to the Yerba Buena campus, allowing Golden's East Hills campus to serve as the site for care for the well-to-do.

Healthcare segregation within health systems has become more visible—and perhaps more intentional—with the recent rapid increase in hospital mergers. The acquisition of a hospital or health system by another hospital or health system can be beneficial in some instances, as when the merger makes it possible for formerly separate and possibly competing hospitals to "share knowledge and best practices with each other."[23] A merger might also produce cost savings through economies of scale, especially when the newly expanded health system achieves "efficiencies by purchasing goods and supplies in greater volume."[24] A merger might also allow a smaller hospital to access the resources of the larger health system that acquires it, thus enabling the hospital to hire staff, purchase needed equipment, upgrade its technologies, and make improvements to its physical plant.[25]

However, hospital mergers can be harmful, as when a health system acquires and soon shutters a hospital that primarily serves a disadvantaged community, making it difficult for people living in the community to access healthcare.[26] Hospital mergers also can be harmful when they increase a health system's market share of healthcare consumers, thereby increasing the system's negotiating power with commercial insurers. As explained later in the chapter, when healthcare providers have the upper hand in negotiations with commercial insurance companies, they are able to demand higher insurance reimbursement rates for the services that they provide to insured patients.[27] Ultimately, insurers pass on those higher reimbursement rates to their members in the form of higher premiums, deductibles, and copayments or a smaller universe of covered services. In short, hospital mergers can be harmful when they result in higher healthcare costs.[28]

In many instances, hospital mergers do not result in cost savings due to economies of scale, knowledge sharing that results in improved quality of care, or resource sharing that results in the provision of better healthcare to the communities that the acquired hospitals serve. Instead, many hospital consolidations follow the "'model in which a health system puts its name on a hospital, raises the rates, and doesn't do much else.'"[29] In these cases, the formerly separate, smaller hospital—which may have a high proportion of low-income patients—is part of the resource-rich health system following the merger. In practice, however, the acquired hospital remains severed from the larger health system's resources. As it relates to healthcare segregation, an acquired hospital usually continues to serve its former population—the poorer, Medicaid-insured patients that it had been serving prior to the merger—while the other hospitals in the health system continue to serve a wealthier, commercially insured patient population. This merger model "operationally [results in] two separate hospitals."[30] However, the health system is able to include the patients cared for at the acquired hospital in its overall patient demographics. This move obscures the segregation within the hospital system, concealing the fact that some of the system's hospitals have nearly no low-income patients while others are bursting at the seams with poor patients. Thus, when Synoptic Health claims that its hospitals "compassionately care for more low-income Medi-Cal patients in Northern California than any other health care system, serving 14 percent of the 2020 Medi-Cal discharge population in Northern California,"[31] it may be appropriate to ask which of Synoptic Health's hospitals are caring for low-income Medi-Cal patients and which are not. Likewise, when Golden Health similarly claims that it is "proud to serve all members of our community, regardless of illness severity, income level or residential area" and that "Medicaid patients represent more than 23 percent of our total patient services,"[32] it may be appropriate to wonder whether some Golden campuses are seeing most of those Medicaid patients, while Medicaid patients are few and far between at other Golden campuses.

Healthcare Segregation Between Departments

The statistics describing Medi-Cal-insured patients as comprising 29 percent and 16 percent of Golden inpatient and outpatient populations hide the fact that some departments within the health system care for many low-income patients, while other departments care for very few. This was made apparent to me when I was first considering whether to conduct my research for this book at Golden. When a research program manager at the health system responded to my request for the demographics of the pregnant patient population, I learned that in September 2021, 95 percent of the *pregnant* patient population at Golden Health was commercially insured, while only 4 percent was Medi-Cal-insured.[33] The statistics describing the percentage of Medi-Cal patients that Golden cares for in general obscures the scarcity of Medi-Cal patients within the obstetrics department in particular. In this way, we may wonder what disparities *between* departments are hidden when hospitals and health systems provide statistics describing their overall patient populations.

Additionally, the fact that only 4 percent of Golden's pregnant patient population was Medi-Cal-insured in 2021 increases the significance of the Young Women's Clinic's location on the Yerba Buena campus. Because the Young Women's Clinic on the Yerba Buena campus cared for *large*—that is, disproportionate—numbers of Golden's Medi-Cal-insured pregnant patient population, we can conclude that *fewer* than 4 percent of the pregnant patients seen on the East Hills campus were Medi-Cal-insured. Thus, a Medi-Cal-insured patient in the obstetrics clinic on the East Hills campus was a rarity. At East Hills, class-privileged people enjoyed their prenatal care alongside mostly other class-privileged people.

THE GENERAL VERSUS EVERYONE ELSE

Although the General's status as San Francisco's "poor people's hospital" enables other hospitals in the city to see relatively few indigent patients, nonprofit hospitals—such as Golden Health, Synoptic Health, Mercy Medical Center, and Brighton Leary Foundation—have an obligation to provide care to indigent patients. Nonprofit hospitals are exempted from paying federal taxes and also some state and local taxes. According to one report, $24 billion in taxes went uncollected nationally due to these valuable exemptions.[34] In exchange for tax exemptions, nonprofit hospitals are supposed to bear the cost of caring for the uninsured and the underinsured. They can fulfill this obligation in a number of ways. They may allow patients' unpaid medical bills to go uncollected,[35] provide healthcare to uninsured people with no expectation of payment,[36] or, crucially, care for substantial numbers of Medicaid-insured patients (as serving these patients results in a financial loss to hospitals and providers due to Medicaid's low reimbursement rates).

Many observers have noted that nonprofit hospitals are doing a terrible job of earning their tax exemptions. One study shows that for-profit hospitals provide as much charity care as nonprofit hospitals.[37] The *New York Times* ran a series of articles that documented some of the often sordid ways in which nonprofit hospitals "have become virtually indistinguishable from for-profit companies, adopting an unrelenting focus on the bottom line and straying from their traditional charitable missions."[38] It reported that "[g]iant hospital systems illegally sent exorbitant bills to Medicaid patients. They used hospitals in poor neighborhoods to qualify for steep drug discounts, funneling the proceeds into wealthier neighborhoods. Others cut staff to dangerously low levels."[39] Nonprofit hospitals adopted these harmful practices to maximize profits—despite the fact that profit maximization sits in tension with a tax-exempt status that is intended to allow these institutions to serve the most vulnerable in their communities. The consequence is that nonprofit and for-profit hospitals have become practically identical insofar as they both structure business operations with the aim of making as much money as possible.

Golden Health is like Synoptic Health, Mercy Medical Center, and Brighton Leary Foundation because they all are failing to truly earn their tax exempt status by caring for substantial numbers of the city's uninsured and underinsured. That is, Golden, like the nonprofit hospitals and health systems that are its competitors, may depend on the General to be the city's "poor people's hospital" so that its class-privileged patients can be relatively insulated from poor people and can have the experiences that their affluence has permitted them to expect from their healthcare providers. However, an important characteristic distinguishes Golden from the other nonprofit hospitals serving San Franciscans: Golden Health, like the General, is a public institution. Golden, like the General, is not privately owned and operated. Thus, the fairly small percentage of Golden patients that are Medicaid-insured—and the even smaller percentage of Golden *pregnant* patients that are Medicaid-insured—is even more striking. In many places around the country, healthcare segregation occurs because public hospitals predominately care for low-income people, while private hospitals predominately care for higher-income people. Consequently, healthcare segregation commonly occurs along the lines of public versus private hospitals. However, in San Francisco hospitals, healthcare segregation occurs along the lines of the General versus everyone else.

There is a great degree of intentionality behind this set of circumstances. The General has consciously directed itself toward serving San Francisco's dispossessed. It is one of many hospitals in the country that are "uniquely organized and oriented to the special needs of low-income and uninsured populations."[40] This explains why the General's home page proudly states that "[e]veryone is welcome here, no matter your ability to pay, lack of insurance, or immigration status."[41] When patients enter the physical doors of the General, they will see flyers that provide phone numbers for services that can connect them with housing, benefits from the Supplemental Nutrition Assistance Program (SNAP) (the program formerly known as food stamps), Medicaid, treatment for substance use disorders, and benefits from Cal-WORKs (the program that provides cash assistance to indigent families). When patients arrive at the General's OB/GYN department in particular, they will see signs advertising programs like Team Lily, a "roving care team providing wraparound services to pregnant people experiencing significant barriers to engagement in clinic-based prenatal care. We primarily serve pregnant people with housing insecurity, active substance use, and/or mental health diagnoses."[42]

At the same time that the General is orienting itself toward the most marginalized people living in San Francisco, the hospital is making itself unattractive to those with commercial insurance. In fact, the General does not contract with most commercial insurance plans.[43] Its first contract with a commercial insurer—which allowed subscribers to the insurer's plan to receive in-network obstetric and midwifery care from the hospital—was signed in 2019.[44] The result is that the hospital is out-of-network for most commercially insured people.[45] Thus, if a commercially insured patient happens to be drawn to the General and wants to receive care from the hospital, they likely will reconsider when they learn that the facility is out-of-network for them, making medical bills appreciably higher if they are cared for at the hospital.[46]

While the General is focusing on vulnerable people, the other hospitals in San Francisco seem to be averting their gaze. Although Golden advertises that it accepts Medi-Cal insurance, it will not help patients sign up for the benefit if they are not already enrolled. Thus, when uninsured, low-income pregnant people call the Golden obstetrics clinic to make an appointment for prenatal care, they will be told that they should call back after they sign up for Medi-Cal. Complicating things is that Golden will not accept new pregnant patients after their first trimester. So the clock is ticking for an uninsured poor person who wants to receive their prenatal care at Golden. They have to find a Medi-Cal office, demonstrate their presumptive eligibility for Medi-Cal, receive official notice that they have been approved for temporary benefits pending their submission of a formal application,[47] and, with that notice in hand, call Golden to make an appointment for prenatal care—all before the end of their first trimester. Alternatively, instead of jumping through these hoops, patients can just go to the General, which will enroll uninsured pregnant patients in Medi-Cal at their first prenatal care appointment.

In failing to enroll presumptively eligible patients in Medi-Cal, Golden erects a barrier for uninsured, low-income patients who would like to receive their prenatal care within its health system. It is not unreasonable to conclude that this barrier may be a major reason that Medi-Cal–insured patients comprised only 5 percent of Golden pregnant patients in 2021 and only 10 percent of all pregnant patients in 2024. Further, those savvy low-income patients who have the wherewithal and know-how to surmount the barrier might experience the barrier as a message that Medi-Cal-insured people are unwelcome—or not as welcome as others—in the health system. As Dr. Sitara Davani, a high-energy, generous woman who was known throughout Golden's obstetrics department for her commitment to caring for low-income people, put it, "If I were one of those patients, I would be like, 'Why *would* I go to Golden?'"

Dr. Brianna Turner, a Golden Health obstetrician who worked at both Golden and the General as part of her residency, described Golden as a "byzantine bureaucracy" that *all* prospective patients likely would find difficult to navigate: "Golden is not patient-centered for anyone." According to Dr. Turner, while Golden assists no patient in deciphering its complex system, those with class privilege are much more likely to figure out how to navigate the complexity and access care. Those without class privilege, on the other hand, more frequently find the system inscrutable and, consequently, the care inaccessible. Dr. Turner explained this issue by using the example of health insurance:

> There are so many times that a patient will say, "Oh, I have insurance," and we [at Golden] will respond, "Your insurance is not active." Now, a healthcare-savvy patient will call their insurance company. They will figure it out. But Golden will not figure it out for them—or even help them figure it out for themselves. This matters a great deal when you're talking about low-income people, who often are un- or underinsured. If we really wanted to help them, we would say, "Oh, let's figure out how to activate your insurance" or "Let's get your insurance transferred to this locale." Or something like that. Instead, we essentially say, "Not my problem." So even though anyone, technically, can get care at Golden, it is exceedingly difficult to do so if you don't know how to navigate the system.

Dr. Turner also raised the issue of scarce prenatal care appointments. During my fieldwork, the demand for prenatal care appointments far outstripped the supply. In a context of scarcity, do poor patients or class-privileged patients receive the resource? She concluded the latter:

> Who gets these appointments? How many times do you have to call to actually get an appointment before the end of your first trimester? Of course, in a space of limited resources, the scarce resource goes to the people who assert their power and their privilege and who call ten times demanding things. The resource goes to the people who have the *time* to call ten times. Those are the folks who get those appointments. Low-income people, unprivileged people just aren't able to advocate for themselves in that way.

Consider as well that at the General, advertising for services designed to assist the poor—people who are housing-insecure, food-insecure, or healthcare-insecure—cannot be avoided. In glaring contrast, Golden's walls are not papered with flyers announcing services that can connect patients with basic necessities. This absence subtly communicates that Golden is not the place for people who might need these services. Indeed, the absence might send the message that people with those kinds of needs might be better served elsewhere. As Dr. Davani explained it,

> Golden is not a place that screams, "We're here for you no matter who you are." It doesn't say that at all, right? In San Francisco General, for all of its extreme frustrations—the waiting times, the fact that it is hard to get in touch with people on the phone—when you walk in, I think there is the vibe of "We're going to figure this out for you. It may not be pretty. [laughs] We have our issues. But we're going to figure this out for you."
>
> I believe that, if you want to bring in Medi-Cal-insured people—*more* Medi-Cal-insured people—you have to intentionally design your services for the needs of Medi-Cal-insured people. So if you're like, "We're open to Medi-Cal-insured people," and you do nothing else. . . . Sure, your doors are open. And you're going to get what you're going to get.

And, in 2024, Golden Health—a self-professed progressive public institution in a self-professed progressive city in a self-professed progressive state—was getting a Medi-Cal-insured pregnant patient population that constituted just 10 percent of its total patient population.

Further, in failing to design their services to meet the needs of vulnerable, low-income patients, Golden and its competitors in the San Francisco healthcare market have become *bad* places for vulnerable, low-income patients to receive healthcare. While Golden and its competitors might be able to offer exceptional medical care to the indigent patients they see, they are unable to offer these patients the other services—such as assistance with securing housing and help in signing up for food benefits—that patients need if they are to become and remain healthy. A scenario is created wherein dispossessed patients might be better served at the General, as Golden and its competitors are unable to care for multiply marginalized people in the holistic way that they may need. As an example of this phenomenon, Dr. Marie Clarke, an obstetrician at Golden, explained to me that because only 5 to 10 percent of Golden's pregnant patients are Medi-Cal-insured, the birth center is ill-prepared to provide low-income patients with "the right support in ancillary services"—that is, assistance with securing benefits from social safety-net programs: "We're just completely caught off guard—and it is *because* our number [of Medi-Cal-insured patients] is 5 percent, or 10 percent or whatever it is now. So for the past four or five years, we've really been working hard to beef up [the provision of ancillary services]. But we're still nowhere near what our colleagues at San Francisco General offer." In this way, it may be wise for pregnant patients with significant nonmedical needs to receive their prenatal care from the General instead of Golden.

Dr. Davani agreed that the General's existence as the city's safety-net hospital allowed all of the other hospitals in San Francisco—for-profit and nonprofit—to become sites where more affluent people receive their healthcare. However, she was ambivalent about whether a system of truly integrated healthcare actually would be better for the city's most marginalized:

> I think that San Francisco General enables a lot of the other hospitals in the city to not pay attention to Medi-Cal patients. San Francisco General is definitely an enabler. Part of me feels that if you shut the hospital down, other hospitals are going to rise to the occasion. They won't have a choice. But the other part of me knows that that's not the right answer. Because while I think that other hospitals will rise to the occasion [and serve low-income patients if the General were to close down], I have questions about *how high* they will rise. They'll do more. They'll sign people up for presumptive eligibility. They'll do the basics. But I know the breadth and the depth of what a place like San Francisco General does for the truly marginalized. And these other hospitals are never going to do that. Golden is never going to do that.

THE QUESTION OF QUALITY IN SEGREGATED HOSPITALS

Many might not think that healthcare segregation—poor people and wealthier people relying on different institutions for care—is problematic. They may believe that healthcare segregation becomes concerning only if the places to which poor people turn for healthcare offer substandard care. For them, the stakes of healthcare segregation would increase dramatically if relative affluence meant that affluent people received superior care while poverty meant that impoverished people received inadequate healthcare.

So we must ask the million-dollar question: Do safety-net hospitals provide lower-quality healthcare? As it turns out, the answer is complicated, partly because quality is a nebulous concept. Does it refer to health outcomes alone? Does it also refer to patient experience? Does it refer to the ability of the institution to meet the needs of the patient that impact health but are not strictly medical?

As a general matter, hospitals that care for large numbers of uninsured or underinsured patients run at a deficit, unable to cover their operating costs by billing patients and their insurance plans for care. As a consequence, many of these hospitals rely on government subsidies to remain solvent.[48] When those subsidies are not adequate or are less than the revenue that institutions *without* a large uninsured or underinsured patient population generate from billing commercial insurance plans for care, these hospitals "may provide lower-quality services" relative to their counterparts serving wealthier people.[49]

Consistent with this possibility, my previous book contains an interview with a chief resident who proposed that the quality of the healthcare offered at one of New York City's General-like safety-net hospitals, Alpha Hospital, was inferior to the care offered at the private hospital next door, Omega Hospital, that served large numbers of commercially insured patients. She described it as follows:

> Anywhere from the actual machine for a CAT scan to the X-ray machine is better at Omega than it is here [at Alpha]. It has a higher resolution. So, for example, if we're ruling out a pulmonary embolism—which we do a lot, because in pregnancy, people are at an increased risk for getting blood clots—they will often call it a poor study here, whereas at Omega, they never do. One time, I asked the radiologist why that was so, and he just said that the actual scanner [at Omega] is a better-quality machine. So there is just the equipment level. And then there's the number of scanners and the number of staff—so that makes it easier to scan, or MRI, or whatever, over at Omega than to do it here. And it's not always true that one is going to be better than the other. It's just that, in terms of the overall, it's easier to get a scan there. And it's better quality. . . .

> Another procedure, for example, that we could do at Omega is a procedure called endometrial oblation. There are all different types of techniques to do it. And we don't have all that technology [at Alpha] to do that. . . .
>
> If you compare what is here [at Alpha] versus what is at Omega, there are just more restraints here—because it's all based on budgets.⁵⁰

This chief resident indicates that healthcare segregation in New York City results in the have-nots receiving second-rate care. Thus, we might safely conclude that at least some safety-net hospitals provide inferior care relative to their counterparts that serve the more affluent.

But what about the General? There was intense disagreement among the obstetricians that I interviewed about whether the General offered the same excellent healthcare as Golden. Part of this disagreement was because the physicians had different definitions of what quality care was. However, most intriguing to me was when a physician disagreed *with herself* about the quality of the healthcare provided at the General relative to Golden. Consider Dr. Juliette Chalifour, a Golden-based obstetrician who had spent many years caring for patients at both Golden and the General. When I asked her whether she thought that the General provides "the same quality of care" to its pregnant patients, Dr. Chalifour responded as follows:

> Yes. I think the [obstetric] care is really good. [pause] Yeah, I think their [obstetric] care is really exceptional. There's a lot of cross talk between Golden and San Francisco General in terms of providers. So San Francisco General still has that academic flavor. For example, our [maternal-fetal medicine specialists] work over there; our high-risk [obstetrics] doctors go there. Their midwives are really good, really seasoned. Their C-section rates are really good, too. They're doing well.
>
> In answering this question, what is going through my mind is: what would happen at San Francisco General if shit hits the fan? Let's say that someone is hemorrhaging, and you need to act quickly. San Francisco General has interventional radiology, which is what we would use to save somebody's life. They have doctors that can do—God forbid that you need to do—a [Cesarean-hysterectomy]. They have all the medications. Their anesthesiologists are Golden anesthesiologists. I think they're good.

Dr. Chalifour made these statements just minutes after she had explained to me that when she stopped working at the General many years ago, she tried to take with her as many of her low-income patients as possible: "I really wanted to encourage patients to come over to a more resourced setting and get the care that they deserve, regardless of their insurance status." So in one breath, Dr. Chalifour believed that the General was offering "the same quality of care" found at Golden, and yet in another breath, Dr. Chalifour believed that patients at the General were not getting the care that they "deserved"—care that could be found in a "more resourced setting."

Dr. Turner also seemed torn on the question of whether the General offered the same quality of care as Golden. She initially shared her view that Golden possessed strengths that the General lacked, and vice versa. Her sense was that while the General is better at "dealing with the larger structural forces that affect people's ability to parent," Golden is better at caring for medically "complex cases." But then she thought better of what she had said and offered an amendment: "Well, actually, I think the surgeons are very strong in their care at the General. They have more experience with, like, abnormal placenta—like, very crazy cases." She concluded, "Yeah, I think, generally speaking, you can get very good care from both hospitals. Maybe subspecialty strengths may differ slightly. But both places provide very good care."

Later in the interview, however, Dr. Turner made an observation that contradicted her original claim that the General, like Golden, offers "very good care." A residency at Golden Health is highly coveted because residents care for patients at both Golden and the General. But she frequently noticed a shift in some Golden residents over time. At the outset, many residents were excited to practice medicine in a safety-net hospital. Indeed, the opportunity to help marginalized people at the General often initially drew them to Golden's residency program. However, Dr. Turner reported that while many residents had a "really beautiful experience," others had "a very complicated relationship with the General and their training":

> I think that working at the General makes them ask the question, "What does it mean to work at a safety-net hospital? What does it actually mean on the day-to-day? Are you part of a system that is not set up to best support

patients?" I think it's hard for some residents. Some people really struggle with it. It causes them a real moral distress. They came to medicine with the spirit of service. But then they arrive at the General, and it just feels *wrong* that they are supposed to provide care without the same resources—although the need is the same. It is inequitable. The care that you can provide at the General is *different* than what it would be elsewhere. And is that difference fair? Just? I remember sitting in on a class meeting with [first-year residents], and they were just. . . . They had created a moral distance between themselves and what they were doing. They thought that they were providing care that was suboptimal.

It is difficult to reconcile Dr. Turner's original claim that the General offers "very good care" with her subsequent claim that the care that it delivers is, at times, "suboptimal."

One way to resolve the tension is to recognize the bipolarity that characterizes the way that observers understand the General. On the one hand, the General does many things right in its quest to care for San Francisco's most marginalized. Consider Dr. Turner's glowing evaluation of the General:

> Now the General has a brand-new building—a beautiful building with gorgeous art. And I think it's very clear that people feel that physical spaces reflect investment in them. I think the new building is a powerful statement that the city cares about the patients. I also think that there is increasingly activated leadership at the General and other key people who have tried to create more enduring structural solutions to the inequity that we see in prenatal and obstetric care. They have Team Lily. They have a CPS [child protective services] timeout, which is designed to counter the incredible bias in CPS reporting that is so prevalent. Our [residents] have also diversified, as well as the midwives. They started the black-centered [group prenatal care program] at the General. So there are really great things going on over there.

On the other hand, while the General is getting many things right in how it provides healthcare to a population that is ignored by other institutions in San Francisco's healthcare ecosystem, it also fails this same population—by offering resource-constrained care that is just *different* from that dispensed by the institutions that care for those with class privilege. Thus, the General ricochets in the estimation of providers between being the praiseworthy equivalent of a highly esteemed institution like Golden and being subpar, subject to all of the fiscal limitations that restrict what safety-net hospitals can offer their vulnerable patients.

Two additional things are clear about the General. First, the respect that the General deserves for caring for the city's disregarded is neither here nor there to class-privileged San Franciscans who have options when it comes to their healthcare. The General does not ricochet in *these* onlookers' estimation. Instead, it tends to exist in their perception as a bad place that provides substandard healthcare. Because wealthier San Franciscans of all races have no reason to resign themselves to receiving inferior healthcare, they invariably avoid going to the General. However, wealthier *black* San Franciscans avoid going to the General because, for them, the stakes of possibly receiving substandard healthcare are higher. For at least half a decade, we have been told that we are in the middle of a black maternal health crisis. Because pregnant, class-privileged black people are attempting to escape this crisis, they choose not to receive healthcare from the General. Fascinatingly, they make this choice although an argument can be made that institutions like the General that are intended for people of color are better for people of color—even when these institutions lack the resources possessed by their rivals. The analogy to historically black colleges and universities (HBCUs) is instructive. Although the endowments of HBCUs are generally a small fraction of those of the predominately white colleges and universities that are their competitors,[51] many black students may be better served if they attend an HBCU—especially if they aspire toward a career in a science, technology, engineering, or mathematics (STEM) field.[52] Even so, scores of black students elect to attend predominately white institutions for college because they seek the benefits that they imagine accrue to those who matriculate at better-resourced places with largely white student bodies. Something similar may be happening in the context of the General and Golden Health. The General might be better for black people because, in many important respects, it is intended for people who are marginalized along various axes, including race. Nevertheless, high-income black people avoid the General and turn to health systems like Golden because they are seeking the benefits that they imagine accrue to those who receive their healthcare from better-resourced institutions with predominately white patient populations.

Commercially insured black people are convinced that one of the benefits that flow from the receipt of healthcare at places like Golden is a better chance of avoiding maternal death or severe injury. So in dodging the General, they are attempting to dodge a race-based harm and a particular manifestation of antiblackness. Importantly, in steering clear of the General for this reason, commercially insured black patients are simultaneously steering their health insurance—with its high reimbursement rates—toward places like Golden and its competitors. Thus, from the perspective of hospitals that predominately serve commercially insured patients, *the black maternal health crisis is good for business.* The crisis effectively eliminates any of the General's remaining capacity to compete for commercially insured black people's business.

A second thing that is clear about the people's perceptions of these two healthcare institutions is that the quality of the patient experience at the General is inferior to the one offered at Golden. Indeed, individuals who have not been disciplined to accept a certain level of frustration in their encounters with the institutions that are supposed to serve them would find it maddening to receive healthcare at the General. As Dr. Davani puts it:

> San Francisco General cares deeply, but they do not have their shit together enough. They can't pull it off. They don't provide really high-quality care in many ways. In some ways, they do. In terms of patient-centeredness, they provide great care. But there are some basic fundamentals that they lack. Like, people shouldn't have to wait an hour or more for their appointment. They shouldn't have to wait an hour to talk to someone on the phone. They should be able to *reach* their provider—whether by phone or email or otherwise. I mean, Golden is not knocking it out of the park when it comes to some of this stuff either. But at the General, it is *unforgivable.*

MAXIMIZING PROFITS BY MINIMIZING THE NUMBER OF MEDICAID-INSURED PATIENTS

So why are most hospitals satisfied with allowing the local "poor people's hospital" to care for Medicaid-insured patients? Why are most hospitals and health systems not clamoring to increase their market share of the

Medicaid-insured population in the areas that they serve? For some healthcare institutions, the answer is easy. For others—namely, academic medical centers, like Golden, that have a more formal relationship with the local safety-net hospital—the answer is more complex.

Let's start with the easy answer. Many hospitals and health systems do not want to care for large numbers of Medicaid-insured patients because Medicaid reimburses at a fraction of the rates paid by Medicare and commercial insurers. With an eye on the budget, state governments set the reimbursement rates for the state's Medicaid program. In contrast, the federal government sets the reimbursement rates for Medicare. This helps to explain why Medicaid reimburses at lower rates than Medicare: State budgets tend to be subject to more constraints than the federal budget.[53] Further, the low-income people who benefit from states' Medicaid programs have less political power than the senior citizens who primarily benefit from Medicare.[54] Meanwhile, the government is not involved in setting commercial insurance reimbursement rates. Instead, those rates are a product of negotiations between individual providers and the insurance company. As a result, commercial insurance reimbursement rates vary widely from provider to provider, with the providers that enjoy more market power—and therefore greater negotiating power—being able to secure higher rates.[55] Although there is great variability in commercial insurance reimbursement rates, it is generally safe to assume that those rates are going to be moderately higher than Medicare rates[56] and considerably higher than Medicaid rates. Thus, from the perspective of a hospital or health system, a commercially insured patient is a more lucrative proposition than a Medicaid-insured counterpart.[57]

Further, Medicaid rates tend to be so low that they often do not cover the provider's cost of delivering the care. The University of California "estimated that Medi-Cal reimbursement covers between 50 to 60 percent of the cost of services per patient."[58] Accordingly, institutions stand to *make* money when they see a commercially insured patient and to *lose* money when they see a Medicaid-insured patient.[59] As discussed earlier, because most hospitals and health systems are engaged in the project of profit maximization, they typically try very hard to increase the proportion of their patient population with commercial insurance—which leads to a corresponding decrease in the proportion of their patient population covered by Medicaid. As Dr. Davani put it, "It is not in Golden Health's strategic plan to increase the Medi-Cal-insured population. It *is* in their strategic plan—and it has been very clearly in their strategic plan for many, many years—to increase the commercial market share." This explains why most profit-seeking hospitals and health systems in the San Francisco healthcare marketplace—including Golden—focus on competing for commercially insured patients while leaving it to the General to see Medicaid-insured patients.

But things are slightly more complicated when we consider Golden Health and similarly situated academic medical centers across the nation. For over a hundred fifty years, Golden has had a partnership with the General whereby Golden's physicians, residents, and interns care for patients and conduct research at the General.[60] This partnership benefits the General, which can boast that "having [Golden] physicians and scientists in house means that top-notch care and cutting-edge research is available to all San Franciscans."[61] Meanwhile, the partnership benefits Golden as well, as it makes Golden's residency programs highly coveted and competitive. On its website, Golden quotes a resident as saying, "Being at the General is exciting and rewarding: pretty much anything you can think of—and some things you'd never imagine—can happen."[62] Moreover, the partnership leads the General to send patients requiring tertiary or quaternary care—extremely complex cases that exceed the General's capabilities—to Golden instead of one of Golden's competitors. Patients requiring this higher level of care—very young babies requiring intensive care, pregnant people whose fetuses require surgery, pregnant individuals in need of surgery themselves—are the patients that Golden wants the most.

The partnership has led Golden to consider the General when it is making decisions about its own operations. The partnership inclines Golden, more than any other San Francisco healthcare institution, to pursue courses of action that would benefit—or, at least, would not harm—the General. Thus, part of the reason that Golden avoids seeing significant numbers of Medi-Cal-insured patients is that it would hurt the General. Caring for these patients would be tantamount to pilfering the client base that the General needs to survive.

With this in mind, consider a story that Dr. Chalifour recounted to me. Many years ago, she met a black Medi-Cal-insured patient who was in the second trimester of her pregnancy and was being triaged in the labor and delivery (L&D) department at Golden. (Golden's L&D also serves as an emergency room for pregnant patients who require urgent medical care related to their pregnancies.) The patient had been receiving her prenatal care from the General, but she liked the way Dr. Chalifour had cared for her during her visit to Golden's L&D, and she wanted to continue to see Dr. Chalifour for prenatal care throughout the rest of her pregnancy. This would have required the woman to become a Golden patient. Now, there should have been no issue with having the patient transfer her care from the General to Golden: Golden accepts Medi-Cal insurance, after all. In reality, things were not that simple. As Dr. Chalifour recalled:

> A couple of weeks after I saw [the patient and her partner] in the L&D at Golden, I got an email from them telling me that they were having difficulty getting into my clinic [at Golden]. They said that they were told that they need to be seen at San Francisco General Hospital because of their insurance status. . . . [T]he first time that happened, I thought it was a one-off. But through my time at both Golden and the General, I saw that it wasn't a one-off. I never got a satisfactory answer about this, but the folks who were answering the phone were directing Medi-Cal patients to the General. . . . I eventually learned that the number of births in San Francisco is fairly low for a city. There are four main institutions that fight over those small numbers of births—Golden, Synoptic, Mercy, and San Francisco General Hospital. And San Francisco General was losing. So what I gathered was that, at least at that time, the folks who were answering the phone [at Golden] were told to send Medi-Cal patients over to San Francisco General Hospital so their numbers would go up—so that they would be a solvent division.

Dr. Davani's analysis was consistent with that of Dr. Chalifour. I asked Dr. Davani whether she was disturbed by the low numbers of Medi-Cal-insured pregnant patients at Golden:

> Given the volume issues that we've had at San Francisco General, you can argue—and I would argue—that we don't want Golden to go after San Francisco General patients. It's definitely not advantageous to San Francisco General

to try to take those patients. [If Golden were to aggressively pursue Medi-Cal-insured patients in San Francisco], it would actually threaten the sustainability of San Francisco General because, right now, it is already teetering on the threshold of safety to run a labor and delivery unit. So having a low volume of Medi-Cal patients at Golden is actually allowing San Francisco General to sustain its base—to sustain itself. And to be clear, San Francisco General has been very clear with Golden about that. They've very clearly said, "We need a higher volume." So I think that Golden *should* keep that in mind when deciding whether or not to aggressively pursue Medi-Cal patients.

Dr. Chalifour, Dr. Davani, and the other Golden physicians who spoke with me all doubted that Golden continued to explicitly direct Medi-Cal-insured patients to the General. But there was a widely shared belief among Golden's providers that *the policy of guiding Medi-Cal-insured patients away from Golden and toward the General lived on in the form of Golden's decision to refrain from trying to meet the nonmedical needs of low-income patients.* The policy lived on in Golden's choice to be bad at helping vulnerable people. The effect of this decision is to render Golden more inaccessible to those Medi-Cal-insured patients who, like the class-privileged patients to whom Golden caters, might want to receive their care from the health system.

Some people may be disturbed to learn that separate hospitals for the haves and the have-nots exist in a country that purports to value equality. It may be even more disturbing to learn that this separation results, in part, from a reduction in poor people's autonomy.

HOW THE GENERAL ALLOWS GOLDEN TO COMPETE FOR COMMERCIALLY INSURED PATIENTS

Medical anthropologist Ellen Lazarus observed over three decades ago that in the peculiar world that is the United States' market-based approach to healthcare provision—a world that makes the country atypical among other industrialized nations—providers have adopted a market orientation that leads them to vie for patients in ways that are practically indistinguishable from the ways that any other purveyor of goods or services competes for consumers.[63] As Nike promises that its sneakers will help the (aspiring) athlete jump higher and run faster and as Apple's Beats by Dre assures that its headphones will deliver exceptional sound quality while making the wearer look cool and on trend, physician groups, hospitals, and health systems pledge a certain quality of experience that will appeal to the healthcare consumer with options. As Lazarus writes:

> A market orientation has led hospital management to deal with competition with comparable institutions through public relations and image enhancement. Marketing has become a hospital priority . . . in what has been called the "corporatization" of medicine. With a surplus of doctors and hospital beds in areas that serve the middle class, competition for patients is fierce. For that reason, hospital administrations . . . announce through slick mailings and newspaper advertisements how their hospitals use the latest technological marvels in an atmosphere of compassion and emotional support. (A typical newspaper pronouncement was headlined "We don't just look at you as a human body, we look at you as a human being.")[64]

A hospital with a large Medicaid-insured patient population will be disadvantaged in this competition for commercially insured patients insofar as Medicaid's lower reimbursement rates will leave the institution without the funds necessary to woo healthcare consumers who have their pick from a menu of different providers. Indeed, Medicaid's paltry reimbursement rates will deny the hospital with a large Medicaid-insured patient population the ability to offer the experience that class-privileged people expect from the institutions with which they interact.

Lazarus writes that one of the people she interviewed described the offerings that different providers advertised to "lure" patients to their offices and hospitals as "'unbelievable yuppie things."[65] Golden's offerings may be described similarly. In the obstetrics clinic on the East Hills campus, patients can help themselves to a cup of herbal tea from the tea station in the waiting area. On the Yerba Buena campus, patients can wander through the building that houses the obstetrics clinic and admire the art on the walls—installations that rotate periodically and are created by local artists. On both campuses, patients can sit in beautifully maintained outdoor spaces that take advantage of the perpetually pleasant Bay Area weather—a lawn with park benches situated alongside a running path on the East Hills campus, a wooded atrium with a cobblestoned walkway on the Yerba Buena campus. Golden's postpartum recovery rooms offer meals that seek to match the options found in San Francisco's better restaurants. One patient who keeps a vegan diet told me about her three-day stay after delivering her baby via Caesarian section: "Usually vegan options at places are just blah. But the hospital food was so good! I didn't want to go home. And it wasn't just because I was going to have to start cooking for myself. [laughs] Whatever I was going to make was not going to be as good as what they were giving me in the hospital." Medicaid reimbursement rates will not permit hospitals to offer these kinds of amenities to their patients.

Medicaid's low reimbursement rates disadvantage hospitals in the fierce competition for commercially insured patients, not only with respect to the extras that an institution might offer but also with respect to the experiences that middle-class and upper-middle-class people demand from the institutions that serve them. For example, during my fieldwork, Golden's administration replaced the furniture in the waiting area of the obstetrics clinic on the East Hills campus. Administrators presumably made this investment because the furniture had become fairly worn and some chairs had ripped upholstery. However, administrators likely considered this investment a wise one because most of their patients are middle-class or affluent, and class-privileged people do not expect to sit on shabby furniture in the institutions with which they engage.

Consider as well that low Medicaid reimbursement rates prevent providers from hiring staff members who can contribute positively to patient experience. One set of researchers describes a study showing "an unsurprising correlation between provider rates and the wages providers pay."[66] The researchers conclude that "[h]ealth providers that rely principally on Medicaid revenues face greater workforce recruitment challenges than those primarily serving commercial patients. Relatively low Medicaid base payment levels put providers who primarily serve Medicaid and uninsured patients at a disadvantage . . . with respect to attracting and retaining a robust and qualified workforce."[67]

When I started my fieldwork at Golden Health, I immediately noticed the caliber of the obstetrics department's nonclinical staff—that is, the women who worked behind the front desk and greeted patients, the people who answered the phones and made appointments, and the managers of the various clinics. Their desire for patients to have a positive experience was always apparent.

One incident is representative of this focus on the patient's experience. Golden's obstetrics clinics have a fifteen-minute grace period. If patients are less than fifteen minutes late for their appointment, they will be seen; if they are more than fifteen minutes late, they will be rescheduled. One afternoon, a patient—a brown-haired white woman with a slight eastern European accent and the brown and tan Louis Vuitton tote bag that was popular with women in San Francisco's monied class—arrived more than fifteen minutes late for her 1 p.m. appointment. She became upset when Gloria, a Latine temporary worker, informed her she could not be seen that day and would need to reschedule her appointment. Raising her voice above the low tones used by most patients in the clinic, the patient shouted, "I did everything that I could to get here on time! It's not fair!" She began to cry. "I'm always on time. I've never been late. I don't want to be rescheduled. It's not fair." Gloria offered the patient a tissue and asked her to sit down while she conferred with her supervisor. A few minutes later, the obstetrics clinic manager emerged from behind the secured doors that separated the waiting area from the exam rooms. Stella, a dynamic black woman, knelt next to the patient so that she could be at eye level with her. She explained that Gloria had relayed what happened. She went on to say that although the clinic does limit its grace period to fifteen minutes, she would ask the care providers who were in the clinic that day if anyone was able to add the patient to their schedule. Slightly mollified, the patient nodded, and Stella hustled off to the exam rooms. About ten minutes later, Stella returned and informed the patient that a nurse practitioner, Bryce, would be able to squeeze the patient into her schedule in about three hours—at around 4 p.m. Surprisingly, the patient still was not pleased. She raised her voice again and said, "But I can't wait around all day! I have to be on a conference call—a Zoom—in an hour and a half." When she asked if there was any way that she could be seen earlier than 4 p.m., Stella apologized and said no but offered the patient an empty exam room where she could have her video meeting. This satisfied the patient, resolving the conflict.

The incident demonstrates Stella's orientation toward patient satisfaction—indeed, *customer* satisfaction. I saw this orientation in most members of the clinic staff. Their goal appeared to be to work out disputes in a way that left the patient happy. The staff was not uniformly exceptional in this regard; some staff members were better than others. However, it was always clear to me that the decision-makers in the hospital sought to hire people who, like Stella, would be attuned to patient satisfaction and could deliver in this regard. Large numbers of commercially insured patients—and the high reimbursement rates that come with them—enable the administration at Golden to offer the wages that can secure this level of talent.

When I asked Dr. Davani about Golden's obvious concern for the satisfaction of the patient as customer, she emphasized that Golden prioritized patient satisfaction because Golden needed to compete for patients. The administration at Golden considered the health system to be in a struggle to win the business of people who were seeking healthcare in San Francisco and had options, so it operated its health system accordingly. In contrast, Dr. Davani said, the General did not prioritize patient satisfaction. The hospital could not afford it, and, equally importantly, the General's administrators did not feel that the hospital was competing for patients. They considered their patients to be a captured audience, their poverty preventing them from leaving. As Dr. Davani explained:

> I think that places like San Francisco General are just like, "Whatever." [laughs] They don't treat patients like they have a choice. They are more like, "Of course you're going to come here. You're poor, and you need healthcare." Now, the folks at San Francisco General will probably say, "Well, things are more chaotic here than at Golden. And that's because we are serving a more vulnerable population over here. So we can't concern ourselves with patient satisfaction." But I think, "Of course you could do it. Of course you can." You can have chaos. You can have chaos *and* be really intentional about creating a space that feels like a really nice space to be in. Things can be chaotic in the clinic *and* you can give patients an experience that treats them like they have a choice about where to receive their healthcare.

Dr. Davani's point about "chaos" raises an additional facet of appealing to class-privileged patients that becomes more difficult when an institution cares for substantial numbers of low-income patients. This is the minimization of wait times. At Golden and its competitors, wait times generally are insignificant. Golden patients usually can expect that within minutes after arriving for their appointment—provided that they arrive on time—they will be ushered to an exam room where their vital signs will be taken. A short wait, typically no more than ten minutes, then separates them from their encounter with the provider that they are scheduled to see that day.

In contrast, one of the most expected features of receiving healthcare from "poor people's hospitals"—and public institutions, generally—is stultifying, infuriating wait times. In my first book on maternal healthcare in the United States, I engaged with the "hideously long waiting periods" that were a deeply ordinary aspect of the obstetrics clinic at Alpha Hospital.[68] Because patients had to meet with several different professionals (including a social worker, nutritionist, and health educator) during their first prenatal care appointment, the wait times on that day, called the Prenatal Care Assistance Program (PCAP) appointment day, typically were exasperatingly long. I wrote:

> [T]he PCAP day teaches women that public institutions (which Alpha exemplifies) are frequently too understaffed to effectively and efficiently meet the needs of those who depend on them. Insofar as the poor are compelled to rely upon public institutions more than their non-poor counterparts, the length of the PCAP appointment day might be understood as educating PCAP patients about how the poor are commonly treated and the expectations the poor should have when negotiating these institutions. More forcibly, it communicates to women that their time is not highly valued; the exorbitant length of the PCAP day, and the excessive waiting periods that can be expected more generally within the Alpha [Women's Health Clinic, or WHC], abundantly demonstrates the state's conception of their time as being something utterly negligible.[69]

If the very long wait times that are an expected part of the experience at safety-net hospitals communicate to the indigent people who rely on these institutions that "their time is not highly valued," then a lot is riding on Golden's and its competitors' success in guaranteeing that pregnant patients will have trivial wait times at their appointments. That is, nonexistent or insignificant wait times communicate that *these institutions highly value the time of the class-privileged people who receive their healthcare from them.* Short wait times convey the respect that the institution has for its patients. They impart the message that the institution holds its patients in high esteem.

In my first book, I attributed the lengthy wait times at safety-net hospitals to a staffing shortage. I concluded that patients have to wait hours for their appointments at places like Alpha and the General because safety-net hospitals are unable to hire the appropriate number of providers and nonclinical staff to care for the large number of patients who turn to these institutions for healthcare.[70] Medicaid's low reimbursement rates certainly contribute to this phenomenon, leaving institutions with a large Medicaid-insured patient population less likely to have the revenue that would enable them to hire the staff and providers that would meet patient demand. Institutions with a large commercially insured population, on the other hand, are more likely to have the funds that they need to staff their clinics in a way that matches patient demand. In this way, Golden's small Medicaid-insured population allowed Golden to minimize the wait times in its clinics, helping to ensure that the class-privileged patients who sought care from it had experiences that aligned with their expectations.

However, another aspect of this issue deserves mentioning. At Alpha's Women's Health Clinic, clinic administrators double-booked or triple-booked appointments, scheduling two or three patients in one fifteen-minute slot. I once thought that patient demand was so high that the only way the clinic could meet it was to double- or triple-book appointments—a solution that also guaranteed that patients would have long waits. I assumed that the problem could be solved if the clinic simply hired more providers to meet patient demand. However, I eventually learned that many safety-net hospitals, including the General, double- and triple-booked appointments because they expected that many patients would not show up for their scheduled appointment.

Any institution that serves low-income people should anticipate a relatively high rate of no-shows and tardiness. And this is simply because the daily lives of low-income people are more contingent—less predictable—than the lives of their more privileged counterparts. The buses and trains that poor people depend on are often late or do not come at all, or the older cars that they drive have mechanical issues that make them unreliable. The shifts at low-wage jobs change from week to week, and financial precarity makes low-wage workers feel compelled to pick up shifts at the last minute. The friends and family members who help poor people with childcare must navigate the contingency in their own lives, making them undependable caretakers. Poor people themselves might be called on to care for the children of friends or family members when such care is needed.

The tardiness and no-shows among low-income patients, then, are functions of the uncertainty that poverty produces. As a result, the institutions that serve low-income people have to figure out ways to contend with this phenomenon. We might understand double- and triple-booking appointments as a technique that safety-net hospitals deploy to respond to the high rate of no-shows while simultaneously helping these institutions meet the demand for healthcare. The problem is that long wait times ensue when both of the double-booked or all three of the triple-booked patients show up for their appointments. The problem is further compounded when patients arrive late for their appointments, and the clinic attempts to squeeze the tardy patients into the schedule.

Because institutions that serve low-income people tend to be cash-strapped, *not* seeing patients often is not an option. A clinic with a 50 percent no-show rate certainly could schedule one patient in a fifteen-minute slot, but it would run the risk of earning half the revenue that it might have expected—half the revenue that it might need to remain solvent. The more fiscally responsible decision may be to double-book appointments. Even though there would be long wait times if all of the scheduled patients show up, the risk might be worth it. If half the patients do not come, as the historical data might suggest, the clinic will still meet its revenue goals.

To return to the initial point: The tardiness and no-shows among low-income people are functions of the uncertainty that poverty produces. When institutions like Golden and its competitors in the San Francisco healthcare ecosystem find themselves serving a relatively small number of low-income people, they insulate themselves from having to develop techniques to manage tardiness and no-shows. The fact that their patients are mostly *not* poor and have the predictable, noncontingent daily lives that class privilege makes possible means that late arrivals and no-shows will be few and far between. Golden's obstetrics clinics can schedule four patients every hour and expect that in that hour, four patients will be seen—and their care reimbursed. The clinic can implement a policy that requires the rescheduling of patients who arrive more than fifteen minutes late for their appointment and not fear the loss of revenue such a policy may produce. That is, hospital administrators can make decisions about how to operate the clinics that facilitate the minimization of wait times and, consequently, the clinics' appeal to class-privileged people seeking a particular experience of healthcare.

Interestingly, Dr. Davani remarked that the various barriers, discussed earlier in the chapter, that made it difficult for Medicaid-insured people to be seen at Golden also functioned to ensure that only the most sophisticated, least vulnerable of Medicaid-insured people made it into the clinic and achieved the status of "Golden patient." She stated, "My Medi-Cal-insured patients at Golden are predominately English-speaking. They are savvy. They are on MyChart.[71] They're technologically inclined. They generally seem to have transportation." She continued, "My Medi-Cal-insured patients at Golden very rarely are late. I never get no-shows."

The barriers that impede low-income people's access to healthcare at Golden function as a sieve, allowing those indigent patients who manage to get through to be the people who "fit right in" at spaces designed for the class-privileged. They are the most fortunate among the poor: They have managed to reduce some of the chanciness that comes with poverty. At the very least, their lives are predictable enough to permit them to be on time for their doctor's appointments, allowing the healthcare institutions that serve them to be the efficient, ordered spaces that communicate the respect that the institution has for its patients.

NEW YORK CITY–STYLE HEALTHCARE SEGREGATION

There is nothing uncommon about San Francisco's healthcare ecosystem. Indeed, healthcare segregation exists in most cities in the nation. An examination of New York City's hospitals reveals a dynamic between "poor people's hospitals" and their counterparts that closely mirrors the dynamic found in San Francisco's healthcare ecosystem.

The New York City Health and Hospitals Corporation (HHC), a quasi public agency, operates the "poor people's hospitals" in the city. Currently, HHC's hospital system, New York City Health and Hospitals (H&H), consists of eleven hospitals with a total of 5,000 beds alongside "five post-acute/long-term care facilities with nearly 3,000 beds, 6 diagnostic and treatment centers, and more than 70 community-based healthcare centers and extension clinics."[72] At present, H&H is the largest system of municipal hospitals in the country.[73]

Like the General in San Francisco, H&H hospitals have affiliations with elite medical schools, which allow the city to promise the patients who turn to these hospitals that they will be cared for by the nation's best physicians.[74] These affiliations reciprocally allow the medical schools that partner with H&H hospitals to promise medical students considering the schools' residency program that, as residents, the students will benefit from "a valuable learning experience in urban public hospitals and community health settings."[75]

Most of the patients cared for by H&H annually are indigent, and very few of the hospital system's patients have commercial insurance. As one report notes, "The relatively small population of commercially insured patients typically visit the system's trauma center, burn center, snakebite center, and behavioral health programs."[76] In other words, absent these particular exigent circumstances, commercially insured New Yorkers do their best to avoid going to an H&H hospital for healthcare.

New York City's healthcare ecosystem is slightly different from the one found in San Francisco insofar as New York City has a number of safety-net hospitals that are distinct from both the public hospitals that the city operates and the nonprofit hospitals and health systems that primarily care for commercially insured patients. These safety-net hospitals are privately owned and operated institutions that, like H&H hospitals, dedicate themselves to providing care to New York City's poor.[77] While this additional category of private safety-net hospitals makes the two cities slightly different from each other, the cities are alike insofar as the private hospitals that do not have an explicit mission to care for the indigent offload the city's poor to private safety-net hospitals and H&H hospitals, allowing these private hospitals to become sites where those with class privilege (and the commercial insurance that comes with it) receive their care.

Consider the following citywide numbers from 2019. While only 21 percent of the patients at the hospitals that serve more affluent people were Medicaid-insured, 55 percent and 48 percent of patients at H&H and safety-net hospitals, respectively, had Medicaid insurance.[78] Further, while 47 percent of the patients at the hospitals that serve more affluent people were commercially insured, only 7 percent and 14 percent of patients at H&H and safety-net hospitals, respectively, had commercial insurance.

It matters greatly that H&H and safety-net hospitals have high numbers of Medicaid-insured patients and that the other hospitals in the New York City healthcare ecosystem have high numbers of commercially insured patients. The high number of Medicaid-insured patients at H&H and safety-net hospitals means that these institutions provide care to a large percentage of their patient population at a loss. This explains why New York City gives more than $1 billion to HHC annually just to keep H&H hospitals solvent.[79] Meanwhile, the high number of commercially insured patients at the other hospitals in the New York City healthcare ecosystem means that the care that they provide to a large percentage of their patient population will be reimbursed above cost. To be precise, these hospitals earn surplus revenue when caring for close to half of their patients, and they can use this surplus revenue to invest in their facilities' physical plant, purchase new technology, and hire the best staff. That is, they can use the surplus revenue that they earn from a near majority of their patients to acquire the features that will appeal to their predominately middle-class and upper-middle-class clientele.

Although wealthier people's hospitals in New York City largely leave H&H and safety-net hospitals to care for the city's indigent, they still claim to be dedicated to ensuring that the most vulnerable people receive the healthcare that they need. Indeed, they make these declarations even though their nonprofit status obligates them to provide care to the indigent. Consider the pseudonymously called Franklin Medical Center. In an annual report highlighting some of its many achievements, Franklin states that, in the previous year, it provided close to $370 million in unreimbursed care to Medicaid-insured patients[80] and that 26 percent of its patients were Medicaid-insured.[81] Further, when a *New York Times* story reported that Franklin's emergency room tended to favor rich donors and friends of the institution—prioritizing their care and allowing them perks like private rooms for triaging—a Franklin spokesperson noted, "'We treat undomiciled persons every day and give every effort to do so with dignity, respect and compassion. . . .'"[82] The spokesperson then "pointed to data showing that [Franklin] treats thousands of Medicaid-eligible patients."[83]

Many of the hospitals that serve a wealthier clientele in New York City display the same characteristics as the hospitals and health systems that serve a wealthier clientele in San Francisco. Consider Franklin once again. While Franklin publicizes that close to a quarter of its patients are Medicaid-insured, this number likely obscures the fact that most of the health system's facilities are largely devoid of Medicaid-insured patients. Franklin consists of three campuses—in Manhattan, on Long Island, and in Brooklyn. The Brooklyn campus was added after Franklin acquired a struggling hospital in a disinvested, disadvantaged neighborhood in the borough. As one feature on the merger described it, "Franklin–Brooklyn serves a community with the highest percentage of Medicaid patients in the nation."[84] We can reasonably conclude that a substantial portion of the patients cared for at Franklin's Brooklyn campus are Medicaid-insured. Further, Franklin also operates more than three dozen federally qualified health centers (FQHCs) in Brooklyn.[85] FQHCs are federally subsidized clinics that serve communities whose healthcare needs would otherwise go unmet.[86] Franklin's network of FQHCs is the largest network in the country.[87] Thus, we can reasonably conclude that a substantial portion of the patients cared for at Franklin's network of FQHCs are indigent and Medicaid-insured. So when Franklin says that close to a quarter of its patient population has Medicaid insurance, we can safely assume that a *significant* portion of that number is cared for at the Brooklyn campus and in the FQHCs; we can also safely assume that an *insignificant* portion of Franklin's Medicaid-insured population is cared for at Franklin's Manhattan and Long Island campuses. Accordingly, the class-privileged patients who receive their healthcare at these locations can anticipate an experience that aligns with their expectations as middle-class and upper-middle-class people.

Although Franklin accepts Medicaid as a formal matter, Medicaid-insured prenatal patients will have a difficult time receiving their prenatal care on Franklin's Manhattan campus. I found that *few of the individual obstetricians who worked at Franklin's Manhattan campus accepted Medicaid*, and fewer still were accepting new Medicaid patients. In April 2024, when I called the obstetrics clinic on the Manhattan campus to ask whether a Medicaid-insured patient would be able to be seen there, the kind and patient call center employee informed me that only *one* physician at the location who accepted Medicaid insurance had available appointments. When I asked what a Medicaid-insured patient should do if their schedule did not align with that one physician's availability, the woman cheerfully responded, "We have a lot of other locations. She should probably try Brooklyn."

* * *

Healthcare segregation is such a mundane feature of American life that most find it unremarkable. Nevertheless, it is astonishing that in the United States, something that is so intrinsic to life—healthcare—is provided in separate institutions that serve either the haves or the have-nots. When this fact intersects with racial disparities in maternal mortality, a black person's decreased odds of surviving pregnancy, childbirth, and the postpartum period pull class-privileged, commercially insured black people seeking to survive pregnancy to places that cater to the haves. Moreover, when this pull happens inside of a profit-generating healthcare system, places like Golden Health benefit from the "business." In this way, the black maternal health crisis is profitable for institutions that serve the haves.

While most people will be able to discern healthcare segregation in their city or town, this chapter has tried to show that healthcare segregation goes beyond the simple fact that in any given location, some hospitals serve low-income people, and other hospitals serve those with class privilege. The chapter also offers the insight that the hospitals that serve those with some degree of class privilege *are made possible* by the existence of the hospitals that serve low-income people. "Poor people's hospitals" care for those who, because of their Medicaid insurance or lack of insurance altogether, would prevent the hospitals that care for the class-privileged from earning the "surplus revenue" that allows them to "reinvest in staff, modern facilities, and new technology."[88] Further, "poor people's hospitals" serve those who, because of the irregularities that characterize their lives, impede a clinic manager's plans for the smooth flow of individuals through the space—from intake through checkout. With these patients offloaded onto "poor people's hospitals," other hospitals can provide the features that middle-class and upper-middle-class people expect from the institutions that serve them, such as aesthetically pleasing physical spaces, short wait times, an emphasis on customer service, and a concern about patient satisfaction.

It is not just that within market capitalism in the United States, there are desirable places for the rich and undesirable places for the poor. It is that *the undesirable places for the poor enable the places for the rich to possess the characteristics that make them desirable.* The ambiguity that characterizes the quality of the healthcare dispensed at safety-net hospitals makes possible the indisputably exceptional nature of the healthcare dispensed at wealthier people's hospital. The chaos found in "poor people's hospitals" makes possible the order found in wealthier people's hospitals. The discomfort and inattentiveness experienced by those without class privilege in the healthcare institutions they rely on make possible the comfort and attention that those with class privilege experience in the healthcare institutions with which they interact. In essence, poor people make it possible for wealthier people to have nice things.

Healthcare is far from the only aspect of American life that is segregated along the lines of the haves and have-nots. If Golden Health can offer concierge-like care to its overwhelmingly middle- and upper-middle-class patients at least in part because the General provides care to the most vulnerable in San Francisco, then we might consider how this phenomenon might show up in other contexts.

For example, if the neighborhoods that wealthier people call home have clean air, pristine water, and soil devoid of lead and other contaminants, how might those features of their communities be made possible by the toxic air, polluted water, and lead-infused soil found in the communities that poor people call home?

If the schools that wealthier children attend have well-maintained buildings, instructors with advanced degrees, state-of-the-art technology, new books, and low teacher-to-student ratios, how might those features be made possible by the crumbling physical plants, uncredentialed instructors, outdated (or nonexistent) technology, old books, and high teacher-to-student ratios found in the schools that poor children attend?

If the jobs that wealthier people have pay generous wages and come with benefits like health insurance, sick days, employer contributions to retirement plans, paid time off, and annual inflation-adjusted increases in salary, how might those features be made possible by the meager wages, lack of benefits, and overwhelming *insecurity* that characterize the jobs held by the poor?

If wealthier nations have strong economies, political stability, and abundance, how might those features be made possible by the struggling economies, political instability, and scarcity found in poor nations?

Indeed, *how might the ease enjoyed by those who are not poor depend on the poor's suffering?*

In this chapter, we have seen how racial disparities in maternal mortality accrue to the benefit of healthcare institutions like Golden Health, which are promised a patient population that includes commercially insured (that is, profit-generating) black people who turn to them as a strategy to survive the black maternal health crisis. By continuing to examine how the deprivation and distress that some groups endure might be beneficial to other groups, the next chapter invites us to consider how racial disparities in maternal mortality might benefit defenders of the racial status quo. When these disparities are explained in terms of concepts that are familiar to the lay public—like genes and culture—they legitimate racial inequality across myriad domains of American life.

3 The Many Contributors to Racial Disparities in Maternal Mortality

In June 2023, Elaina Boone was admitted to her neighborhood hospital in the Bronx in New York City, where she delivered her first child, a son named Zion, through an emergency Caesarian section.[1] She died less than three months later, succumbing to complications that she developed after Zion's birth.[2] Shortly after Elaina's death, her sister, Talissa, posted a sixty-second video to her Instagram page[3] showing the entrance to the hospital, an unremarkable brown and tan building with neon blue and white letters spelling the hospital's name. Talissa narrates from off-screen, her voice cracking with rage and sadness:

> Y'all see this hospital right here? Don't bring nobody here. . . . Do *not* bring your black ass here. They will kill you. My sister was fine when she came here. She was healthy when she came in here. She had a baby in here. They knew she was sick and sent her home with the wrong medications. They killed my thirty-six-year-old sister, bro. I'm letting you know . . . that I'm suing the shit out of you. Stop killing our black women! Stop killing us. My sister was thirty-six, healthy. She had a C-section. Y'all knew she was sick and sent her home. Y'all killed my sister![4]

It is hard to watch the video without feeling the heat of Talissa's anger and the weight of her grief. Her pain is palpable. It is tempting to believe that Talissa is right—that Elaina Boone would still be alive and caring for her son if the hospital had provided her with competent healthcare. If Talissa is right, then we can explain the higher rates of maternal mortality and morbidity among black people in the United States in terms of inadequate hospitals that offer inferior care. If this is the problem, then the solution would be for black people to avoid receiving care from these hospitals. Problem solved.

However, many factors contribute to the appalling fact that black people are twice as likely as their white counterparts to suffer a severe, potentially life-threatening condition during pregnancy and three to four times more likely than their white counterparts to die from a pregnancy-related cause. The problem will not be solved if black people simply avoid certain problematic hospitals.

This chapter explores five contributors to racial disparities in maternal deaths and severe injuries—the disproportionate burden of poverty that black people bear in the United States, black people's epigenetics, the stress and weathering that black people endure as racial minorities in a racially hostile country, inferior healthcare provided to black people at the systems level and the individual level, and black patients' distrust of healthcare providers and institutions. This chapter provides an introduction to these factors for those who may be unfamiliar with them and a deeper, critical engagement for those already fluent.

However, before beginning the exploration, we must look at genes and culture—two explanations for racial disparities in maternal mortality and morbidity (and for racial disparities in health, more broadly) that some scholars and scores of laypersons believe account for the phenomenon. Many people are convinced that black people have poorer maternal health outcomes—and, on the whole, are sicker and die earlier than nonblack people—because they either have genes or a culture (or both) that are killing them. This chapter begins by looking at these two mythical contributors to racial disparities in health before turning to the five actual contributors to racial disparities in maternal deaths and severe injuries.

GENES

Science has established that there is no genetic uniformity within the groups that we think of as races.[5] In fact, research has shown that there is more genetic diversity *within* racial groups than there is *between* racial groups.[6]

Because of the genetic diversity that characterizes the groups that we consider to be races, unrelated individuals who share a racial identity or ascription should not be assumed to share the same genes. As biological anthropologist Christopher Kuzawa and sociologist Elizabeth Sweet put it, "[O]ver three decades of research consistently show[s] between-group genetic differences to be small compared to the genetic variation found within continental regions."[7] That is, there is more genetic variations *among* Africans (and more genetic variations *among* Europeans) than there are *between* Africans and Europeans. Nevertheless, the idea that race reveals something significant about a person's genetic composition lives on.

When the issue is racial disparities in health, many observers intuitively believe that people of color are sicker and die earlier than their white counterparts because people of color possess genes that predispose them to death. This intuition is based on the assumption that "human genetic variation can be differentiated into conventional racial clusters, and that disease-causing alleles are likely to be among those variants that segregate between these groups."[8] This assumption, however, has no basis in reality.

Despite the thirty years of research showing that "traditional racial categories [are] poor predictors of gene frequencies,"[9] studies regularly pop up that offer to explain racial disparities in health in terms of the illness-causing genes that people of color are imagined to have. Consider a recent study that investigated why black survivors of childhood cancers are more likely than their white counterparts to develop cardiomyopathy, a disease that affects the heart muscle and is a precursor to heart failure.[10] The authors begin the article by noting that "[s]tudies of racial/ethnic differences among childhood cancer survivors are limited but have reported a higher prevalence of cardiovascular risk factors and an elevated overall risk for cardiovascular disease among survivors of African ancestry. Adjustment for socioeconomic and cardiovascular risk factors[,] while modifying the risk in some studies, has not consistently abrogated the risks, suggesting potential genetic factors."[11] These researchers make a mistake that is common to those who propose that black people's genes are killing them. They assume that because identified nongenetic factors cannot explain increased morbidity or mortality among black people, an *unidentified genetic* factor must be the cause.

The cardiomyopathy researchers suppose that because "socioeconomic and cardiovascular risk factors" have been ruled out as explanations of black cancer survivors' higher incidence of cardiomyopathy, black people's genes must be the culprit. However, the conclusion does not follow from the premise. Perhaps some as yet unconsidered nongenetic factor explains the higher rates of cardiovascular disease among black cancer survivors. Perhaps decades of enduring structural and interpersonal racism and experiencing the stresses associated with that burden explain the higher rates of cardiovascular disease among black cancer survivors. Nevertheless, the authors, without explanation, dismiss the possibility that an unidentified nongenetic factor is responsible for racial disparities in cardiomyopathy rates among cancer survivors.

Ultimately, the authors conclude that their study provides support for the claim that a genetic factor causes higher rates of cardiomyopathy among black cancer survivors: "[W]e identified an increased risk for cardiomyopathy among survivors of African ancestry compared with those of European ancestry and, importantly, identified genetic variants significantly associated with this disparity. . . . Two genetic loci on chromosomes 1p13.2 and 15q25.3 conferred significantly increased risk for survivors of African ancestry."[12] This conclusion is unsurprising in light of the researchers' failure to even the mention the fact of racism—despite all that is known about the ways social environments affect the body. We are reasonable to wonder whether the researchers permitted their commitment to the idea that the races are genetically distinct groupings of individuals to guide their interpretation of the data they received.

The proposition that genes explain racial disparities in health has been debunked by research showing that black people who have not been exposed to racism enjoy levels of health that match their white counterparts. Consider the studies documenting that the health outcomes of US-born babies of African immigrants are much better than the health outcomes of US-born babies of African Americans.[13] If black people, as a race, possessed genes that incline them toward death, then US-born babies of African immigrants would suffer the higher rates of morbidity and mortality that US-born babies of African Americans endure: Both groups, being part of the black race, would share the same race-based genes and suffer the same gene-determined rates of sickness and death. But that is not what these studies reveal. Instead, the research demonstrates that black people who have not been exposed to years of racism and race-based discrimination (such as new immigrants to the United States) give birth to babies that are much healthier than the babies born to black people who have had to sustain a lifetime of antiblackness in the United States.

Devastatingly, the research shows that as black people's exposure to the race-based hostility found in the United States increases, their birth outcomes suffer. When US-born babies of African immigrants grow up and themselves have babies in the United States, their babies' health outcomes tend to look more like the poor outcomes found among African Americans' babies and less like the enviable outcomes found among white babies.[14] Tellingly, the reverse is true for white immigrants to the United States. The birth weights of white immigrants from Europe "were originally lower than the mean for US whites, but increased with each generation."[15] In other words, while birth outcomes improved across the generations for white people who immigrated to the United States, they decreased across the generations for black people who immigrated to the country. Further, as Kuzawa and Sweet emphasize, "It goes without saying that these opposing biological responses were far too rapid to be due to changes in gene frequencies."[16] Differently stated, the health outcomes that these studies documented have nothing to do with imaginary race-based genes and everything to do with actual racist environments.

As legal scholar Dorothy Roberts has written, "It is implausible that one race of people evolved to have a genetic predisposition to heart failure, hypertension, infant mortality, diabetes, and asthma. There is no evolutionary theory that can explain why African ancestry would be genetically prone to practically every major common illness."[17] In essence, it is exceedingly unlikely that black people possess genes that incline them to all manner of death, including pregnancy-related deaths. Insisting that this is a possibility permits us to avoid addressing the systems, processes, and institutions that are actually shortening the lives of black people and other marginalized groups.

CULTURE

Another frequently heard explanation of why black people have higher rates of illness is culture—the idea that black people possess beliefs and engage in behaviors that cause them to be sicker and die earlier than other racial groups. For example, one might hear that black people have higher rates of hypertension and diabetes because a key part of "black culture" is soul food, which is comprised of high-fat, high-sodium, high-sugar foods that cause various states of unhealth. One might hear that black people do not exercise as often as they should because exercise is not an element of "black culture," and a sedentary lifestyle causes a wide range of negative health consequences. One might hear that black people do not go to the doctor as often as they should because medical mistrust is a feature of "black culture," and the failure to receive healthcare is bad for health. (The issue of black patients' distrust of healthcare institutions and providers is discussed later in the chapter.) The examples are numerous.

I encountered a tiresomely common cultural explanation of racial disparities in health in the early days of the COVID-19 pandemic. In April 2020, I was invited by National Public Radio to discuss the fact that, at the time (this was before the development and distribution of the vaccines that greatly reduce the risk of dying from COVID-19), black people were being killed by the disease at a much higher rate than their nonblack counterparts.[18] I explained that because of structural racism—the environmental injustices in the segregated neighborhoods that black people call home, the inaccessibility of quality healthcare providers, the voter suppression and vote dilution that prevent people of color from electing lawmakers who will protect their communities—black people suffered from diseases like hypertension, heart disease, lung disease, asthma, diabetes, and kidney disease at higher rates than nonblack people. These conditions increase the odds that a SARS-CoV-2 infection will be fatal. I explained that when the novel coronavirus infected bodies that structural racism had already damaged, the result was exactly what was seen in the first year of the pandemic—higher rates of COVID-19 deaths among black people.

That evening, I received an email from a woman who had listened to the program—a self-described "white, sixty-four-year-old registered nurse who has worked in critical care for 40 years." She reprimanded me for failing to address the "fact" that black people are sicker than other racial groups because of "black culture":

> You will hate this comment, but blacks are usually overweight if they are in the healthcare system. This clearly means they are not eating right and not exercising. There is a CULTURE of great food, family fun . . . but not physical fitness. These people have made THEMSELVES SICK. There is no excuse as to why anyone would not be fit and eats a poor diet. The food is there. Turn off the t.v. and go walk. Stop eating fattening food, go to the food bank and eat vegetables not fast food and fried chicken.
>
> I believe the black CULTURE increases the likelihood of blacks not being taken care of as well as whites. It is a choice of their own. Also, in the traditional black Christian religious culture there is much talk about God healing and not taking meds. This happens frequently in the black CULTURE. Who in the black community is leading by example? It's an internal intimate cultural issue.

Cultural explanations of health behaviors have been around for a long time, and they undeniably will persist into the future. Even physicians subscribe to these beliefs. One set of researchers surveyed several hundred undergraduate students at a selective university who were planning to apply to medical school.[19] When asked why black people have higher rates of cardiovascular diseases and obesity, many of the students offered "black culture" as the answer. The researchers report that one student theorized, "Their background consists of slavery so they may eat less healthy food like biscuits and gravy. . . ."[20] Another student offered that "[p]erhaps the cultural norm is to try to tolerate more pain, including chest pain."[21] Another student proposed that "[t]here is more of a cultural influence on African American men than white men. The culture surrounding food intake is less healthy."[22] The idea that white men are less susceptible to cultural influences than African American men was so apparent to this student that they did not bother to defend, explain, or justify the proposition. But why does this student (as well as scores of others) believe that some groups (usually nonwhite people) are mired in their cultures in a way that other groups (usually white people) are not? Why do white people enjoy a relative immunity from culture while black people find "black culture" impossible to escape?

Behavior undeniably impacts health. Individuals who eat unhealthy foods, smoke cigarettes, drink alcohol, and fail to exercise regularly are more likely than others to become sick. However, this simple truth becomes more problematic when health behaviors are imagined to constitute a culture that dictates the beliefs and actions of racialized groups (again, usually nonwhite people).

There are at least three fundamental problems with cultural explanations of racial disparities in health. The first problem relates to the culture concept itself. The concept might erase the differences within the group of people who are imagined to belong to the culture. As a personal example: I am a black person who keeps a vegan diet and exercises daily. In making these lifestyle choices, have I rejected "black culture"? If so, how did I come to exist outside of my own culture? I am not unique, though. Millions of other black people also avoid eating high-fat, high-sodium, high-sugar foods, and millions of other black people also exercise regularly. If millions of black people do not subscribe to "black culture," what makes it accurate to describe it as *black* culture? Further, eating high-fat, high-sodium, high-sugar foods did not originate with black people, and black people are not the only folks eating these kinds of foods today. Indeed, black people's dollars alone have not made McDonald's into a multi-billion-dollar corporation. If millions of black people—alongside even more millions of nonblack people—subscribe to behavior that some call "black culture," what makes it accurate to describe it as *black* culture?

The second problem with cultural explanations of racial disparities in health is that attributing black people's health-damaging behaviors to a culture erases the structural conditions that constrain the choices available to them. If black people eat unhealthy foods at higher frequencies than nonblack people, it may be because black people disproportionately live in food deserts—"areas characterized by poor access to healthy and affordable food."[23] If black people do not exercise as often as they should more frequently than nonblack people, it may be because black people disproportionately live in neighborhoods that lack parks, fresh air, nonviolent streets, and areas where the residents can be active outdoors safely. "Culture" erases the larger forces that reduce the choices that people can make around their health behaviors.

Finally, the third problem with cultural explanations of racial disparities in health is that the evidence does not support the claim that the engine behind these disparities is racial differences in health behaviors. In the words of one set of researchers who conducted a survey of the literature, "As observed ten years ago, . . . health behaviors can be potent contributors to disease risk; there is little evidence, however, that alone or in combination[,] health behaviors can explain racial and ethnic health disparities."[24]

As problematic as cultural explanations of racial disparities in health are, they may be strengthened by a framework that the medical community has embraced for over forty years in hopes that it will help to *diminish* disparities. This is the concept of cultural competence, which chapter 6 analyzes.

Before this chapter turns to an exploration of the actual contributors to racial disparities in health, we should think about how genetic and cultural explanations of these disparities work to legitimate the status quo. If racial disparities in health are caused by black people's genes or "black culture," then society has not produced these disparities—which, in turn, means that society does not bear responsibility for eliminating them. In other words, if black people's genes or "black culture" is killing them, then society can wash its hands of the issue of racial disparities in health, essentially telling black people, "That's a you problem."

The average person likely is more familiar with the idea that genes and culture distinguish the races than with the idea that racial groups are genetically arbitrary groupings of individuals. Similarly, the average person likely is uncritical of the concept of culture and unfamiliar with analyses that understand it to be an amorphous concept that imperfectly describes a group's behavior, worldviews, and ways of life. Accordingly, when confronted with the fact that people of color have shorter, sicker lives than their white counterparts, people are more likely to understand this fact in terms of concepts they are familiar with (genes and culture) than in terms of unfamiliar concepts (epigenetics, stress, and weathering). In this way, the undisputed fact of racial disparities in health works to reaffirm the false belief that the races are fundamentally different from one another and that genes and culture lie at the heart of this fundamental difference.

Further, if genes and culture explain why black people have poorer health outcomes than nonblack people, might genes and culture also explain why black people have higher poverty rates than nonblack people—perhaps because black people's genes or "black culture" causes them to be unsuccessful within market capitalism? Might genes and culture also explain why black people have higher incarceration rates than nonblack people—perhaps because their genes or culture propel them to commit crime more frequently than nonblack people? Might genes and culture explain why black people are admitted to competitive colleges and universities at lower rates than nonblack people—perhaps because their genes or culture has made them less intelligent and less hardworking than their nonblack counterparts? Essentially, if racial groups have distinct genes or cultures, then the dramatic racial inequality that we witness across American life is not the result of unfairness. Instead, the inequality would be *inevitable*. In this way, the statistics describing black people's poorer chances of surviving pregnancy and childbirth—when invoked in a society that is convinced that genes and culture distinguish racial groups—are beneficial to justifiers of racial inequality. Racial disparities in maternal mortality work to reaffirm that the other racial disparities that we see across society—in poverty rates, within the criminal legal system, in higher education—are also inescapable and are not the consequences of injustice at all.

POVERTY AND ACCESS TO HEALTHCARE

Researchers have long established that poverty compromises the lives of those compelled to live in it.[25] Being poor means that you are less likely to have access to fresh fruits and vegetables and other healthy foods. Being poor means that you are more likely to live in a neighborhood with polluted air, contaminated soil, and toxic water. Being poor means that you are less likely to have health insurance and, therefore, access to preventative healthcare and the means to manage any chronic conditions that you might have. Even if you have health insurance, being poor means that you may have a harder time making it to your doctor's appointments. You may have to rely on public transportation, take time off from a job that does not provide sick or personal days, and arrange childcare that is not readily available.

When trying to understand racial disparities in health—and racial disparities in maternal mortality and morbidity, specifically—we have to consider the fact that black people endure higher rates of poverty than other racial groups. In 2022, the poverty rate among black people was more than twice that of white people.[26] (The only group that had poverty rates higher than those of black people was American Indian/Alaska Native people.)[27] But poverty, on its own, cannot explain the higher rates of maternal mortality and morbidity among black people. If poverty explained these disparities, then wealthier black people would have health outcomes that were similar to those of their wealthier white counterparts. But this is not true. As the introduction to this book notes, racial disparities in maternal mortality and morbidity persist across incomes levels. In the words of one set of researchers, "Poverty is linked to a higher risk of maternal mortality, but the risk of pregnancy-related death for Black women spans income and education levels."[28] Indeed, "[t]he increased risk of maternal mortality for African American women cannot be explained away by known risk factors, such as advanced maternal age, inadequate prenatal care, low education, or socioeconomic status. Controlling for these known factors has only resulted in a small reduction in [the] odds ratio for pregnancy-related mortality (3.07 to 2.65)."[29] In essence, *factors independent of poverty* are making it difficult for black people to survive pregnancy, childbirth, and the postpartum period.

EPIGENETICS

Recent research in the field of epigenetics offers an account on the level of the molecule for the persistence of racial disparities in health across socioeconomic statuses. The epigenome is distinct from the genome. The genome is the complete set of genes that an organism possesses, and the epigenome influences how genes will be expressed. As one set of researchers explains, "If we consider genes as the body's hardware, then the epigenome is the software that instructs them how to work. Essentially, the epigenome is the instruction guide on top of the genome, and it serves as a dimmer switch that promotes a gene to turn on slightly, turn on fully, or turn off completely."[30] For example, if a person possesses a gene that suppresses the formation of tumors, the epigenome will determine whether the tumor-suppression gene is expressed and can work to prevent the development of tumors in the person. Conversely, the epigenome may quash the expression of the tumor-suppression gene, preventing it from stopping the development of tumors in the person—which makes the person vulnerable to cancer.

The science of epigenetics is, as one might expect, quite complicated. At a basic level, scientists have identified three mechanisms by which epigenetics alters gene expression. The most frequently studied mechanism involves methylation, or the attachment of methyl groups to areas on DNA called "CpG islands."[31] The methylation of a gene generally impedes the gene's expression, while the acetylation of the gene contributes to gene expression.[32] Researchers have shown that black and Latine people tend to have higher rates of methylation of stress-related and inflammation-related genes,[33] which may impact "such functions as glucose metabolism, blood pressure regulation, fat deposition, and the physiologic response to stress."[34]

An individual's genome is inherited at conception, and it will not change during a person's life course absent a mutation—that is, an alteration in the gene's nucleotide sequence. However, the epigenome is more easily transformed, and research has demonstrated that the environment can transform it. In this way, individuals inhabiting healthy, supportive environments will develop epigenomes that permit their genes to be expressed in a way that conserves their health. In contrast, individuals inhabiting adverse, hostile environments will develop epigenomes that cause their genes to be expressed in ways that are incompatible with health and, ultimately, life.

Further, research has shown that not only do the environments that individuals inhabit during their infancy, childhood, adolescence, and, to a lesser extent, adulthood, produce health-impacting epigenetic changes, but *prenatal* environments also can affect an epigenome. Thus, when pregnant persons are forced to withstand physical or psychological stress, these pressures may impact the epigenome of the fetus. After birth, the baby's epigenome would carry the "biological memory" of the parent's deprivation.[35] Their health would suffer as a consequence.

Perhaps most significantly, epigenomes can be transmitted across generations. That is, individuals can pass their epigenome down to their children. Researchers have documented that the babies born to women who were pregnant during the Dutch famine of 1944–1945, which occurred after Nazi Germany cut off food supplies to the western part of the Netherlands, possessed genes that were methylated differently from the genes of their siblings who did not have prenatal exposure to the famine.[36] Further, these differently methylated genes play a role in the regulation of weight and cholesterol levels, among other developmental processes—causing the famine-exposed fetuses to have health issues related to obesity, heart disease, and diabetes after they were born, grew up, and became adults.[37] Researchers have found that when these adults—who had been exposed to the famine as fetuses—had children of their own, their babies also had health issues relating to obesity.[38] In other words, the *grandchildren* of the women who endured the Dutch famine of 1944–1945 were affected by their grandmothers' food insecurity. Thus, epigenetics explains how individuals transmit the health-damaging conditions that they inhabit to future generations —identifying the precise mechanisms for that transmission at the molecular level. Individuals may bear the consequences of the adverse environments that their recent ancestors endured, even though the individuals themselves inhabit more health-conserving environments.

Consider my grandmother, a black woman who was born and raised in the Jim Crow South and worked as a maid her entire life. She suffered all of the hostility and deprivation that white supremacy was designed to inflict on black people. This hateful environment undoubtedly produced epigenetic changes in her, leading to the expression of genes that predisposed her to cardiovascular disease, high cholesterol, diabetes, stroke, and cancer—all of the ailments that are found in black people at higher rates than their white counterparts. Significantly, the children that she bore—including my mother—undoubtedly were born with health-compromising epigenomes due to prenatal exposure to the vile environment that my grandmother inhabited while pregnant with them. Further, although the civil rights movement forced the nation to grant black people formal equality and provided my mother with the opportunity to scramble her way into the middle-class during her young adulthood, she likely passed her health-compromising epigenome to her children—my siblings and me. Thus, in a way, the violence of the Jim Crow South lives on in me. I, the grandchild of a woman who survived antiblackness in one of its most repugnant forms, have been affected by the inhumanity my gorgeous, fierce, resilient grandmother endured. This is true even though I have class privilege by virtue of the high levels of education that I have acquired and my status as a tenured professor at a selective law school. If I and other black people in the nation have a predisposition toward dying during pregnancy, it is not because black people, as a race, possess genes that kill them. That account of biological race and genetic determinism is too simplistic and empirically unsupported. It is more plausible that black people have higher rates of morbidity and mortality because this country's history of antiblackness has become embedded in black people's epigenomes.

STRESS AND WEATHERING

In the 1980s, public health researcher Arline Geronimus observed that black people who bore children when they were in their mid-twenties had pregnancy outcomes that were poorer than their black counterparts who bore children when they were teenagers.[39] However, when white people bore children in their mid-twenties, their pregnancy outcomes were better than their white counterparts who bore children when they were teenagers.[40] Delaying childbearing improved white people's pregnancy outcomes and compromised black people's pregnancy outcomes. Geronimus questioned why this was so.

She proposed the concept of "weathering" to explain the phenomenon.[41] The idea behind weathering is that stress—which Geronimus describes not as the normal stresses of everyday life but rather as a "physiological process" that is "chronic and repeated through [the] whole life course"—has an impact on people's bodies.[42] This unrelenting stress taxes the body systems of the individuals who experience it. Geronimus theorized that black people are exposed to chronic stress due to structural and interpersonal racism. Consequently, their body systems deteriorate at a faster rate than their nonblack counterparts. This would explain why she observed that black people in their teenage years—who had endured fewer years of racism-associated stress than black people in their mid-twenties—have better pregnancy outcomes than older black people. And this would explain why the bodies of white people, who are not exposed to the chronic stress of antiblackness, would be conserved such that delaying childbearing would be beneficial to them.

Weathering—the corrosion of body systems that have sustained "a continuous low-grade inflammatory response" due to existing in a "state of chronic stress"[43]—goes a long way toward explaining why racial disparities in health exist. It also goes a long way toward explaining why racial disparities in maternal mortality and morbidity persist across income levels—that is, why even wealthier black people die from pregnancy-related causes more frequently than wealthier white people. Living at the higher ends of the socioeconomic ladder does not immunize black people from racism-associated stress.

Initially, Geronimus's weathering hypothesis was dismissed. (She explains that when she first published her research around weathering, "Many in the medical community really seemed to think that there was just something intrinsic or genetic: that black-white differences in health must be [caused] by some hypertension gene." Meanwhile, "sociologists sensed that there was an essential pathological culture that led to bad behaviors and weak families."[44] In essence, the twin faith in genes and culture as causes of racial disparities in health had a stranglehold on the imagination of scholars and thinkers of the day, leading them to refuse to take Gerominus's scholarship seriously.) However, people began to give the weathering hypothesis the respect that it deserves when other researchers provided further empirical support for it. In a widely read and cited paper, neurologist Bruce McEwen and psychologist Eliot Stellar proposed that stress's impact on the body could be quantified through a measure called "allostatic load."[45] They explained that when an individual is exposed to a stressor, the body releases hormones, which cause changes in the brain, kidneys, immune system, and other body systems. Allostatic load measures the fluctuations that body systems have undergone in response to these hormones and, in so doing, quantifies the damage that stress has inflicted on individuals' bodies. McEwen and Stellar's work—which described how individuals with high allostatic loads were more susceptible to disease than their counterparts with lower allostatic loads—provided a physiological explanation for what Geronimus had observed about black and white people's pregnancy outcomes. Due to racism-related stress, black women in their mid-twenties are more likely to have a high allostatic load, which harms their pregnancies. In contrast, due to the absence of racism-related stress, white women in their mid-twenties are more likely to have a lower allostatic load, which benefits their pregnancies.

More than two decades after first proposing the weathering hypothesis, Geronimus and a few colleagues measured the allostatic load scores of black and white women of varying degrees of class privilege. They found that the black women in the study were most likely to have high allostatic load scores *regardless of socioeconomic status*.[46] The research provided evidence that class privilege does not entirely protect wealthier black people from the effects of racism. While class privilege may allow high-income black people to escape some phenomena that shorten the lives of low-income black people—such as food and housing insecurity and lack of access to healthcare—it does not allow high-income black people to escape being black.

QUALITY OF CARE: SYSTEMS LEVEL

When people think of racial segregation in the contemporary United States, they often think of residential segregation—white neighborhoods, black neighborhoods (frequently called "the ghetto," "the hood," or, simply, a "bad" neighborhood), and neighborhoods known as "Chinatown," "Little Havana," "Japantown," "Little Haiti," and "Koreatown." However, racial segregation also exists in hospitals today. While chapter 2 explores healthcare segregation primarily in terms of class, *class* segregated hospitals frequently are also *racially* segregated hospitals because of the enduring relationship between socioeconomic status and race in the United States.

In the United States, 75 percent of black people deliver their babies in just 25 percent of the nation's hospitals.[47] This means that some hospitals care for incredibly large numbers of pregnant black patients and other hospitals care for preciously small numbers of them. The literature has termed these institutions "high-black-serving hospitals" and "low-black-serving hospitals."[48] Predictably, the rates of maternal mortality and morbidity in high-black-serving hospitals tend to be much higher than the rates in low-black-serving hospitals.[49]

High-black-serving hospitals provide substandard care to *all* who enter, regardless of race. As one set of researchers found, "[B]lack and white patients who delivered in black-serving hospitals had a higher risk of severe maternal morbidity after accounting for patient characteristics" than black and white patients who delivered in low-black-serving hospitals.[50] While all patients risk receiving substandard care when they enter high-black-serving hospitals, the black people who disproportionately rely on these hospitals bear the brunt of the poor-quality healthcare that these institutions provide. As one set of researchers explained, "If black . . . mothers delivered in the same hospitals as white women, . . . they would experience 940 fewer severe morbid events, leading to a reduction of black severe maternal morbidity rates by 47.7 percent. . . ."[51] This means that to save black people from death or severe injury during pregnancy, childbirth, and the postpartum period, we have to improve the quality of the care dispensed at the *de facto* segregated hospitals where black pregnant patients disproportionately receive their healthcare.

QUALITY OF CARE: INDIVIDUAL LEVEL

There is a wealth of research that shows that healthcare providers give inferior care to people of color. This certainly contributes to racial disparities in health—and racial disparities in maternal mortality and morbidity, specifically.

Studies conducted in emergency rooms have revealed that when black patients present with chest pains, providers are less likely to order testing—like "EKGs, cardiac monitoring, oxygen saturation measurement, and chest X-rays"[52]—that could reveal the pain's cause. Black patients in emergency rooms are also less likely to receive treatment for pain, less likely to be admitted to the hospital, and less likely to be given an antidote when suffering an acute drug overdose.[53] Other studies have shown that healthcare providers are more likely to amputate the lower limbs of black patients when they have diabetic foot ulcers,[54] less likely to perform surgical interventions for lung cancer on black patients,[55] less likely to treat depression in black patients,[56] less likely to offer flu vaccines to black patients,[57] and less likely to refer their black patients for cardiac catheterization (a procedure that can diagnose and treat some heart conditions).[58]

Unsurprisingly, racial disparities in quality of care are present in the realm of reproductive healthcare as well. Providers are less likely to perform minimally invasive hysterectomies on black patients and more likely to subject them to more extreme procedures that involve large abdominal incisions.[59] Providers are less likely to prescribe antenatal steroids to pregnant black people at risk of preterm birth, thereby increasing the likelihood that their infants, if born prematurely, will have poor health outcomes.[60] Providers are less likely to screen their pregnant black patients for lipid disorders, which can result in preeclampsia and eclampsia, gestational diabetes, and preterm birth.[61] Providers are less likely to counsel their pregnant black patients about the importance of abstaining from drinking and smoking during pregnancy.[62] Providers are more likely to surgically remove black people's ovaries before menopause, increasing the risk that these patients will suffer a stroke or develop a heart condition.[63]

Consider as well that physicians are less likely to perform surgical interventions on black people suffering a hemorrhage after childbirth.[64] At the same time, physicians are more likely to perform Caesarian sections on their black patients.[65] Clinical factors cannot explain black people's increased likelihood of undergoing a C-section. A black person is more likely to have a C-section than a white person who is identical in terms of age, weight, parity, education, insurance status, and comorbid conditions.[66] Moreover, as legal scholar Colleen Campbell explains, "[T]he disparity is visible even for low-risk pregnancies, i.e., those pregnancies for which there is no medical complication. In other words, perfectly healthy Black women who do not need a C-section are also receiving this major surgery."[67]

When confronted with these studies, few observers have contended that providers *intentionally* give inferior care to their black patients. Instead, most observers have asserted that this inferior care is a function of providers' implicit biases.

Implicit bias has long been a topic of conversation in the United States, and most people are familiar with the concept. As law professor Osamudia James describes it, "Societal understanding of implicit bias is now so commonplace that presidential candidates are expected to raise the issue in debates."[68] The science of implicit bias proposes that people are not consciously aware of many of their associations and aversions. For example, some people may unconsciously associate black men with criminal activity or black women with welfare dependency, and because of these negative associations, they may have an aversion to black men and women. Since these associations and aversions happen outside of people's awareness, they do not know that they hold black people in such low esteem. When asked, they actually may say that they like black people and do not think of them as criminals or drains on society.

Researchers have shown that many people, including healthcare providers, have prowhite and antiblack implicit biases. According to one set of researchers, years of studies have shown that "similar to the general US population, most [healthcare providers] across multiple levels of training and disciplines have implicit biases against Black, Hispanic, American-Indian and dark-skinned individuals."[69] More crucially, research shows that providers act on their implicit biases. Many of these studies begin by giving providers the Implicit Association Test (IAT) on race, which measures the existence and extent of the test taker's implicit biases around race by asking test takers to match positive and negative words with black and white faces under intense time constraints. These studies have shown that providers whose IAT scores reveal them to have prowhite or antiblack implicit biases are less likely to prescribe narcotics to black children who have just undergone surgery, less likely to prescribe appropriate treatment to black people presenting in the emergency room with acute coronary syndrome, and more likely to have poor communication (including being more verbally dominant) with black patients.[70] While the research has not established that providers' implicit biases *cause* poor health outcomes in patients on the receiving end of the biases, it has established that possessing these implicit biases correlates with negative outcomes.[71] As one set of researchers summarizes the state of knowledge, "[T]he literature demonstrates an association between [implicit bias] and decision making, treatment recommendations, nonverbal communication, and adverse birth outcomes."[72]

The concept of implicit bias has been at the forefront of the nation's thinking about racism and racial inequality. Until the murder of George Floyd by police officer Derek Chauvin on May 25, 2020—an event that sparked prolonged nationwide protests and then a swift, enduring racial backlash—the way that most people talked in public about racial inequality in the United States was with the language of "implicit bias." People did not use the language of explicit bias—the possibility that some people in the post–civil rights era were well-aware of their aversion to nonwhite people and had no problem acting on it. People did not talk about structural racism or institutional racism. Instead people cited implicit bias to explain all manner of racial inequities witnessed in contemporary life—from mass incarceration and the disproportionate warehousing of black and Latine people in the country's prisons and jails to punitive and draconian immigration laws.

An excellent example of this is the approach that Starbucks took to a highly publicized incident in 2018 involving an employee who asked two black men to leave the store because they had not purchased anything. When the men refused to leave, explaining that they were waiting for a third person to arrive for a business meeting, the employee called the police. After a video documenting the arrest of the two men sparked widespread protests, Starbucks closed all of its locations in order to provide its employees with a training session about implicit bias, among other topics.[73] It is curious that the decision-makers at Starbucks concluded that the incident involved *implicit* bias. Indeed, it is odd that the Starbucks front office supposed that the employee who called the police to remove two black men who were doing what many people do in Starbucks stores (sit, wait, pass the time) fell victim to an *unconscious* association of black men and criminal activity. It seems more likely this this employee *consciously* associated black men and criminal activity. That is, following conscious deliberation, the employee chose to call the police (the actors charged with dealing with criminals) to remove the black patrons. In response to commercially damaging protests,

Starbucks certainly could have chosen to close its stores to host conversations with its employees about the choices that we have made as a society that have resulted in so many people in the United States associating black men with crime (and black women with welfare dependency, and Latine people with illegality, and Muslim people with religious violence, and Asian people with antisocial levels of intelligence, and Native people with barbarity . . . and white people with *none* of these attributes). Instead, Starbucks chose to close its stores and talk to its employees about implicit bias.

Critical thinkers of race have tried to understand why implicit bias has been such an attractive way to discuss racial inequality and why it has been such an appealing explanation of enduring racial stratification in the post–civil rights era. They have come up with two explanations.

The first explanation for the popularity of using implicit bias to talk about racial inequality is that scholarship often describes implicit biases as being inevitable and expected—indeed, natural. Consider a description of implicit bias that one pair of scholars offers:

> The existence of these biases is consistent with the conclusion of more general research that we automatically and unconsciously use heuristics to cope with the enormous amount of information that bombards us. Implicit racial biases facilitate our ability to "manage information overload and make decisions more efficiently and easily" by "filtering information, filling in missing data, and automatically categorizing people according to cultural stereotypes."[74]

Other researchers have described implicit bias "as a universal human trait."[75]

If implicit biases are "automatic" and "universal," then the people who have them—which is everyone—cannot be faulted for having them. If implicit biases are a function of the way that our brains work, then people should not feel guilty for harboring them. Indeed, even if people have harmed others after acting on their implicit biases, they should be forgiven. Implicit bias releases everyone from culpability. It proposes that the dramatic racial inequalities in the United States have been created and sustained by entirely innocent actors. And this is why implicit bias is an attractive way to talk about racial inequality: It explains continuing racial injustice without identifying bad actors or blameworthy parties.

Of course, people should not be blamed for possessing prowhite or antiblack implicit biases. However, the impulse to describe implicit biases as inevitable products of the way that our brains work obscures the fact that *there is nothing inevitable about having prowhite and antiblack implicit biases in particular.* There is nothing inherent to neurological function that makes our brains automatically associate white people with positive characteristics and black people with negative characteristics. If our brains have those associations, then it is because they—and we—exist in a society that has made it so. For example, nothing in the way that the synapses fire in our brains creates an association between black men and criminal activity. Instead, most people associate black men with criminal activity because this nation has warehoused black men in prisons and jails at disproportionate rates. Society has chosen to use the criminal legal system (police, prosecutors, prisons, and probation officers) to respond to the challenges faced by black communities. *This* choice has created the association between black men and criminal activity. The way that we have organized society has made our brains associate blackness and crime.

The ways that most people talk about implicit biases ignore the societal choices that are responsible for the shape that our implicit biases have taken. Conversations about implicit biases typically leave these essential background facts invisible. Instead, these conversations usually invite us to work on ourselves and learn how to have different unconscious thoughts about marginalized people. Left uninterrogated are the structural conditions that have molded these thoughts in the first instance.

The second explanation for the popularity of using implicit bias to talk about racial inequality is that implicit bias—in the ways that it is typically conceptualized—is an individualist phenomenon. It is about individual actors, the (unconscious) thoughts they have in their individual brains, and the actions that they individually take. We should note how this framework resembles traditional understandings of racism that propose that racism happens when racist individuals think racist thoughts and then do racist things.

Of course, racist individuals continue to think racist thoughts and do racist things. However, critical scholars of race propose that in the post–civil rights era, most of the heavy lifting in creating and recreating the country's racial hierarchy is done by *structural racism* and not by the actions of individual bad actors.[76] These thinkers propose that in an age of formal racial equality, enduring racial inequality is mostly the result of institutions and structures operating in a race-neutral manner that nevertheless perpetuates historical racial disadvantages and produces new forms of racial disenfranchisement. In essence, critical thinkers of race encourage people to think big—to think in terms of systems, macro processes, and large-scale forces. Yet the framework of implicit bias, in its typical formulation, keeps us focused on individuals, their problematic thoughts, and their harmful behaviors.

This might be unsatisfying—especially to people who think critically about race. First, a narrow focus on the individual may suggest that government and society, more generally, are not responsible for enduring racial inequality. It may suggest that government and the society that it regulates are not answerable if they fail to take steps to undo racial stratification in the nation. It may suggest that responsibility lies solely with individuals, who are encouraged to learn how not to act on their "automatic" and "universal" biases. Second, the focus on the individual is unsatisfying to critical thinkers because it permits us to do nothing about the conditions in which individuals operate. We can continue to exist in a country in which schools are more racially segregated today than they were in 1954, when the United States Supreme Court held in *Brown v. Board of Education* that racially separate schools were inherently unequal. We can continue to conceptualize healthcare as a commodity that must be purchased in the market—as opposed to a right to which everyone, by virtue of being human, is entitled. We can continue to attempt to solve all of our social problems with prisons and jails, which further impoverish the already impoverished communities from which most incarcerated people hail. We can leave all of these things in place. All we have to do is ask individuals to attend an implicit bias training or two.

For these reasons, the prevalence of implicit bias in the national conversation about racial inequalities has led some scholars to wonder what we are *not* talking about when we talk about implicit bias. That said, it would be misguided to entirely dismiss the role played by implicit bias in creating racial disparities in health. The elimination of providers' implicit biases—or the creation of conditions that make it more difficult for providers to act on their implicit biases—should be considered an important part of a multifaceted, multipronged program to eradicate racial disparities in health in the United States.

PATIENT MISTRUST

Scholars have proposed that patients of color bear at least some responsibility for racial disparities in health. This proposed responsibility stems from the fact that, on the whole, black people distrust medical institutions and personnel more than their nonblack counterparts do. This well-documented mistrust may cause black people to avoid seeing their doctors as often as they should, delaying the healthcare that could prevent illness or conserve life. This mistrust may lead black people to refuse to share personal information with their providers, even failing to disclose facts about their symptoms or their lives that would help their provider care for them. Mistrust may also lead black patients to refuse to follow their providers' recommendations, making it difficult for their healers to actually heal them. Additionally, mistrust may lead black patients to decline to participate in clinical trials of drugs or devices, making it impossible to know whether the trials' findings are true with respect to black people.

Studies have consistently shown that black people score higher than other racial groups on measures of medical mistrust.[77] While the fact of black medical mistrust is not easily disputed, the question of *why* black people distrust medical institutions and actors has several possible answers.

Many observers have located the origins of contemporary black medical mistrust in historical events—most notably, the Tuskegee Study of Untreated Syphilis in the Negro Male (also known as the Tuskegee Experiment). In the forty-year study, which began in 1932, government researchers from the United States Public Health Service and the Centers for Disease Control and Prevention sought to observe how syphilis affected black people.[78] Assuming that the disease would impact black and white bodies differently, researchers enrolled in their study close to four hundred black men with syphilis, telling them that they had "bad blood" and promising them treatment for their condition.[79] The researchers failed to tell the men that they were research subjects, that they had an infectious disease, and that they could pass the disease (which causes blindness, deafness, heart disease, and death) to their sexual partners and, congenitally, to their children.[80] Cruelly, the researchers failed to provide the men with treatment for syphilis even after an effective therapeutic, penicillin, was discovered and became widely available by 1947.[81] Instead, they monitored the men as the disease ravaged their bodies and the bodies of their sexual partners and children. The government terminated the study in 1972 only after a whistleblower came forward to report the abuse.[82]

The Tuskegee Experiment has been a popular explanation of black medical mistrust. Indeed, most discussions in popular media of black distrust of healthcare providers and institutions mention the Tuskegee Experiment. Indeed, the Tuskegee Experiment was frequently cited as the reason that many black Americans initially were hesitant about receiving the vaccine for COVID-19. One local news station's headline was "Combatting Vaccine Hesitancy after Mistrust Caused by Unethical Study."[83] The story began, "Medical mistrust is deeply rooted, particularly in the Black community. A big reason for that is because of the Tuskegee study."[84]

There are two major problems with claiming that the Tuskegee Experiment is the origin of black patient mistrust. First, explaining black medical mistrust by pointing to the Tuskegee Experiment—a lone, albeit abhorrent, event that ended over fifty years ago—suggests that black people who refuse to trust healthcare institutions today are acting *irrationally*. The study ended over half a century ago, after all. If black people refuse to receive potentially life-saving healthcare today because they have anxieties about an unethical research study that was terminated before many of them were born, then it suggests that black people are acting unreasonably or even foolishly.

Second, attributing contemporary black medical mistrust to the Tuskegee Experiment ignores the fact that large numbers of people of color have had *personal* experiences with healthcare providers and hospitals that have led them to distrust healthcare institutions. Consider Jenna, a thirty-five-year-old black woman who was about thirty-two weeks pregnant with her first child when I met her at Golden Health. Jenna, who owned a business and described herself as an entrepreneur, received her undergraduate degree from Yale University and her master of business administration degree from Harvard University. She revealed that her mother, who had a bachelor's degree from the University of California at Berkeley, had passed away the year before after coping with "one significant health challenge after another" since Jenna was eight years old. Even though her mother was a well-educated woman with money, Jenna had to advocate on her behalf to receive quality healthcare. After decades of interacting with healthcare systems with her chronically ill mother, Jenna said, "I've just seen—and experienced—that it's just different for black people":

> My mother contracted COVID at the top of 2022, and her experience was so negative in the hospital. I had to get involved. I was calling and trying to figure out what was going on. We were fortunate because we had folks on the inside who were able to get in there—to get my mom the care that she needed. But even they admitted that what happened to her was not okay. Anyway, my mother was so traumatized by the experience that when she needed to get more healthcare for another condition, she decided she'd rather just stop all of her treatments and die. She preferred death over being pulled back into any medical facility. [long pause] Yeah. She had navigated the healthcare system for thirty years. Her final experience was so traumatic that she decided she'd rather just die. And that's what she did.

There is nothing particularly unusual about Jenna's story of her mother's experiences with the healthcare system. I interviewed dozens of black women who told me similar stories of medical neglect and mistreatment. There was Fortune, whose medical providers repeatedly dismissed her reports of severe abdominal pain, telling her that she should see a psychologist, as the agony that she was experiencing was all in her head. When she went to the emergency room during a particularly severe bout, the providers refused to give her any pain medication, assuming that she was lying to get drugs. Fortune was later diagnosed with endometriosis, which occurs when uterine tissue grows outside of the uterus and often causes debilitating pelvic pain.

There was Nikki, who suffered a miscarriage of a very wanted baby and underwent a dilation and curettage (D&C), a procedure that removes any fetal tissue remaining in the uterus after a miscarriage. On the way home after the D&C, Nikki began to bleed profusely, so she returned to the hospital. After waiting hours for follow-up care because the hospital insisted on ensuring that her insurance would cover the surgery that she needed, Nikki's bleeding subsided, which led the hospital to deprioritize her case. In the end, Nikki waited over thirty-six hours to receive her surgery. "The whole time, they were so unkind to me," she told me. "They insisted upon searching my purse when they admitted me to the hospital and took me to my room. They didn't give me any food. Because of COVID, they wouldn't let me husband wait with me. They treated me like an inmate. Like a prison inmate. And I had just lost my baby. No one said, 'I'm sorry for your loss. Do you need anything?'"

There was Giselle, who needed to have a cervical biopsy after she tested positive for a virus that causes cervical cancer and a routine Pap smear came back abnormal. She said, "I had some either German or Russian doctor—just some movie villain doctor who slut-shamed me while taking biopsies of my cervix. He's asking me, 'How many sexual partners have you had? This is why women should not. . . .' You know, just being miserable. He was really old and obviously white. And he was taking chunks of my cervix for biopsies with no anesthesia and making me feel like shit as he did it."

While Jenna, Fortune, Nikki, and Giselle—and the numerous other black women I interviewed who told me infuriating stories about the substandard healthcare that they had received—did not develop a distrust of medical institutions as a response to their experiences, such a reaction would have been understandable. And this is why the Tuskegee Experiment is a poor explanation of why black people are more likely to mistrust medical institutions than other racial groups. The Tuskegee Experiment explanation of black medical mistrust denies that, in many cases, black people's refusal to trust healthcare institutions makes all the sense in the world. As sociologist Ruha Benjamin puts it, when we acknowledge the myriad ways that institutions across society—including healthcare institutions—continue to fail people of color, medical mistrust might be a "perfectly rational, even incisive, disposition toward biomedicine in a socially stratified society."[85]

In addition to denying the reasonableness of black medical mistrust, the Tuskegee Experiment explanation ignores the poor treatment that black people receive in doctor's offices and hospitals *today*. This contemporary mistreatment does a better job of explaining black people's unwillingness to place their trust in the healing professions. According to one set of researchers, "Every day, Black Americans have their pain denied, their conditions misdiagnosed, and necessary treatment withheld by physicians."[86] The Tuskegee Experiment explanation of black medical mistrust conceals these present-day instances of violated trust. It implies that when black people enter doctor's offices and hospitals today, they, like their white counterparts, will invariably receive ethical, respectful, high-quality care. It suggests that we need to look in the dustbin of history if we want to find healthcare institutions that betray their black patients.

Finally, the Tuskegee Experiment explanation of black medical mistrust proposes an insufficient solution to the problem. If black people do not trust healthcare providers and institutions solely because of an unethical research study that happened in the mid-twentieth century, then the answer to the problem of black medical mistrust is to apologize for those long-ago events and then educate black people by making them aware of the world-class care that can be found inside the doors of their neighborhood hospital. However, consider how the solution changes if we reframe the problem. If black people do not trust healthcare institutions because these institutions continue to betray them, then *the solution is to make the institutions worthy of black people's trust*. As Benjamin writes, we ought to "reorient ourselves . . . away from a fixation with distrust and towards the problem of institutional trustworthiness."[87] In essence, we should ensure that black people receive the healthcare that *everyone* should expect to receive in one of the wealthiest nations in the world.

* * *

In chapter 2, we saw that racial disparities in maternal mortality are beneficial to healthcare institutions that cater to the commercially insured because the disparities guarantee that their client base will include commercially insured black people who are trying to purchase an exit from their increased likelihood of dying from a pregnancy-related cause. In this chapter, we have seen that when racial disparities in maternal mortality exist within a society that is inclined to believe that racial groups are genetically or culturally distinct, such disparities work to reaffirm the truth of the genetic or cultural distinctiveness of the races—a reaffirmation that is highly beneficial to defenders of the racial status quo. In the next chapter, we will see that racial disparities in maternal mortality are beneficial to yet another part of society—media outlets. Indeed, the black maternal health crisis can be quite lucrative to the journalists who are covering it.

4 Covering the Black Maternal Health Crisis

There is nothing new about the fact that black people die from pregnancy-related causes much more frequently than their white counterparts do. Indeed, racial disparities in maternal mortality might be described as a hoary, hackneyed feature of American life. In the early 1900s, epidemiologists began documenting the frequency at which people died during pregnancy, childbirth, or the postpartum period. These first statistics revealed something that ought to have been completely unsurprising to those turn-of-the-century researchers: Pregnancy and childbirth were much deadlier for black women than for white women.[1] What was true during the early twentieth century remains true in the early twenty-first century.

Although there is nothing particularly new about racial disparities in maternal mortality, these disparities recently have become news. As journalist Helena Andrews-Dyer wryly puts it, "[B]lack women and their wombs have been trending."[2] Media outlets of all sizes, ranges, and varieties have covered what has been styled the "black maternal health crisis." Headlines announcing that it is not safe to be black and pregnant have become constant in the last few years:

> Black Maternal Mortality Is Still a Crisis[3]
> "I Don't Want to Die": Fighting Maternal Mortality among Black Women[4]
> Childbirth Is Deadlier for Black Families Even When They're Rich, Expansive Study Finds[5]
> "I Knew How Dangerous Things Could Become": The Perils of Childbirth as a Black Woman[6]

The Rates of Death for Pregnant Black Women Have Doubled [in] the Last 20 Years[7]
Nothing Protects Black Women from Dying in Pregnancy and Childbirth[8]
I Survived the Black Maternal Health Crisis. My Friend Didn't[9]
We Must Treat the Black Maternal Health Crisis with the Urgency It Deserves[10]
She was a Black Pediatrician But Still Died after Giving Birth to Her 1st Child[11]
Black Women Are Dying during Childbirth and No One Seems to Care[12]
The Quiet Crisis among African Americans: Pregnancy and Childbirth Are Killing Women at Inexplicable Rates[13]
US Olympian Dies from Pregnancy Complication That Disproportionately Impacts Black Women[14]
Regardless of Income, Black Women Face Death to Give Birth in America[15]
Maternal Mortality Is Shockingly High in the U.S.—Especially If You're Black[16]
We Should All Be Talking About America's Black Maternal Health Crisis[17]

A study by communications scholars Denetra Walker and Kelli Boling shows that prior to 2005, virtually no articles about black maternal mortality appeared in newspapers in the United States.[18] Beginning in 2007, however, there was a sharp uptick in reporting on the issue such that by 2010, over four thousand articles on the topic were being published every year.[19] Then, in 2017, National Public Radio and ProPublica collaborated on their "Lost Mothers" series,[20] which did not focus on black maternal deaths but observed time and again that black people's maternal mortality rates were worse than those of their white counterparts. Further, one article in the series—titled "Black Mothers Keep Dying after Giving Birth"—told the story of Shalon Irving, an epidemiologist at the Centers for Disease Control and Prevention whose research focused on racial disparities in health.[21] Three weeks after the birth of her daughter, Irving died from complications from high blood pressure—a condition with notable racial disparities in prevalence.[22] The number of articles about black maternal mortality skyrocketed after the publication of the "Lost Mothers" series.

The number of articles on black maternal deaths spiked again in 2018 after one of the most decorated athletes in the world, tennis phenomenon

Serena Williams, shared with *Vogue* magazine that she developed pulmonary emboli after the birth of her first daughter and that her healthcare providers initially dismissed her concerns when she reported her symptoms:[23] "The nurse thought her pain medicine might [have been] making her confused."[24] The emboli caused Williams to develop a severe cough, which caused her Caesarian-section incision to rupture. When her doctors repaired the incision, they discovered a large amount of collected blood.[25] Williams's postpartum ordeal left her—an extremely wealthy woman at the peak of physical fitness—bedridden for six weeks.[26]

Feminist scholar Jennifer Nash also attributes the increased attention to black maternal mortality that began in 2018 to journalist Linda Villarosa's article published in the *New York Times Magazine* that year. Nash notes that Villarosa's piece, which examined why "America's Black Mothers and Babies Are in a Life-or-Death Crisis,"[27] was "picked up by Public Broadcasting Service (PBS), National Public Radio (NPR), *Truthout*, *Mother Jones*, and *Democracy Now*; was cited by state legislatures as they formed task forces to respond to the crisis of Black maternal health; and also inaugurated a year of significant coverage of Black maternal health in nearly every major US newspaper."[28] In 2019, one of the most famous women alive, Beyoncé, ensured that the media's attention would stay on black maternal mortality and morbidity when she released her documentary *Homecoming* and revealed that she had suffered from preeclampsia, a potentially fatal hypertensive disorder, during her second pregnancy.[29] Activist Derecka Purnell's opinion piece in *The Guardian* represents the tenor of the media coverage that followed the cultural icon's revelation, asking, "If even Beyoncé had a rough pregnancy, what hope do other black women have?"[30]

The murder of George Floyd, a black man, by Derek Chauvin, a white police officer, during an arrest in May 2020 led to widespread demonstrations and a short-lived "racial reckoning."[31] It also worked to ensure that black maternal mortality remained in the news. Explains one set of researchers, "As the protests grew into a movement, mainstream outlets picked up the story, moving from 'episodic' event reporting toward 'thematic' coverage of the reasons underlying the protests, including systemic injustices highlighted by activists."[32] Black maternal mortality and morbidity comprised an integral part of the thematic coverage of the protests that summer. As Nash theorizes, the figure of "the pregnant mother battling obstetric violence in her quest to literally birth Black life"—alongside the figure of the lifeless young black man, slain at the hands of a white cop—came to symbolize the Black Lives Matter movement.[33] Media outlets published stories about black maternal deaths, proposing that black people were much less likely than white people to survive pregnancy and childbirth because of the structural and interpersonal racism that Floyd's brutal murder on the streets of Minneapolis had made unavoidably visible.

In this way, black people dying or nearly dying during pregnancy, childbirth, or shortly thereafter had become a "spectacle"[34]—much like the appalling videos of black people being killed by police officers that circulate on the internet. The extensive media coverage of black maternal mortality and morbidity transformed black people who failed to survive the process of childbearing into something to gawk at, to consume, to click on, and to share with others who need to be informed about what antiblackness looks like.

Activists who worked to secure resources to make pregnancy, childbirth, and the postpartum period safe for black people welcomed the media's sustained attention on black maternal mortality and morbidity. The transformation of black maternal deaths into a spectacle was a welcome change from the days when these deaths were invisible—when advocates and surviving loved ones were essentially screaming into the void when they spoke about black people's high rates of dying from preventable pregnancy-related deaths. Judging by the abundant media coverage, the nation now seemed ready to give a damn. Activists hoped that the coverage—the headlines, op-eds, explainers, long-form essays, quick takes, podcast episodes, primetime features, and think pieces—would let everyone know that an avoidable tragedy was taking place in the United States. They hoped that this attention would ultimately lead to the policy changes and interventions that have been demonstrated to save the lives of pregnant and recently postpartum people.[35]

And so the media's interest in black maternal deaths can be understood as a good thing. However, although many aspects of this media attention are positive, it still can be looked at critically. We can commend the existence of coverage of black maternal death and injury while also being attentive to the coverage's harmful, exploitative, and extractive aspects.

As an initial matter, we might ask why this particular health issue has been so interesting to people. Racial disparities in health exist across numerous domains. Black people's rates of hypertension, diabetes, asthma, kidney disease, and lung disease (just to name a few) are higher than nonblack people's. Of all the excess sickness and death across all the domains, why have racial disparities in maternal mortality and morbidity been the racial health disparity that has captured the media's attention?

Anthropologist Haile Eshe Cole offers a disturbing possibility. She theorizes that the media—and the masses who consume it—are drawn to black people's deaths and near-death experiences during pregnancy because the dying black maternal body makes intuitive sense to people in the United States. Cole reminds scholars that the figure of the "pathological Black mother" is a common trope in American life[36]—existing since the dawn of the nation. During the era of chattel slavery and the period of Jim Crow that followed, there was "Mammy" a black mother who was so devoted to the white children that she was tasked with caring for that she neglected her own children.[37] In the 1960s, sociologist Daniel Patrick Moynihan gave us the "matriarch," a black mother whose fierce independence alienated the black men who would otherwise head her household and led to the collapse of the black family—a collapse that, in turn, led to intergenerational poverty, violence in black neighborhoods, and the failure of the black race.[38] Two decades later, President Ronald Reagan popularized the figure of the "welfare queen," a black mother who bore children in order to obtain generous government benefits, enabling her to parasitically live off of the labor of the taxpayers who supported her lavish lifestyle.[39] Further, the welfare queen's ineptitude as a mother made it inevitable that her children would become the nation's future social problems—criminals and second-generation welfare queens. The crack cocaine scare during the 1980s yielded the figure of the "crack mother," a black mother who selfishly smoked crack cocaine while pregnant, injuring the fetus that she carried. The babies that these black women birthed were understood to be the nation's "newest horror"—"a bio-underclass, a generation of physically damaged cocaine babies whose biological inferiority is stamped at birth."⁴⁰

These kinds of narratives about black mothers' incompetence have circulated in the United States for many generations. Cole invites us to wonder whether the contemporary figure of the black mother dying from a pregnancy-related cause has secured the interest of the masses because it is the latest chapter in a longstanding narrative. Stories about black people who have found pregnancy to be deadly "fall in line not only with historical narratives of blackness, disease, and illness[,] but also with the illegitimacy and pathology of Black motherhood."⁴¹ Might this explain why media outlets have been so keen to cover the tragedy of black maternal deaths? Is the phenomenon comfortably consistent with what we in the United States have come to expect from black mothers?

Cole's provocation may also explain why so many who care deeply about pregnant black people—advocates, activists, and allies alike—have welcomed the extensive media coverage of black maternal deaths. Representations of pathological black motherhood throughout history have consistently faulted black women for their pathology. Mammy's preference for her white charges over her biological children was due to her own internalized white supremacy and antiblackness. Moynihan's matriarch ruined the black family because of her perverse independence and vicious disrespect of black would-be patriarchs. The welfare queen's capitalization of her reproductive capacities was due to her own laziness, cunning, and un-American will not to work. The crack mother gave birth to the nation's future social ills not because she lacked access to healthcare that could help her overcome her dependence on cocaine but rather because she was sociopathic, sadistic, and evil.

While the black woman who struggles to bring a new life into the world might be like these other figures insofar as there is something pathological about her motherhood, she is unlike these other figures insofar as she may not be to blame for the pathology. Rather, the healthcare system that fails her is to blame. Nash writes that "Black motherhood is now cast as suffering . . . rather than pathological, as tragic rather than self-destructive, as traumatized rather than deviant."⁴² For perhaps the first time, black mothers and mothers-to-be have been granted a reprieve from being perpetrators. They are now victims, subject to "attacks" that unfold "in hospitals and institutionalized medical spaces that practice noncare and disregard Black mothers and their families."[43]

We should bear in mind, however, that both of these things can be true: Modern understandings of the black maternal health crisis that conceptualize black mothers as victims might simultaneously conceptualize them as blameworthy and as bearing some responsibility for their own injuries and deaths. As chapter 3 explores, many laypersons (and some experts) believe that the increased morbidity and mortality among black people are functions of black people's genes or culture. These explanations lay the blame for black people's higher rates of maternal deaths and severe injuries firmly on black people. These accounts—which assert that black people are to blame for dying or nearly dying during pregnancy, childbirth, or the postpartum period—contradictorily exist alongside assertions that healthcare institutions and providers are needlessly failing black people who are bringing new life into the world.

After centuries of black mothers being portrayed as clearly "the problem," the ambiguity contained in the media's recent representations of black people who are felled on the path to motherhood has been a breath of fresh air to many. While current discussions of the black maternal health crisis might presuppose that black mothers are pathologically frail due to their genes or culture, they simultaneously presuppose that black mothers are being victimized within medical spaces. This willingness to understand at least some portion of the excessive pregnancy-related deaths that black mothers endure as *not their fault* has been welcomed. Those who have been critical of black people's historical and contemporary subordination have found the recent media attention to a tragedy that is depicted, at least in part, as being inflicted on victimized black mothers to be "seductive."[44]

Yet this attention is not outside of critique. The next section evaluates the media coverage of black maternal deaths, concluding that many of the news stories about black people who die or nearly die during pregnancy or childbirth simply are not very good. Much of the coverage is mediocre, at best. After analyzing why this is so, the chapter turns to an exploration of how black maternal deaths are profitable to the media companies that cover them, generating revenue from patrons and accolades from prize boards. The chapter then focuses on the consumers of media coverage of black maternal mortality and morbidity, asking whether accounts of black maternal deaths and near-death experiences are as ubiquitous as they are because consumers are, at least in part, enjoying black suffering. The chapter ends by examining how black people who are pregnant or desire pregnancy experience being constantly bombarded with the fact that they are less likely than their non-black peers to survive the event.

EVALUATING THE COVERAGE

Much of the media coverage of racial disparities in maternal mortality and morbidity simply is not well done. Subpar reporting often occurs when a media outlet sees its competitors and major media outlets cover the issue and consequently feels the need to publish *something* on the topic. In this type of check-the-box journalism, reporters with no background in health or race or the intersection of the two are given assignments to write articles about the sad state of black maternal health in the United States. The stories that they deliver usually repeat familiar statistics (such as black women are more than three times as likely as white women to die from a pregnancy-related cause) while offering few insights into the processes, institutions, discourses, and policies that have led to this statistic.

One journalist who was reporting on maternal health before the nation began to take an interest in it has said that many of the journalists writing about black maternal mortality and morbidity are "not equipped to handle th[e] topic, and they do not have the time or resources to properly nuance the story."[45] Indeed, many of the recent articles about black maternal mortality and morbidity were written by "general assignment reporters" who have "never reported on maternal health" but have found themselves writing something on this "specialized beat."[46] Further, the ascension of social media platforms has led to the downsizing of traditional media companies and reductions in the number of reporters that they employ. As legal scholar Martha Minow explains, "Smaller staffs mean fewer resources for journalists who are specialists in fields such as science[.]"[47] Thus, in an era of Facebook, Instagram, TikTok, and X (formerly known as Twitter), media outlets are less likely to employ journalists with the expert knowledge in obstetrics, public health, or epidemiology that would allow them to competently cover black maternal mortality and morbidity.

The problem with check-the-box journalism is that audiences learn little about racial disparities in maternal mortality and morbidity beyond the simple fact that they exist. They walk away from the coverage knowing about the phenomenon; but, the lackluster reporting leaves them not knowing what they need to know about the phenomenon. As communications scholar Safiya Umoja Noble notes, issues like black maternal mortality and morbidity are complex, and reporting on such issues "requires knowledgeable people who have studied history and critical theories of race, feminism, and power. It requires expertise and commitment to help us contextualize race in the United States[,] and it takes intentional reframing."[48] Because reporters doing check-the-box journalism lack the expertise necessary to do that reframing, their reporting gives audiences nothing new, leaving them to fit the phenomenon within familiar frames, such as those that blame racially subordinated people for their own racial subordination and locate the source of problems within individuals as opposed to the structures within which those individuals exist. In this way, check-the-box journalism invites the public to conclude that something is wrong with black people—their genes or their cultures—that leads them to die more frequently from pregnancy-related causes. People who care deeply about racial justice may suppose that if this is what the public concludes when the media talks about black maternal death and injury, then it is best for the media to stop talking about it altogether.

PROFITING FROM BLACK MATERNAL DEATHS

It probably is not an overstatement to say that the news is essential to democracy, providing voters with information about public affairs and enabling them to hold public officials accountable for their actions and inactions. Neither is it an overstatement to say that if democracy in the United States is weakening, as some credible observers have concluded, one contributor to its demise is the sustained attack being inflicted on the news industry. Politicians have intentionally sowed distrust in the "mainstream media," and ideologically committed outlets that reject traditional journalistic values have been cosplaying as real news channels. Those of us who are terrified by the languishing of American democracy might be tempted to view media outlets that remain committed to truth and objectivity as doing something truly noble.

While the news is essential to the political health of the country, it does not exist outside a capitalist global economy. According to journalist Wesley Lowery, the news has "never liberated itself from the constraints of American capitalism. Our press remains first a *business*."[49] With the exception of news gatherers and reporters that are nonprofit or public—such as National Public Radio (NPR), the Public Broadcasting Service (PBS), and ProPublica—generating profits is one of the many purposes of media outlets. Thus, when a news source like the *Washington Post* or a local NBC affiliate runs a story on black maternal mortality and morbidity, we can safely assume that it seeks both to inform its audience about a public health disaster that is currently taking place and also to make money. Moreover, the news industry is making *a lot* of money, with revenue between $63 billion and $65 billion every year.[50]

A short primer on the business of the news might be helpful here. Media outlets—including print journalism (such as national outlets like the *New York Times* and the *Wall Street Journal*, as well as local newspapers like *Oaklandside* in Oakland, California, and the *Sun Sentinel* in Fort Lauderdale, Florida), cable news outlets (like CNN and MSNBC), network news outlets (like ABC and CBS), and commercial news and talk radio stations—rely on the same income streams. Although significant changes have occurred in the business of the news over the last couple of decades, the two most important streams of income for media outlets remain advertising revenue and audience revenue (from, for example, subscriptions to both digital and print versions of newspapers, cable fees that subscribers pay to their cable providers,[51] and donations from individuals).[52] Of the two streams, advertising is the biggest revenue source, representing close to 70 percent of the industry's income.[53] Advertising revenue is so important to media outlets that one observer declared that the entire point of commercial media "is 'to attract and hold a large audience for advertisers.'"[54]

Whenever a person reads a story in a print or digital newspaper, watches a segment on a cable or network news program, or listens to a podcast episode or radio broadcast, that engagement represents an opportunity for the media outlet to make money. A story in a newspaper may inspire readers to purchase a subscription to the newspaper or to renew the subscription for yet another year if they are already a subscriber. A cable news segment may lead viewers to purchase or to continue paying for a package from their cable provider that includes the cable channel. Thus, coverage that consumers find informative, interesting, or compelling generates audience revenue for media outlets. Further, news coverage that, in one way or the other, lures audiences to the print, television, or radio media outlet generates advertising revenue, as purveyors of goods or services want to advertise their wares with outlets that have large numbers of readers, viewers, or listeners. Thus, at least one reason for the media's recent interest in racial disparities in maternal mortality and morbidity is that *coverage of black maternal deaths has been drawing audiences and is, therefore, profitable.*

An analogy can be drawn to the extensive coverage of black people's deaths at the hands of police officers (or citizens who have deputized themselves as law enforcement)[55]—an illuminating analogy to which this chapter repeatedly returns. The homicides of Trayvon Martin, Eric Garner, Michael Brown, Tamir Rice, Walter Scott, Freddie Gray, Sandra Bland, Alton Sterling, Philando Castile, Elijah McClain, Ahmaud Arbery, Breonna Taylor, George Floyd, and Tyre Nichols dominated the news cycles when their deaths first occurred. This inundation of media coverage is a triumph in many ways, as it ensures public awareness of the killings, which might be a prerequisite for the social and structural changes that would prevent the recurrence of such violence. At the same time, media outlets understand that killings of black people by police (and private citizens) are good for business, as individuals turn to their preferred news source to learn details about the circumstances surrounding the deaths, follow the drama of the court cases (or nonindictments), get information about any protests that the deaths spark, and listen to pundits opine about the social meaning of the homicides. Because such killings help make money for news sources, some scholars have conceptualized homicides as commodities that media outlets sell in order to make a profit.[56] Further, media outlets are making *handsome* profits from these race-based commodities. According to information studies scholar Tonia Sutherland, media outlets "are, quite literally, 'making a killing' by inscribing and reinscribing death and trauma."[57]

In this way, coverage of the deaths of black people—whether due to pregnancy-related causes or violence from a police officer—presents a conflict for those who are invested in the project of saving black people's lives. On the one hand, a problem that has always plagued black communities is receiving the attention that might be a precondition to policy changes that might save lives. On the other hand, third parties—media companies, pundits who are paid to talk about the issue, and journalists who are rewarded with raises, promotions, and prizes when they cover the issue well[58]—derive sizeable monetary benefits and social capital from black suffering and pain.

We should also think about the media's interest in black maternal health and unhealth in light of the dramatic shifts that have taken place in the news industry in recent decades. The rise of social media has had a ruinous effect on legacy media, as millions of people who once received their news from legacy media outlets that conform to traditional journalistic values now receive their news from Facebook, Instagram, TikTok, X, and YouTube. There is a lot to lament about the citizenry's growing reliance on social media as a news source. As Minow summarizes:

> Leaders at Facebook and Google have stressed that, as tech companies, they are not in the business of journalism. . . . They focus on keeping consumers' attention, not on covering the news. . . . Judgments once made by a variety of people with diverse aspirations are now made by profit-maximizing algorithms seeking to capture the largest number of "eyeballs" and advertising dollars. Algorithms deploying machine learning and data about individuals determine what each user receives on their Facebook feed, Twitter timeline, and YouTube home page—and the big platforms use them to amplify emotions in order to maximize attention.[59]

Reliance on social media as a news source not only produces citizens who are unexposed to a breadth of issues and perspectives (which is terrible for democracy), but also threatens the financial viability of legacy media outlets, which are losing the advertising revenues that have represented their largest income source. Essentially, corporations trying to sell things want to be where the people are. And if the people are clicking through YouTube videos instead of reading the *Sun Sentinel*, then corporations will prefer to advertise their wares on YouTube instead of in the *Sun Sentinel*.

The loss of audiences and advertising revenues has profoundly affected legacy media and the business of the news, especially print media: "Over the past twenty years, newspapers across the country have lost nearly 40 percent of their daily circulation, and in the past ten years, newspaper advertising revenues decreased 63 percent."[60] This means that newspapers have had to find ways to compete for the attention of readers who can get their news for free through their social media feeds. One way that they have competed has been by publishing stories that are less technical and fact-intensive and are more inviting and "emotional."[61] Some have wondered whether newspapers have covered black maternal mortality and morbidity as much as they have because they are trying to lure people's attention away from their TikTok "For You Page" by pulling at their heartstrings through yet another story about a black person who died during labor.

And then there are twenty-four-hour cable news channels, which have been increasingly popular since their advent in 1980, when the first cable news network, CNN, hit the airwaves.[62] The one thing that twenty-four-hour news channels require is twenty-four hours of news, even though there usually is not enough news to fill that space. According to news veterans Howard Rosenberg and Charles Feldman, these channels solve this problem by finding things to talk about and presenting them as news:

> From the very first, CNN founders recognized the potential problem. There was not enough news they wanted to cover on a given day—barring some catastrophic event—to fill 24 hours. . . . So a smorgasbord of separate units was created within CNN to produce soft, feature-type pieces that although not breaking news were deemed to have some informational value. . . . To be sure, this myriad of units did at times manage to dig up something that

generously could be defined as news in the traditional sense. But for the most part, they produced only "filler"—material designed to consume space, hold an audience and, most important, keep advertisers happy.[63]

When CNN and MSNBC[64] cover black maternal mortality and morbidity several times over the course of a month in the absence of anything particularly new to report about the phenomenon, the coverage might be a product of the search for a story to help fill the twenty-four-hour news cycle. Further, if CNN and MSNBC treat the phenomenon as newsworthy, other media outlets—national and local, print, television, and radio—are more likely to conceptualize it in similar ways, leading these competitors to feel the need to provide their own coverage of the issue. And the glut of stories about black maternal deaths expands.

ENJOYING BLACK SUFFERING

Literary theorist Saidiya Hartman has provided a disquieting account of white people's relationship to enslaved black people's suffering during the era of chattel slavery: White people enjoyed it. Hartman theorizes that not only did enslaved people's suffering provide pleasure to enslavers and other defenders of slavery, it, more surprisingly, also provided pleasure to those who opposed slavery. Hartman writes about northern audiences that were "scandalized *and titillated*" by the "terrifying details" about slavery shared in abolitionist tracts.[65] When opponents of slavery confronted accounts of the rapes, assaults, maimings, and murders that were a banality of the institution, Hartman writes about "the *pleasure* of indignation" that they felt in the face of "the spectacle of sufferance."[66]

What kinds of relationships do modern audiences have to coverage of black maternal deaths—even audiences that are outraged that black people are dying preventable deaths from pregnancy-related causes in one of the richest nations in the world? If Noble is correct when she states that "Black death is so titillating[,] so delicious to consume, to read, to be in the pain and the trauma,"[67] then we might wonder whether those who encounter journalism about black maternal mortality and morbidity are enjoying it.

Do individuals derive pleasure from reading about Serena Williams's pulmonary embolism and ruptured Caesarian-section incision; from watching a segment on CNN about Beyoncé's *Homecoming* and her revelation that she had preeclampsia during her second pregnancy; from listening to a radio broadcast reporting on the high rates of black maternal mortality in many of the states that banned abortion after the United States Supreme Court's reversal of *Roe v. Wade*? Of course, there is something upright about bearing witness to this discomfiting, vile fact of American life. However, asks Hartman, "Is the act of 'witnessing' a kind of looking no less entangled with . . . the extraction of enjoyment?"[68]

Writing about widely circulated videos of police violence against black people, journalist Alisha Ebrahimji describes "trauma porn" as "using other people's trauma to shock our system to galvanize support on the issue of police brutality against Black men and ignite some sort of fire in us, which is essentially what sexual porn does."[69] This description proposes that representations of black suffering may generate the feelings that incite political action *while* generating feelings of enjoyment. People who watch the video of Derek Chauvin kneeling on George Floyd's neck or who read ProPublica's article about Shalon Irving's pregnancy-related death can become incensed about the injustice of these deaths at the same time as they derive pleasure from the coverage.

The analogy to the ever-increasing number of videos of black people being killed by police is incredibly helpful here. Observers have argued that the easy availability of these videos is a positive development because the recordings further the cause of eliminating racist police violence. Many in this camp have found support for this position in the long history of black people's struggle for civil rights in the United States. For generations, documentation of white supremacy's brutality in the form of pictures and videos has served antiracist goals. In the early twentieth century, for example, journalist and civil rights activist Ida B. Wells included horrifying photos of lynchings in the materials that she authored and disseminated as part of her campaign against the practice.[70] When a lynch mob in Mississippi murdered fourteen-year-old Emmett Till after he allegedly whistled at a white woman, his mother, Mamie Till-Mobley, gave him an open-casket funeral so that the world could see how vicious and savage white supremacy could be. The images of the boy's disfigured body lying in his casket were published in *Jet* magazine and other media outlets, transforming the "vigilante murder into a spectacular image of state-sanctioned violence against Black people, helping to spark the Civil Rights Movement."[71] Bloody Sunday is another example. When John Lewis and a group of about six hundred civil rights activists attempted to cross the Edmund Pettus Bridge in Selma, Alabama, as part of a protest to obtain a meaningful right to vote for black people, police beat them, whipped them, and sprayed them with tear gas.[72] Appalling images from Bloody Sunday were televised throughout the country, helping to secure the passage of the Voting Rights Act of 1965.[73] Those who argue that the recent dissemination of videos of police brutality is a good thing point to these incidents and others. They say that the country has made significant progress away from its hideously racist past and toward a more equitable racial future because of the distribution of visual evidence of the barbarity of white supremacy.

While it may be true that viewing images of black people's battered bodies has helped to change viewers' hearts and minds and win them over to the cause of formal racial equality, Hartman reminds us that viewers' politically meaningful disgust can coexist with pleasure. Viewers might have felt both revulsion toward photographs of charred black bodies hanging from nooses in a southern grove and also taken a prurient interest in the pictures. The same analysis applies to recent videos of police killings of black men. Viewers might feel horror while watching George Floyd call out for his dead mother as Derek Chauvin kneels on his neck—a horror that might have inspired them to participate in, or at least be sympathetic to, the fleeting racial reckoning that Floyd's murder sparked. However, that horror can be felt simultaneously with a voyeuristic gratification caused by watching someone die. As critical theorist Rasul Mowatt wonders, "Are we consciously or subconsciously enjoying the aesthetics of torture" when we watch these "snuff films?"[74]

Similarly, are we titillated when we encounter coverage of yet another story about a pregnant black person dying or nearly dying? Unlike many police killings of black people, a viral video usually does not accompany coverage of black maternal mortality and morbidity. However, does the reporting nevertheless appeal to a side of readers, viewers, and listeners that derives pleasure from accounts of death and dying? Consider Linda Villarosa's *New York Times Magazine* article about black maternal mortality and morbidity. Villarosa centers Simone Landrum, a low-income, pregnant black woman living in New Orleans, to ground her reporting. Villarosa writes evocatively of Landrum's prior pregnancy, which ended tragically:

> In the car on the way to drop off [her older children], [Landrum] felt wetness between her legs and assumed her water had broken. But when she looked at the seat, she saw blood. . . . By the time she was lying on a gurney in the emergency room of Touro Infirmary, a hospital in the Uptown section of New Orleans, the splash of blood had turned into a steady stream. "I could feel it draining out of me, like if you get a jug of milk and pour it onto the floor," she recalls. Elevated blood pressure—Landrum's medical records show a reading of 160/100 that day—had caused an abruption: the separation of the placenta from her uterine wall. . . . When a nurse moved a monitor across her belly, Landrum couldn't hear a heartbeat. "I kept saying: 'Is she O.K.? Is she all right?'" Landrum recalls. "Nobody said a word. I have never heard a room so silent in my life." She remembers that the emergency-room doctor dropped his head. Then he looked into her eyes. "He told me my baby was dead inside of me. I was like: What just happened? Is this a dream? And then I turned my head to the side and threw up." . . . When she became more alert sometime later, a nurse told her that she had almost bled to death and had required a half dozen units of transfused blood and platelets to survive. "The nurse told me: 'You know, you been sick. You are very lucky to be alive,'" Landrum remembers. "She said it more than once." A few hours later, a nurse brought Harmony, who had been delivered stillborn via C-section, to her. Wrapped in a hospital blanket, her hair thick and black, the baby looked peaceful, as if she were dozing. "She was so beautiful—she reminded me of a doll," Landrum says.[75]

Landrum's devastating experience reads like the script for a horror movie. And this is not simply because Villarosa is a master storyteller. It is because Landrum's story features several elements common to the horror genre—blood, gore, the doll-like body of a lifeless baby. We should not be shocked, then, if those who are drawn to horror as a genre—because it is bloody, gory, and macabre—derive some enjoyment from Villarosa's recounting of Landrum's near-death experience.

Haile Eshe Cole has written about the possibility that some audiences may take pleasure in accounts of black people dying and nearly dying during the perinatal period, theorizing that black maternal deaths may be a "modern day example of . . . the ways in which abhorrence and enjoyment become affixed around Black suffering."[76] Disgust, sadness, and righteous indignation—the feelings that can provoke political action—certainly can coexist with less honorable, more sordid emotions.

Even if those who *truly* are committed to eliminating preventable black maternal deaths from the nation's landscape are not titillated by the spectacle of black people dying or almost dying from pregnancy-related causes, many are not so committed. We can be more certain that these less invested, more agnostic consumers of the coverage are enjoying stories of black people being felled on the path to childbirth. They might be consuming these reports in the same way that they consume reports about rivalries between sports teams or celebrity romances—that is, as entertainment. Instead of bearing witness to black suffering, these observers might simply be spectators to black pain. They may have no "intended purpose . . . beyond being a voyeur in the lives and fates of other citizens."[77] And it is not unreasonable for people who are protective of black life to be deeply offended by this reality. It is not unreasonable for them to want to shield black people's trauma from this gaze.

Another reason for the mass interest in stories of black maternal mortality might be that these stories make nonblack people feel protected from death.[78] When nonblack people read articles, watch news segments, or listen to radio broadcasts about black pregnant people dying, the coverage might provide them with some pleasure because it may implicitly assure nonblack consumers of these accounts that *they* are safe. The crisis, they are told, affects *black* pregnant and recently postpartum people. The reporting may allow them to assume that they, as nonblack people, are not in harm's way. In this way, engagement with media coverage about black maternal deaths may be gratifying to these audiences who consume it as a reassuring security blanket.

Finally, some individuals engage with the extensive reporting about black maternal mortality and morbidity because they feel that, as people with progressive politics, they are doing "the work" when they expose themselves to representations of black suffering and death. Rasul Mowatt has made this argument in the context of videos of police killings of black people, writing that "non-Black allies" may propose that their viewing of these recordings is "proof of their steadfastness in support."[79] Further, the distressing nature of these videos—the fact that many people find it hard to watch someone die—underscores the strength of the viewers' commitment to the cause. Something similar may be happening in the context of media coverage of black maternal deaths. People who consider themselves allies with black people as they struggle against antiblackness in all of its myriad forms might engage with reporting on black maternal deaths—especially when it is bloody and appalling—because it allows them to feel that they are doing what they should be doing as progressives.

So audiences may have many possible orientations to coverage of black maternal deaths—and some orientations may be more virtuous than others. And it is not entirely irrational if one feels some disdain for media outlets that offer black people's suffering to all those who care to consume it. In essence, media outlets do not require that their customers have a particular relationship to their news offerings. All the varying relationships are equally profitable.

THE COSTS OF BEING A SYMBOL

Jennifer Nash proposes that the dead or dying black mother has become a symbol that is invoked for various purposes.[80] Media outlets invoke her to signal that they have their finger on the pulse of all that is newsworthy. They cover black maternal mortality and morbidity because everyone has been talking about this new–old problem, and their reporting on the new–old problem maintains their legitimacy as a serious news source. Pundits commenting on yet another video of a black person being killed by the police invoke the dead or dying black mother to signal just how ubiquitous antiblackness is in the United States—that even labor and delivery rooms are not safe places for black people in the country. Democratic politicians attempting to win the loyalty and votes of their base invoke the dead or dying black mother when discussing the shortcomings of the country's healthcare system. Politicians refer to her to signal that they, unlike their out-of-touch opponents, are aware of the system's flaws and to identify a site for their future policy interventions (if they are elected).

How has being transformed into a symbol affected living, breathing black people who are pregnant or desiring pregnancy? What are the effects of being understood not as an "embodied position" but rather as a "political subject"—albeit one that is deserving of pity, solicitude, anxiety, and, perhaps, new policy?[81] What are the effects of being repeatedly warned that you are three to four times more likely than your white counterparts to die from a pregnancy-related cause? As Nash asks, "What does it *feel* like to be a pregnant Black person when the pregnant Black body is constructed (again) as a particular kind of problem, when pregnant Black women hear—again and again—that pregnancy can lead to death, that hospitals are death-worlds, that conventional obstetricians neglect black women's pain?"[82]

Helena Andrews-Dyer has reflected on the experience of being black and pregnant at a time when there has been an "onslaught of bad news about black women and pregnancy . . . permeat[ing] the headlines for the past two years":[83]

> You know that feeling you get immediately after clumsily tripping over something but right before actually falling? The throat catching, the stomach diving, the arms airplane-ing. That's how it feels waiting for the medical system to fail you in the way so many articles and anecdotes tell black women it inevitably will.[84]

Andrews-Dyer is describing what it is like to experience stress, which is terrible for maternal and infant health outcomes. Indeed, stress is correlated with preterm birth, low birth weight, preeclampsia, and other pregnancy complications.[85] Thus, the symbol that black mothers have become might have a devasting effect on actual embodied black mothers. Moreover, recall the discussion of epigenetics from chapter 3, which describes how the hostile environment in which the pregnant person exists can cause the fetus's genes to be expressed in a way that is harmful to its health. Epigenetics means that the media's indulgent coverage of black people's life-or-death struggles to birth new life ironically can work to perpetuate the struggle for generations to come.

While many of the black women who spoke with me for this book told me that they did not object to the way that media outlets have covered black maternal health and unhealth, many others were more critical. Loren fell into the latter camp. She worked in marketing at one of the many tech companies located in the Bay Area and was pregnant with her first child when I met her in the obstetrics clinic at Golden Health. Loren described the media coverage of black mothers who die or nearly die during pregnancy as a "drumbeat" that underlay everything that she did as an expectant mother. She found it frustrating and harmful:

> I just want to switch the narrative about black maternal health. I'm so tired of hearing about how much more likely we are to have all of these things. I'm already stressed about doing the best possible job of bringing this life into the world, and then . . . you add this narrative. And I just don't want to hear about that right now. Instead of focusing on what the statistics say and all that, I think that we should be creating things that are uplifting, positive, encouraging. We should be creating tools. . . . I want to shift that narrative so much because it's very. . . . It's just so dark.

Of course, the media's job is not to create things that are uplifting, positive, and encouraging. Its job is to inform the public about events that are happening in the world. In the best-case scenario, after the media informs the public, the public will engage in the political actions that will lead to the creation of things that are uplifting, positive, and encouraging. Loren's frustrations arise not from the media's failure to do its job but from the fact that the nation exists in the space between awareness and action. That is, the country is very aware that black maternal mortality and morbidity are issues, but we, as a society, have not acted. We have not created the tools that will fix this large-scale, systemic problem.

Nevertheless, media coverage might give individuals the information that they need to fashion their own tools to fix a problem as it affects them.

And as the next chapter explores, many of the people who spoke with me have attempted to do this. They have chosen not to receive their prenatal care at the General. They have taken their employer-provided health insurance to the Bay Area hospital that provides the most technologically sophisticated care. They have hired doulas to act as their advocates in the delivery room. They have elected to receive their prenatal care from black providers, midwives, or maternal-fetal medicine specialists. In essence, many of the black women that I interviewed have heard the drumbeat of media coverage about black maternal deaths and have attempted to equip themselves in ways that they hope will help them survive their pregnancies. For this reason, many reported feeling pleased about the recent discourse around black maternal deaths; they experienced it as a reminder to be vigilant about the healthcare that they were receiving.

And so I posed a question to Loren: Did she find at least some aspects of the recent spate of media coverage to be empowering—a reminder to be vigilant about her prenatal care? She responded without hesitation:

> No! No. It makes me more worried than anything. Yeah, there's nothing empowering about it to me. I don't feel more empowered knowing that I'm more likely to die because I'm black. . . . There's *so* much emphasis on all the things that could go wrong—all the things that *have* gone wrong for other people. . . . I wish that there was a way of educating, of informing in a way that's not fear-based. Something that is more tool-based.
>
> This is going to sound like a nonsequitur. [laughs] But I took a workshop with Mom's Against Drunk Driving. [laughs] Anyway, the facilitator was like, "What are you *for?*" And that was just so powerful to me. What are you for? When you say that you're against something, that's fine. We know what you're working against. But *what are you for?* We are against black women bleeding out during delivery and having strokes and having heart attacks. We are against black women not being listened to. We are against black women dying needlessly. But what are we *for?*

Again, the media's job is not to develop a positive program for building a livable world. Its purpose is to report on wars, not to end wars. So Loren was wishing that the media would provide something that it is not designed to provide. But Loren's grievance was born from living in the space between awareness and action. When institutions like the media raise awareness and raise awareness and raise awareness, *and people with the power to effect change do not act*, then the project of raising awareness seems to be nothing more than fearmongering. And individuals are left frustrated as they navigate the problem itself in addition to their fears about the problem.

The inaction is important to underscore. If the country does not pursue the policy changes that will fix the systemic failures that lead to black maternal deaths, then the profits made by media outlets, pundits, and others participating in the public conversation appear to be the major material effect of the discourse that swirls around black maternal health.

This is not to say that absolutely nothing has been done to address maternal mortality and morbidity. Most of the action has been taken on the state level. Recognizing that many fatal pregnancy complications unfold months after the birth of the baby, nearly all states have extended Medicaid coverage to twelve months (instead of sixty days) postpartum.[86] Thirteen states now cover doula services, which have been shown to improve maternal health outcomes, as part of their state's Medicaid programs.[87] Additionally, some states have situated themselves as leaders in the quest to eliminate preventable maternal deaths. California initiated the California Maternal Quality Care Collaborative (CMQCC) to address the state's rising maternal mortality rates.[88] CMQCC developed quality improvement toolkits for several causes of preventable maternal deaths, including hemorrhage, sepsis, and cardiovascular disease.[89] The toolkits compile "best practice tools and articles, care guidelines in multiple formats, hospital-level implementation guide[s], and professional education slide set[s]."[90] Through CMQCC, California has lowered its maternal mortality ratio from 16.9 deaths per 100,000 live births in 2006 to 5.9 deaths in 2016—even as the nation's maternal mortality ratio climbed to 21.8 deaths during that period.[91] (Interestingly, CMQCC was started in 2006, at least a decade before black maternal deaths became "news." Thus, it appears to have been created independent of media coverage of black maternal mortality and morbidity.)

While some states have acted to improve black maternal health outcomes, there have been only overtures of action on the federal level. During the presidential primary campaign in 2020, many Democratic candidates promised to address racial disparities in maternal mortality and morbidity if they were elected. Senator Elizabeth Warren unveiled a plan to financially reward hospitals with low rates of maternal deaths while penalizing their counterparts with higher rates.[92] Mayor Pete Buttigieg pledged to deal with black maternal mortality through implicit bias trainings.[93] Senator Kamala Harris vowed to continue the work that she already had undertaken around the issue, citing the Maternal CARE Act and the Black Maternal Health Momnibus Act, two pieces of legislation addressing black maternal mortality and morbidity that she had introduced during her short time in the United States Senate.[94] Once Harris became vice president to President Joe Biden, the Biden administration pointed to Harris's work while senator as evidence of the administration's commitment to solving the problem.[95] In fact, the administration incorporated aspects of the Maternal CARE Act and the Black Maternal Health Momnibus Act into its Build Back Better Act, a three-part plan to address the economic fallout from the COVID-19 pandemic, the nation's crumbling infrastructure and climate change, and issues that challenged the country's families (such as the absence of paid family and medical leave and the high cost of childcare).[96] While Congress passed the parts of the Build Back Better Act that related to infrastructure, climate change, and the pandemic, it failed to pass the part that tackled maternal mortality and morbidity.[97] So while there has been an "outpouring of attention" to black maternal health, that attention has been met with "political stasis" on the federal level, where it might matter most.[98]

It is useful to return, for the final time, to the videos showing police killings of black people. Some scholars have observed that although dozens of these videos are available online to anyone who cares to view them, there have been precious few indictments and convictions of the police officers who were recorded in the act of taking a life. Most of these videos have not led to accountability within the criminal legal system. For this reason, Safiya Umoja Noble describes them as "an *imagined* means of justice within a legal framework."[99] What purpose have these videos served? Sure, they have prompted some advocates and their allies to take to the streets to demand change. Yes, they have raised consciousness about the existence and persistence of police violence. Absolutely, they have convinced some otherwise disbelieving individuals of what black folks in the United States have been saying since time immemorial: Police do kill black people wrongly, unjustifiably, inhumanely. But that is about the extent of the change they have inspired. In fact, in the two years that followed George Floyd's May 2020 death and the widespread protests that it ignited, the number of black people killed by police actually *increased*: "police killings rose to an all-time high in 2022."[100] In the absence of concrete actions—convictions in individual cases, an overhaul or abolition of the system that makes police violence possible, or even a mere reduction in the number of black people who die at the hands of the police—some might conclude that these ubiquitous videos have done little beyond generating profits for traditional media outlets, *massive* profits for social media platforms, and pleasure for some consumers of the videos.

While left-leaning politicians have not achieved any federal policy successes in addressing black maternal health, talking about it has been quite useful for them. Speaking about black people who die during or after childbirth has served as a credential that establishes the progressiveness of their politics and proves that they have their finger on the pulse of the nation's inequities. It has served as evidence that they know, in the words of Marvin Gaye, "what's going on." In this vein, Jennifer Nash theorizes that the political left in the United States has "transformed Black mothers into a distinct form of . . . political currency."[101] She writes that "suffering Black mothers" have become "a kind of political commodity that, simply by being referenced, can provide moral authority for those who speak their names."[102] Nash's use of the language of "currencies" and "commodities" is helpful, as it invites us to consider how the symbol of the black mother has generated value to those who trade in it. It has been politically lucrative for those with progressive politics to invoke black maternal death. Alongside media companies, politicians have profited from the recent discourse around black maternal mortality and morbidity.

* * *

Many years ago, when I analyzed New York State's prenatal care program for indigent people, I found much to critique. Nevertheless, I remained aware that there was much to celebrate about the program's existence. In a country that is resolutely uncommitted to ensuring that its citizens can access healthcare at all times, New York had erected a system that bucked this trend—at least during pregnancy. And so I recognized that I was in a bind: "As I thankfully acknowledge the radical nature of [New York's prenatal care] program—one midwife I interviewed insisted upon characterizing the program as 'revolutionary'—I find myself in the awkward position of criticizing the revolution."[103]

I find myself in a similarly awkward position in this chapter. I have criticized the attention that actors and entities have given to black maternal mortality and morbidity. I think that much of it is wounding, exploitative, and extractive. At the same time, if everyone began to ignore black maternal deaths—as they did from the dawn of the nation until a few years ago—I would criticize the inattention. I would argue that ignoring disparities between black people's pregnancy survival rates and the rates of their nonblack peers is evidence of black people's profound marginalization.

I will not try to resolve the bind—to free myself from the awkward position in which I find myself. I am satisfied with simply acknowledging it, hoping that we can soon escape from this exhausting, infuriating space between awareness and action. For too long, we have mistaken talking about black maternal deaths with doing something about black maternal deaths. That mistake has become tedious. It is time to stop discussing, reporting, chronicling, recounting, and deliberating and to start engaging in the hard political work of making pregnancy, childbirth, and the postpartum period safe for black people.

In our societal failure to *do* something about the preventable pregnancy-related deaths of black people, we are leaving it to individuals to figure out ways to avoid losing their lives in the pursuit of bringing another life into the world. The next chapter explores some of the many strategies that class-privileged pregnant black people have adopted to try to stay alive within the country's black maternal health crisis.

5 Going to the Doctor in Yale Sweatpants: Techniques for Avoiding Racial Disadvantage During the Clinical Encounter

Jenna, who was introduced in chapter 3, spent much of her life helping her chronically ill mother navigate the United States' byzantine healthcare system. After her mother had a traumatizing experience during a hospitalization, she chose to stop treatment for her condition and died within a year. The incident that led her mother to choose death over trying to live was not her only negative encounter inside of a hospital or doctor's office; it simply was the final one.

Jenna—who spoke to me via Zoom from her home office, where colorful abstract art hung on the walls—felt that her mother's black race was key to understanding why she was treated poorly during many of her dealings with the nation's healthcare system. Jenna also felt that her own blackness diminished her power as an advocate for her mother—her Ivy League degrees be damned. Jenna put it plainly: "A lot of times when I would interact with doctors on my mom's behalf, they would just treat us like we were some niggas." Jenna told me that only after providers saw that she and her mother were educated would they begin to give her mother the care that she deserved: "Once they started to hear the phrases we were using. . . . Once they found out that I went to Harvard and Yale and my mother went to UC Berkeley. . . . It was only after they saw and heard all these indicators that they were like, 'Maybe she's worth a damn.' Or at least at that point, they didn't do whatever the hell they wanted to do to her."

Jenna's experience was not unique among the black people who spoke with me as part of my research for this book. Many interviewees told me stories about receiving inferior healthcare up until the point that they managed to communicate their class privilege to their providers. Indeed, many interviewees were very intentional about performing their high levels of education, relative wealth, or elevated status during medical encounters as a tactic for securing high-quality healthcare.[1] Jenna certainly had adopted this approach. Like dozens of black women who spoke with me, Jenna made a point to "dress up" when she goes to the doctor in order to "send a signal" that the provider ought to give her top-tier care.[2] She said, "Even if I'm casually dressed, then I will casually have on my Yale paraphernalia. . . . I'm wearing sweatpants. But the sweatpants have 'Yale' on them."

This chapter explores the myriad strategies that pregnant class-privileged black people adopt to reduce the likelihood that their race will disadvantage them during their healthcare encounters. It begins by examining high-income black people's popular stratagem of emphasizing through various means during their visits with healthcare providers that they are *not poor*. It then analyzes why many black patients elect to receive their healthcare from black providers as a tactic to avoid experiencing negative health outcomes on account of their race. After turning to an investigation of why some black patients choose to manage their providers' training—electing to be cared for by midwives and not by obstetricians—as a technique for avoiding racial disadvantage during pregnancy-related clinical encounters, it concludes by looking at a fascinating approach that some black patients adopt when interacting with healthcare institutions and providers. This approach consists of denying that race matters and could impact health outcomes, notwithstanding all the evidence to the contrary.

PERFORMING CLASS PRIVILEGE

Time and again, interviewees told me that whenever they walked into a doctor's office or hospital, they tried to emphasize their class privilege in order to diminish any disadvantage that they might experience by virtue of being black. Their collective sense was that if they could get their providers to grasp that although they were black, they were not poor or uneducated, then their providers would give them the same quality of care that they gave their white patients of all socioeconomic statuses and education levels.

Consider Meredith's thoughts on the ability of class privilege to offset the racial disadvantage that comes with being black. Meredith was thirty-four years old and pregnant with her second child when I met her following a prenatal care visit with Dr. Helen Volante at Golden Health's Black Wellbeing Clinic, which offers black-identifying patients the opportunity to be cared for by black-identifying providers. (Chapter 6 takes an in-depth look at the Black Wellbeing Clinic.) Meredith was a San Francisco native who had spent two decades living in Atlanta, Georgia, where she attended college and law school and began her legal career. She had returned to San Francisco the previous year because she wanted to be closer to her mother, who was "getting older."

Friendly, funny, and introspective, Meredith suffered a miscarriage a few months before her current pregnancy. She explained that in light of this loss, she intentionally chose to receive her prenatal care from an all-black care team in the Black Wellbeing Clinic: "Going through the miscarriage and also being pregnant at a later age. . . . I just wanted to have a bit more support. And so I felt like that would happen with a black doctor." I asked whether she had ever felt unsupported when she had received care from nonblack doctors. She replied, "I've definitely had situations where I felt as though my concerns were just being brushed off. But that has tended to happen when I was with male doctors of any race—black, white, or whatever." She paused, collecting her thoughts—presumably trying to reconcile her preference for *racially* concordant prenatal care with her experience of *gender* as the characteristic in her provider that correlated with a positive or negative clinical encounter. She continued: "I think that when you talk to someone who is black—someone who looks like you and has some kind of common foundation with you—the conversation is just a little easier. I don't necessarily have to think about how I'm saying something, or even what I'm saying. It brings a level of comfort that you don't necessarily. . . . Or rather, I should say: It brings a level of comfort that *I* have not had with nonblack doctors." Meredith paused again, this time presumably trying to reconcile that statement with what she was about to say next:

Meredith: Well, now I'm thinking back to some of the doctors that I have had in the past, and there was one gynecologist who was really great. She was a white lady. I feel like our conversations were the same as the ones that I have with Dr. Volante. Talking to her was as easy as talking to a black person. Seriously. I felt like she understood where I was coming from even though she was not black. [long pause] But the other piece to this is that when people know your profession, they kind of interact with you differently based on, you know, what you do, or your level of education, and things like that. And so I feel like with her, the white gynecologist, she knew.

Khiara: She knew what exactly?

Meredith: She knew that I was a lawyer. She had been my doctor when I was in law school. And she was my doctor when I was working as an attorney.... I don't know. I don't know if that had anything to do with it. [pause] I think that it did, though. Because just generally, in life, people will engage with me differently when I say that I'm an attorney versus when I don't mention my occupation.

Khiara: Do you feel like black providers engage with you differently when you say that you are an attorney? Or let me be more concrete. Do you think the fact that you are an attorney matters during your prenatal care appointments with Dr. Volante?

Meredith: [pause] You know what? [pause] I don't even know if Dr. Volante knows that I am attorney. [laughs] I don't even know if I mentioned it to her. I'm not sure. I really don't know. But I will say: I don't think that occupation is a variable that Dr. Volante uses when determining how to interact with a patient. But I definitely think my occupation—my education, the fact that I was not poor—was why I got what I got from my white gynecologist.

Khiara: And what did you get precisely?

Meredith: Um, treated like a human being? Quality healthcare? I don't know.

Jenna, whose story begins this chapter, had expressed something similar about black race, class privilege, and black providers. She told me that although she typically tries to "send a signal" during her doctor's appointments that she is a graduate of Yale and Harvard, she had not been doing that during her pregnancy, as she had been receiving her prenatal care from black obstetricians. She reflected, "I think the only time I have not played up [my education] has been with Dr. Volante at the Black Wellbeing Clinic."

In this way, Meredith and Jenna have similar philosophies about the relationship between class advantage and racial disadvantage. Both Meredith and Jenna believe that their class privilege—their education, the fact that they are not poor—diminished their racial disadvantage when they performed it effectively with nonblack providers. And both Meredith and Jenna believe that their class privilege was irrelevant during their interactions with black providers, as their black race did not disadvantage them during those encounters.

There are two things to keep in mind about Meredith's and Jenna's ideas about class privilege and racial disadvantage. The first is that if Meredith, Jenna, and the dozens of other black women that I interviewed are correct and class privilege does, in fact, reduce race-based disadvantage in clinical encounters with nonblack providers, then this lever is mostly unavailable to low-income black patients who may want to manipulate privilege in an effort to receive higher-quality healthcare. Low-income black patients may wear their best clothes to a medical appointment or use correct grammar when speaking to their provider, in hopes of performing an elevated socioeconomic status and receiving better treatment. But any attempt to convince providers that they possess an elevated socioeconomic status would be thwarted by the fact that they would begin their appointment by tendering their Medicaid insurance card—or no health insurance card whatsoever.

The second thing to keep in mind about Meredith's and Jenna's ideas about class privilege and racial disadvantage is the fragility of the power of class privilege to diminish race-based disadvantage. The capacity of class privilege to contain racial disadvantage may not be as durable as people of color on the higher ends of the socioeconomic ladder may want to believe. The experience of Giselle, a black woman who received her care from one of Golden Health's competitors in San Francisco, may exemplify this.

At the time of our interview, Giselle—an extroverted, beautiful woman whose parents were lifelong members of the black elite in Washington, DC—lived in San Francisco with her husband and three-year-old daughter. Her parents' wealth allowed her to pursue her dream of becoming a painter and sculptor. To that end, she received a bachelor's degree in art history from Howard University and a master of fine arts degree from Columbia

University. Giselle was forty years old when she married and was intent on getting pregnant as soon as possible after her wedding. Things worked as planned, and she was pregnant with her daughter less than a year later. She knew that she wanted a black obstetrician to care for her during her pregnancy because she believed that a black doctor would provide her with the "warmth" that she sought in clinical encounters. So Giselle began her prenatal care with a black female physician who was in her commercial health insurance's network, Dr. Anderson.

Giselle was optimistic that Dr. Anderson's blackness would make her empathetic toward Giselle and willing to engage in a sort of comradery with her. Her hope was that shared black race would lead Dr. Anderson to allay Giselle's worries and make her pregnancy less anxiety-producing than what it frequently is for first-time mothers: "I picked this black woman because I had hoped that as a black doctor and an age contemporary, she would recognize my fears and try to assuage them. And she did *nothing* of the sort. It made me wildly uncomfortable." Black race failed to operate in the manner that Giselle had hoped, and Dr. Anderson disappointed her again and again.

In her third trimester, Giselle discovered that there was a chance that Dr. Anderson would be out of town when Giselle went into labor. She experienced this as a breaking point, and, although she was thirty-four weeks pregnant at the time, she began to search for another provider. She found the obstetrician who ultimately cared for during her labor and childbirth, Dr. Tal, on the recommendation of a coworker. Giselle explained:

> The best way to describe her is an Israeli Mrs. Claus or no, like the Berenstain Bears mom. She's really tall. She's this tremendous woman. Curly blond hair. Has a scar on her lip. She calls you "*bubbale.*" She drops Yiddish phrases when she's talking all the time. She's just fantastic. Really personable, really caring. So when I went in, automatically I felt at ease. And I was like, "Can you please take me?"

Giselle found in Dr. Tal the gentle, big-hearted care that she had hoped that she would receive from her obstetrician during her pregnancy and childbirth. Notably, Dr. Tal was not black, demonstrating what ought to be expected—that a provider's black race only imperfectly correlates with the characteristics sought by black patients choosing racially concordant healthcare.[3]

While Giselle understood Dr. Tal's "warmth" as something that could ease her anxieties around pregnancy and childbirth, she did not believe that this warmth could cleanse Dr. Tal of the racial biases that, in Giselle's view, lead medical doctors to make unnecessary and potentially dangerous interventions on black people. Giselle explained that after she delivered her daughter, her uterus did not promptly expel the placenta. Accordingly, Dr. Tal attempted to remove it manually, with no success. As Giselle colorfully puts it, "Remember, she's a big woman—Berenstain Bear. She had her Berenstain paw elbow-deep in there trying to get the placenta out." After Dr. Tal was unable to remove the placenta, she told the care team in the delivery room that it would have to be removed surgically. Giselle recounts:

> She was like, "Okay, well, it's not coming out. I can't get it. Book an [operating room]." And I looked to [my husband]. . . . This is one of the things I was adamant about: I do not want any unnecessary cuts. I do not want an episiotomy, I do not want a C-section unless it's absolutely necessary to save my life or [my daughter's] life. Do not let them cut me. I told him, "Do *not* let them cut me." Because too often, I know that . . . and Dr. Tal had been awesome. But, again, I had switched to her just six weeks before this happened. A lot of doctors, you know, they try to—they do that. It's like, "Oh, it's a woman of color? This is easier. She's not paying for it anyway."

While many of the high-income black women that I interviewed believed that their class privilege could contain some of the disadvantage that they might experience by virtue of their race, Giselle revealed her understanding that class privilege's power in this regard is not unlimited; it can be overwhelmed in certain circumstances. That is, in the context of an urgent condition in the delivery room, race-based disadvantage will win. Blackness can make class privilege invisible and, in so doing, overpower class privilege's ability to diminish race-based disadvantage.

It is worth making this point especially clear: Even though Giselle had health insurance through her employer and did not have Medicaid insurance, she believed that a provider would forget this fact about her *because she is black*. She supposed that many providers conflate racial disadvantage and class disadvantage and, seeing Giselle's black race, would conclude that she was not paying for her medical care. Any willingness that they might have had to defer to her desires would be abandoned, and they would do what was most expedient. Giselle believed that even Dr. Tal, whom she trusted and liked immensely, was susceptible to these heuristics—these mental shortcuts. Giselle's reflections reveal that she did not believe that these heuristics were insurmountable. She emphasized the relatively short period of time that she was under Dr. Tal's care—an emphasis that suggests that Giselle considered racial disadvantage and class disadvantage to be something that could be delinked in a provider's mind over time or under certain conditions. Giselle judged the six weeks that Dr. Tal had known her to be insufficient for decoupling the association between blackness and indigence or Medicaid. She relied on her husband to be her advocate and to save her from the expedient, unnecessary interventions that she believed low-income Medicaid beneficiaries are forced to endure.

It should be mentioned that class-privileged black patients did not believe that their high socioeconomic status was the *only* tool available to temper their racial disadvantage. Significantly, some black women with white husbands shared that they leveraged their spouse's race privilege and status as a man to their benefit. Recall Annette, whose traumatic pregnancy and childbirth are recounted in the book's introduction. Annette's providers failed to diagnose the potentially fatal heart condition that she had developed during her pregnancy. Although she experienced terrifying symptoms throughout her pregnancy, her providers diagnosed her with the condition only after she had been admitted to the hospital to give birth. Because of this late diagnosis, she was forced to deliver her baby in the cardiac intensive care unit (ICU), a unit that was not designed for labor and childbirth. Annette explained that she was unsure whether having her white husband present while she was laboring and giving birth in the cardiac ICU helped her, but her sense is that "it would have been worse" had he not been there:

> I do know when *he* would advocate, shit would happen. Like, I was begging for ice for my mouth, and they weren't bringing it, and they weren't

bringing it, and they weren't bringing it. Then my husband lost his shit and ran out of the room and was like, "My fucking wife needs ice!" And you know what? Big, tall, white dude in a button-down shows up, and he's like, "Here's ice!" . . . Fucking miraculously. Here's ice.

The ability of her husband's race and sex to diminish Annette's disadvantage along the axis of race (and likely sex, as well) was a lesson that Annette carried with her long after the birth of her daughter. Even five years later, "when I have an important doctor's appointment, I take him with me. Because I'm like, 'Don't just see *me*. He's a white man who's invested in my well-being. A white man cares deeply about me. And maybe knowing that—maybe that will correct whatever bias that you may not even be aware of.'"

WHAT ARE BLACK PATIENTS SEEKING WHEN THEY SEEK A BLACK PROVIDER?

As Jenna's, Meredith's, and Giselle's stories make clear, many black patients attempt to avoid race-based disadvantage during clinical encounters by receiving their care from black providers. We should ask, then: What characteristics do black patients expect correlate with a provider's black race? Beyond a healthy pregnancy and newborn, what are black pregnant patients seeking when they seek a black provider? This section explores some black patients' beliefs that black providers will supply them with comfort and other black patients' beliefs that a black provider will supply them with the relationship with biomedicine that they desire.

On Black Race and Comfort

"Comfort" emerged repeatedly in my conversations with class-privileged black patients who chose black providers to care for them. Although most of the black patients who spoke with me used the language of comfort when describing their experiences of racially concordant care, patients used this term to refer to several different aspects of the patient–provider relationship. For some, comfort meant the absence of a fear that the provider would judge them negatively or refuse to take their concerns seriously. For others, comfort meant a belief that their provider would advocate for them when necessary, fighting to ensure that the patient received the highest-quality care from the institution providing healthcare.

To begin, some patients used comfort to describe the ease that they felt when sharing information with their provider. For example, when Meredith invoked comfort—telling me that having a black provider "brings a level of comfort that [she has] not had with nonblack doctors"—she was describing a freedom from anxiety about how her provider would perceive her. Meredith and other patients who used comfort in this way enjoyed this freedom from anxiety because they believed that they had a shared experience with a black provider—having what Meredith called a "common foundation."[4] As another patient who used the language of comfort to describe the texture of her interactions with black providers put it, "I don't have to translate as much." For black patients, this comfort led to easier conversations and better communication, as patients did not have to exert a great deal of care in making sure that they were saying the right things or saying things the right way.

Other patients used comfort to touch on a different aspect of communication. For them, comfort was not a condition that enabled patients to speak freely with their providers. Instead, comfort was a product of knowing that their providers were not being dismissive of them. As one patient said of Dr. Marie Clark, "She takes my concerns seriously. So I feel comfortable with her. I know that my concerns will be considered. They will be examined."

These two senses of comfort are not mutually exclusive, and many patients likely experience them at the same time—feeling *comfortable* sharing information with their provider and *comforted* by the knowledge that their provider is attentive to their concerns.

Additionally, some patients used comfort to describe their belief that their provider would advocate on their behalf to ensure that they had a positive pregnancy outcome. This usage expressed a sense of security that was born of the confidence that their provider was working behind the scenes, enabling the patient to navigate the healthcare system successfully. Jenna's comments exemplify this sense of comfort. Jenna was aware that although she was receiving her prenatal care from Dr. Volante, there was no guarantee that Dr. Volante would be present when she was admitted to the hospital to give birth: "You never know with timing." However, she believed that

Dr. Volante would ensure that even if she were not present, Jenna would be properly cared for during labor and delivery:

> I'm certain that even if Dr. Volante isn't able to deliver the baby, she has a certain level of advocacy, awareness, care. . . . Even if she isn't there, I know that I won't be just completely left out in the cold, blowing in the wind, right? I won't be just another number in [the labor and delivery room].
>
> My mother was sick most of my life. And I saw the way she was treated within the healthcare system. So it was really important to me that I had a doctor who I felt *comfortable* with—someone who was not, like, colorblind. Colorblindness doesn't do me any good. I wanted a provider who I knew would be an actual advocate for me.
>
> I've always used community to navigate unfair systems. Like, I've always found people, found my tribe, created my tribe. Black people are always just saving ourselves. It has been very rare that I've seen systems just work out for my benefit without my needing to do some real navigating, some real maneuvering. These systems are not set up for my success.

Jenna sought a black provider because she wanted a physician who would go beyond simply ensuring that her and her baby's vital signs stayed within an acceptable range and sounding the alarm if there was any departure from these norms. Jenna wanted a provider who would help her complete the complicated, opaque, bureaucratic task of receiving high-quality healthcare in the United States. Jenna felt that as a black person, she was at a disadvantage in navigating healthcare systems, and she had firsthand experience of what race-based disadvantage looked like in the context of healthcare. For Jenna, comfort described her sense that she had created a "tribe" that was committed to helping her maneuver her way through a system that failed—and felled—black people all too often.

On Black Race and Orientations to Biomedicine

The black patients who spoke with me for this book had a variety of relationships to biomedicine. Some trusted that biomedicine, as a body of knowledge and collection of practices, was superior to other ways of managing pregnancy and childbirth, while others were deeply skeptical of the authority over reproduction that biomedicine has achieved. Intriguingly, black patients who chose black providers to care for them during their pregnancies invariably believed that having a black provider would facilitate the precise relationship that they wanted with biomedicine.

It may be useful to preface this exploration with a brief history of the medicalization of pregnancy and childbirth. Since ancient times, midwives provided care and support to pregnant people. However, in the nineteenth century in the Western world, medicine sought to make pregnancy and childbirth into objects of its expertise. This required the denigration of midwifery and the women, many of whom were black, who practiced it. Physicians frequently invoked sexist and racist tropes to undermine midwifery. As obstetrician and medical historian Irvine Loudon puts it, during the struggle to wrest pregnancy and childbirth from the jurisdiction of midwifery, most physicians would have described midwives as "'not far removed from the jungles of Africa, gin-fingering, guzzling . . . with her brains full of snuff, her fingers full of dirt and her brains full of arrogance and superstition.'"[5] Medicine ultimately was successful in constructing pregnancy and birth as medical events that only doctors could competently supervise: "While almost no women saw physicians prior to delivery in the early [twentieth] century, almost all pregnant women receive such care today."[6] Additionally, 98 percent of all childbirths in the United States today take place in hospitals "under the authority of a physician."[7]

Feminists have been highly critical of the way that medicine has conceptualized pregnancy and childbirth. Anthropologist Robbie Davis-Floyd's critique is emblematic. She argues that we should understand obstetrics to be a "male-dominated institution" exerting "control over women's bodies."[8] Further, she describes obstetrics as having constructed "pregnancy as a dysfunctional mechanical process" to which science and the medical gaze must be applied if the pregnant woman and the infant are to survive.[9] She writes that the creation of childbirth as a pathology

> is accomplished by birth's dissection into components—the stages of labor— and by the application to these components of standardized measurements and rules (e.g. Friedman's curve) that say how each stage should proceed, plus diagnostic technologies (e.g. external and internal electronic fetal monitors) that investigate whether or not these stages are proceeding as they should,

plus remedial technologies (Pitocin, episiotomies, Cesarean sections) to make them proceed as they should if they aren't.[10]

Feminists have argued that medicine's treatment of pregnancy and childbirth as processes that are predisposed to malfunction disempowers the individuals who are actually pregnant and giving birth. Medicine delegitimates the knowledge that pregnant people have about their own bodies. Instead, legitimacy is given to the technology that externalizes individuals' experiences of their bodies, permitting the "experts in the room" who are capable of interpreting the data that the technology yields to claim that they have a superior knowledge of what is happening to, in, and with the pregnant person's body. Philosopher Iris Young, writing in 1984, captures this sense when she says that

> the pregnant woman has a unique knowledge of her body processes and the life of the foetus. She feels the movements of the foetus, the contractions of her uterus, with an immediacy and certainty that no one can share. Recently invented machines tend to devalue this knowledge. The foetal-heart sensor projects the heartbeat of the six-week-old foetus into the room so that all can hear it in the same way. The sonogram is receiving increasing use to follow the course of foetal development. The foetal monitor attached during labor records the intensity and duration of each contraction on white paper; the woman's reports are no longer necessary for charting the progress of her labor. Such instruments transfer some control over the means of observing the pregnancy and birth process from the woman to the medical personnel.[11]

The feminist critique of the medicalization of pregnancy and childbirth has not been without its own critiques. The most compelling criticisms note that feminists like Robbie Davis-Floyd and Iris Young have tended to assume that affluent white women's experience of obstetrics is indistinguishable from that of other groups. In reality, "medicalization provides and denies reproductive choices differentially to women at different social locations."[12] Further, differently situated people might have different desires around medicalization. Anthropologist Gertrude Fraser's study of obstetric and midwifery practices in the South illustrates this point. Women in the impoverished black community in which Fraser did her fieldwork—a community that a classist, racist medical establishment had historically disregarded—very much wanted medically managed pregnancies and childbirths.[13] The black women in this community believed that receiving their prenatal care from obstetricians instead of midwives—and delivering their babies in hospitals with the aid of anesthesia as opposed to delivering at home without pharmaceutical pain management—"signaled [a] symbolic, if not fully realized, inclusion in the field of vision of a health care bureaucracy that had until then largely ignored the health needs [of African Americans]."[14] In my earlier work, I observed a similar phenomenon in the obstetrics clinic of the large, public hospital in New York City in which I conducted my research.[15] Many of the low-income women of color that I interviewed chose to receive their care from this hospital—as opposed to facilities that were closer to their homes—because they had heard that the hospital offered the "best" prenatal care, with "best" being understood as the most technologically intense and most scientifically advanced. Other research similarly shows class differences in the preferences that individuals have around childbirth. For example, anthropologist Ellen Lazarus describes a study showing that "[m]iddle-class women wanted to participate actively in childbirth and to avoid interventions, while working-class women wanted more interventions. Working-class women wanted less pain and reduced labor."[16]

Moreover, the feminist critique of the medicalization of pregnancy and childbirth has been described as "consumerist"[17] inasmuch as it implicitly encourages the class-privileged, race-privileged individuals who have been most receptive to the critique to purchase the prenatal care and birth experiences that they want in the market. It counsels these individuals to exercise their power as consumers to buy the birthing classes, birth coaches, dimmed lighting, mood music, birthing balls, and water births and, in so doing, to purchase the experience of labor and delivery that most aligns with their desires.

The black patients who spoke with me for this book fell on all sides of the critique of the medicalization of pregnancy. Some patients had confidence in medicine's truth and superiority, while others considered medicine to cause harm as frequently as it prevents or eliminates it. Thus, some patients sought prenatal care that was administered perfectly in accordance with the biomedical model of pregnancy and childbirth; others sought as complete an exit from this model as possible.

Patients used different methods to acquire healthcare that matched their orientation to medicine. For example, some chose to receive their care from midwives because they believed that midwifery care provided an escape from medicine's excesses—an effort that is explored later in the chapter. However, black patients both committed to and skeptical of biomedicine often sought a black provider because they believed that a provider's black race would facilitate the relationship with medicine that they wanted. To be clear, some black patients sought a black provider because they believed that medicine was superior and that a provider's blackness would perfect medical practice. Meanwhile, other black patients sought a black provider because they believed that medicine was flawed and that a provider's blackness would protect them from medicine's failures.

Harlow and Ifeoma illustrate these two contrasting relationships with medicine and the deployment of provider black race to access them. The two women had a lot in common. Both Harlow and Ifeoma identified as black. Both attended historically black colleges (in fact, they attended the same college). Both lived in Atlanta, Georgia. Both were friends of Golden Health patients whom I had interviewed. Both were recommended to me by their San Francisco–based friends, who felt that these two women would be interested in sharing their pregnancy journeys with me for this book. Both were solidly middle-class. Both had commercial health insurance. Both married their husbands in their late thirties and became pregnant in their early forties. And both sought a black provider to care for them during their pregnancies. Their similarities end on the issue of what they believed that a provider's black race would deliver to them. Ifeoma believed a provider's black race would shield her from a body of knowledge that constructs pregnancy as a dangerous, potentially deadly event in need of medical management. In contrast, Harlow believed that a provider's black race would decontaminate medical practice. For Harlow, bad pregnancy outcomes occur when medicine is incorrectly practiced. As a result, she sought a black provider because she believed that the provider's race would help to ensure the correct practice of medicine and, in so doing, grant her an easy pregnancy, untroubled childbirth, and healthy newborn.

Forty-two-year-old Harlow was living in Atlanta with her husband and four-year-old son at the time of our conversation in fall 2020. Born and raised in Hartford, Connecticut, she had received a doctorate in education from New York University and was working as an administrator at an Atlanta-area college. Harlow, who was thirty weeks pregnant with her second son when I interviewed her, had no criticisms of obstetrics. She did not see herself and her experience reflected in common critiques that medicine—unnecessarily, unjustifiably, and harmfully—treats pregnancy as a medical condition requiring surveillance, management, and intervention. She understood medicine to be a tool for making pregnancy, childbirth, and the postpartum period safe and pleasant.

> **Khiara:** Do you have a birth plan?
> **Harlow:** Epidural. [laughs] I'm not curious about the natural birth process at all. [laughs]
> **Khiara:** Is that something that is new for you? Or have you always been like, "I trust medicine. Medicine is good. Medicine relieves me of pain?"
> **Harlow:** For the most part, yeah. Luckily, I haven't had—knock on wood—too many major health issues in my life. But when [my oldest son] was born, I was like, "Where is the modern medicine to relieve me of this pain?" [laughs] I'm not a soldier. It's just not me.

Harlow frequently described nonmedical approaches to pregnancy as "not me." For this reason, she sought out obstetricians, as opposed to midwives, for healthcare during her pregnancy. The fact that her "advanced maternal age"—that is, she was over the age of thirty-four—was her only pregnancy risk factor somewhat frustrated her desire for her pregnancy to be viewed and treated through a medical lens. She explained:

> **Harlow:** I'm a high-risk pregnancy because of [my advanced maternal age], but there's nothing wrong with me. So [the practice where I receive my prenatal care in Atlanta] push[es] me towards midwives. Technically, you are supposed to rotate and see whoever is available at the time. Sometimes I see physicians, sometimes I see midwives. Seeing the mix, I have preferred

the physicians over the midwives. I try to make my appointments with the physicians, and they are always like, "That's really for people who have complications with their pregnancies. You don't have any complications, so go to the midwife."

Khiara: What do you prefer about the physicians?

Harlow: I feel like the physicians are more direct. But that's just how physicians are. They hear something, and they want to investigate it immediately. They want to allay your fears. They are more factual. I feel like I get things done with the physicians, whereas the midwives are kind of crunchy to me. Granola. [laughs] They're like, "Oh, did you take some rosehips?" And I'm like, "No. That's just not my. . . ." [laughs]

Khiara: That's not your style.

Harlow: No, no. I'm way more formal than that.

Medicine offered Harlow a "formality" that aligned more with her personality and the way she thought of herself. For Harlow, nonmedicalized ways of thinking and doing are not based in the "facts" that she believed led to positive pregnancy outcomes. Indeed, nonmedicalized ways of thinking were inconsistent with the ways in which Harlow conceptualized herself:

Khiara: Have you ever considered delivering outside of the hospital?

Harlow: Other people have offered. [laughs] . . . My mom's church friends have been suggesting a homebirth. Even my husband was like, "You know we could have a homebirth." I'm like, "Do you want to join my mom at the homebirth? Y'all can sit there in the pool. I am going to the hospital." [laughs] Like, the pool, the whole thing. . . . It's just not me. I respect people, however they want to bring their children into the world. It's just not me.

Significantly, Harlow believed that biomedicine was right to worry about pregnant people. While she never gave me the sense that she thought her pregnant black body was in crisis, she was very aware that things can go wrong during pregnancy. Miscarriages can happen, babies can be born prematurely, people can die or be severely injured during childbirth. Harlow explained her deference to medical authority in terms of the possibility that tragedy can occur during pregnancy. She thought that medicine justifiably understood pregnancy as an event that ought to be managed and monitored closely because "babies are coming, and we can't mess around. Every week counts, and every day is very important."

Importantly, Harlow tended to assume that when tragedy occurred during pregnancy, it was due to the nature of pregnancy—not medical interventions. As noted above, I interviewed Harlow in fall 2020—after the arrival of COVID-19 in the United States but before the development and distribution of vaccines that could reduce the deadliness of an infection. Like most who lived through the pandemic, Harlow described her life as having been turned upside down. She was trying to parent her four-year-old son in a world of school closures, nonexistent childcare, and family that was physically distant by necessity. Upon the onset of the pandemic, Harlow began working remotely, but a midwife in the practice where she was receiving her care initially hesitated to provide Harlow with a note that would allow her to work from home. The midwife—whom Harlow called "the Scottish midwife"—said that Harlow likely would not contract COVID if she wore a face mask and maintained a six-foot distance between herself and others while at work. Essentially, the midwife did not conceptualize pregnancy as a condition that made the pregnant person any more or less vulnerable than anyone else. For her, the same precautions that everyone had been advised to take in order to avoid contracting COVID were sufficient protection for pregnant people. Harlow disagreed and ultimately received a note from a black obstetrician in the practice: "So I mentioned it again to the black physician who I saw that day, and she was like, 'I will get you a letter before you leave this office. You are not going back to work. Period. . . . [Y]ou will have [the letter] before you leave this office today. End of story.' And I appreciated that. She's cautious." I asked Harlow why she thought "the Scottish midwife" had taken this approach to COVID, apparently disbelieving that everyone should try their hardest to protect pregnant people from the risks associated with a new virus that was demonstrating its lethality on a daily basis:

> **Harlow:** I don't know. [laughs] I have no idea. We don't know how that virus affects my unborn child.
>
> **Khiara:** Tell me if you agree with this. I wonder if it's because her approach, as a midwife, is to think of pregnancy as a natural state of the body. So

pregnant people are as vulnerable as everybody else. She might embrace the idea that a pregnant person is healthy. They are healthy unless they are suffering from hypertension or diabetes. Pregnant people do not have comorbidities as a matter of course. And so they are as vulnerable to COVID as everyone else who does not have any comorbidities.

Harlow: Yeah, but they might. Pregnant people might come to have comorbidities. You can develop preeclampsia, you can develop gestational diabetes, you know. I don't have it, thank God. But you can. That's possible.

For Harlow, then, the nature of pregnancy was such that pathologies could develop at any time. She viewed medicine as a tool for managing the inherent risks of pregnancy.

Harlow sought a black obstetrician for her prenatal care because she believed that a physician's black race would help to ensure that medicine was practiced as it should be practiced. In her experience, a provider's nonblack race frustrated the provider's ability to recognize the information that Harlow provided as valid. In Harlow's experience, nonblack providers—specifically, white providers—did not "hear" her or "listen" to her. In Harlow's view, when a doctor's white race frustrated their ability to register the proper inputs from a patient, medicine should be expected to deliver improper outputs.

Harlow was clear that she believed that managing a provider's race was more important than managing a provider's sex when trying to find a provider who would "hear" her. While she typically preferred women gynecologists, she found that she was still unheard when the gynecologist was a white woman. As a case in point, Harlow pointed to the "the Scottish midwife" who refused to provide Harlow with the documentation that she needed to work from home. She also cited her experience in receiving ultrasounds during this pregnancy: "There are two male doctors, and at first, I was a little concerned. But there's one doctor there—the black one—that I really, really like. He heard me when I was speaking. He could understand, and we could dialogue. And I just felt understood." These encounters reaffirmed for Harlow that womanhood does not typically enable a provider to "hear" her. Black race, however, does.

Compare Harlow's understanding of medicine and a provider's black race with Ifeoma's, who was also pregnant with her second child when I interviewed her. While Harlow sought a black healthcare provider because she believed that the provider's black race would ensure the correct application of medical truths to her pregnant black body, Ifeoma sought a black healthcare provider because she believed that a provider's black race would immunize her from a medicalization of pregnancy that she felt was entirely unwarranted.

Ifeoma scheduled our interview for 1 p.m., a time when her husband would still be at work and her daughter, Adelayo, would still be in school. The doula training course that she was taking (a course she had enrolled in before she discovered her current pregnancy) would have ended an hour before, and her business partner would not yet have arrived at her house to help design labels for their skin care products, which they were planning to introduce to the market in a few months. When she answered my phone call at the designated time, she laughingly said, "I forgot to schedule time to eat!" and apologized for eating her kale salad and drinking her probiotic smoothie during our conversation.

When Ifeoma was pregnant with Adelayo nine years earlier, there was "no question" that she would try to have "as natural a pregnancy experience as possible." This was consistent with her general approach to medicine: "I've never been someone who runs to the doctor at the first drop of a hat. I've never been someone to pop a pill—to take somebody's medication, somebody's prescription—whenever I feel sick. I've always been receptive to other ways to heal the body." She described herself as "living her medicine" through a healthy diet, exercise, her faith (Ifá, a traditional Yoruba religion from West Africa), a meditation practice, and a commitment to shielding herself from "toxic people, places, and things."

When Ifeoma was pregnant with Adelayo, she found her midwife, a black woman, through a friend. When I asked her whether she intentionally sought a black provider, she paused and said, "The thought of going to someone who isn't black never even crossed my mind. [laughs] I mean, I live in Atlanta. [laughs]" She elaborated: "My approach towards my health is kind of wrapped up with my faith—which is wrapped up with my race. Like, I can't tease them apart. So for me, to find a provider who shares my orientation towards health would be to find a provider who is black." Because

Ifeoma and I had developed an easy rapport, I felt comfortable pressing her a bit:

> **Khiara:** So you don't think there are nonblack providers in Atlanta who share your orientation towards health?
>
> **Ifeoma:** Probably. Definitely. But the care would be different. I feel like . . . What I'm doing when I look for healthcare that is not so clinical and sterile and poking and prodding and "measure this" and "weigh that"—I'm trying to benefit from the knowledge that my ancestors had. A white midwife who is not poking and prodding and measuring—they will not be trying to bring that knowledge to bear on me. They would be doing something different.
>
> **Khiara:** Perhaps. But the care would look the same.
>
> **Ifeoma:** Maybe it would look the same. But it would be different.

In this way, Ifeoma conceptualized blackness and an embrace of natural approaches to managing health as simultaneous. For Ifeoma, when nonblack providers offered care that was outside of the medical paradigm, they were offering only a copycat of what black natural providers delivered. Because Ifeoma did not need to accept anything less than the real thing (she "live[d] in Atlanta" after all), she sought and found a black provider who could provide this implicitly racially informed care.

Ifeoma's pregnancy with Adelayo progressed without complications, and she was able to have the homebirth that she very much wanted. During her first pregnancy, the only complications that she had were a function of the complexities of the US healthcare system. For her midwifery care and her homebirth, Ifeoma paid out of pocket because her "insurance had made it very clear that they were going to cover no parts of that." However, to avoid paying out of pocket for the expensive laboratory work that she needed throughout her pregnancy, she saw an obstetrician for "the milestone visits." She describes the obstetrician as having "a hard time understanding the whole homebirth thing. She didn't know what I was doing outside the office with the midwife if I was coming to her for care periodically." Ifeoma tells me that she had to repeatedly explain the arrangement to the obstetrician: "Every visit."

With her second pregnancy, Ifeoma planned to replicate the experience that she had with Adelayo—even though she was nine years older and, technically, now at an "advanced maternal age." As soon as she discovered she was pregnant, she called the midwife who had cared for her during her pregnancy with Adelayo to make an appointment to see her:

> [The midwife said,] "You know, Ifeoma, this isn't rocket science. [laughs] You've done this before. You weren't a high-risk pregnancy. There is no reason to think that you're high risk now." She said, "Technically, I don't see a reason to see you before the end of the first trimester." She said, "Usually new moms are pretty excited and want to come in right away. But I have no need to see you until after your first trimester." Which I was fine with. It made a lot of sense to me.

At the time of our interview, Ifeoma had begun having "the milestone visits" with an obstetrician. Entering a space where pregnancy was conceptualized and treated as a precarious medical condition reaffirmed for Ifeoma that she had made the right decision when she had opted into a paradigm that approached pregnancy as a natural state of the body:

> So now we have started with all of the other visits. And I had to go to a perinatal whatever. And they had to tell me all of the things that could possibly go wrong during this pregnancy. [laughs] . . . What's sad is that the information that people are being fed at this place is just insane to me. It feels really crazy. And if you don't have a certain knowledge or experience to work from, all you're being told is what's *not* going to happen—what could go wrong. We were waiting to get the ultrasound the other day, and they had this video running in the background. And it was, like, everything that could go wrong. Everything you need to be worried about. I was like, "God! They are really selling fear up in these hospitals!"

So Harlem and Ifeoma thought of pregnancy in ways that were diametrically opposed to one another—with one woman conceptualizing pregnancy complications as things that are "possible" and the other conceptualizing those complications as things that are "not going to happen." Nevertheless, *both* women sought a black provider because they believed that a provider's black race would facilitate the relationship with medicine that matched their understandings of and expectations around pregnancy.

RACE, MIDWIFERY, AND SKEPTICISM OF MEDICINE

While Harlow and Ifeoma managed their providers' *race* as a way to obtain the relationship with medicine that they believed would result in good outcomes for their babies and themselves, other black patients managed their providers' *training* to secure the same. The account given by Annette, whose providers failed to diagnose the potentially fatal heart condition that she had developed during her pregnancy, is representative. When Annette discovered that she was pregnant, she immediately knew that she wanted to receive her prenatal care from a midwife, as she believed that a providers' training as a midwife would protect her from a medical discourse that pathologized her body size. According to medicine's norms, Annette is obese. Her expectation was that a midwife would view her outside of medical conventions and understand that her larger body was not in a state of unhealth but rather was unproblematically within the normal range of shapes and sizes of healthy humans.

Annette was very conscious of her desire that a midwife would act as a shield against fatphobia. That is, she was very aware that her interest in the training of her provider was linked to her desire to find an exit from the medical gaze with respect to weight. While she also was critical of medicine's approach to pregnancy as a general matter ("I have doulas in my family, and so I kind of grew up feeling that the medical industrial complex had taken over birth"), most of her wish to avoid medicalization of her pregnancy was related to her body size:

> I felt like I would be in safer hands as a fat woman [with a midwife] because there is so much stigma around weight in medicine. And it's so common, I think, for doctors to see a higher body weight as a problem—as a medical condition—as opposed to just part of body diversity. So I wanted to protect myself against that during my pregnancy since I knew I was going to be gaining weight and I was already going into it at what the medical profession would call an obese body weight.

Importantly, Annette's race was bound up with her experience of her weight. Annette, who identified as both multiracial and black, said that the nonwhite side of her family accepted her larger body size, finding it unremarkable.[18] However, the white side of her family often criticized her because she was overweight. Because her white family members apparently loathed her large body, Annette came to loathe her large body when she was around them. Annette explained that when she was in the company of these white family members, she felt different from them in terms of both race and body size. That is, in her white family's presence, Annette felt both nonwhite and fat, in the pejorative sense. As a result, her negative feelings about her body size were bound up with her experience of herself as nonwhite—as black. Thus, when anyone—medical providers or otherwise—made Annette aware of her body size, they simultaneously made her aware of her non-whiteness. Insults about her body size became insults about her blackness. In other words, Annette experienced fat bias as antiblackness.[19] Consequently, Annette's choice to receive prenatal care from a midwife was not solely an attempt to secure an exit from a medical discourse that pathologized larger bodies; it was also an attempt to protect herself from racism. Thus, managing her provider's training allowed Annette to manage her racial disadvantage as a black woman attempting pregnancy.

Because Annette imagined that midwifery training itself would perform antiracist work, she did not have desires around the race of her specific midwife. This distinguishes Annette from many other black people who also believe that midwifery care will shield them from antiblackness during their pregnancies. That is, many black people who believe in the latent antiracism of midwifery do so because of its origins in black, Native, and immigrant communities' ancestral practices.[20] Black folks who turn to midwifery to call on black, Native, and immigrant people's historical knowledge are, like Ifeoma, likely to seek care from a black midwife—a task that has been made more difficult by the underrepresentation of black people among licensed midwives today.[21]

But Annette sought only a midwife—not specifically a black midwife—and she ultimately received her care from a practice that had two white midwives. Unfortunately, her expectation that she would feel comfortable with a midwife—both in her blackness and in a body that medicine had marked as overweight or obese—went unmet. This was largely because the midwife who provided most of Annette's care was stereotypically white.

Annette described her with a series of adjectives and nouns: "thin, blond, ponytail, vocal fry." As Annette explained, "I was very self-conscious around her—about my weight and my race. I did a lot of code-switching with her, as I recall. . . . I felt like I just had to kind of de-race myself around her." Annette's perception of the midwife as "very" white left Annette feeling vulnerable—both racially and as a large woman. Indeed, Annette felt that her midwife's overwhelming whiteness left the midwife's training unable to negate racism and fat bias.

As noted above and in the introduction, Annette had a terrifying pregnancy, labor, and delivery—in part because her care team dismissed her symptoms of a dangerous heart condition. I asked her if she thought that she had erred in deciding against managing the race of her provider and whether she would choose a provider of color if she decided to have another baby. Annette explained that because she had such serious complications during her pregnancy with her daughter, she would not be able to be cared for by a midwife if she ever became pregnant again. The heart arrythmia that she developed during her first pregnancy would mean that any subsequent pregnancy would be considered to be high risk. If she chose to receive her care from a nonwhite provider during any future pregnancy, it would have to be a nonwhite obstetrician. For Annette, the whiteness of the discipline of obstetrics would negate the nonwhiteness of the provider who practices that discipline:

> I would probably feel safer, probably, with a black OB [obstetrician]. It would depend on the person. But at the same time, I know that the black OB would still be functioning within a white system of medicine. So given how full of intervention another pregnancy would be for me, I'm not confident that [the race of the obstetrician] would make a big difference at that point.

Compare Annette's understanding of the relationship between black race and medicine with Harlow's understanding of the same. Whereas Harlow theorized that a provider's black race would *perfect* biomedicine—allowing it to operate as it should and producing the positive outcomes that it claims that nonmedical approaches cannot deliver—Annette theorized that a provider's black race would be *defeated* by medicine and its insistence upon regulating, disciplining, and intervening.

The failure of Annette's providers to diagnose her heart condition earlier in her pregnancy is not the only potentially lethal oversight committed by her care team. When Annette was in her second trimester, she started having chest pain that was so intense that it caused her to vomit, become incontinent, see double, and writhe on the floor. She described it as "truly the worst pain I've ever had." The pain occurred every week and lasted for fifteen or twenty minutes—"long enough to be really awful." Every time the pain began, Annette went to the emergency room. And every time that she went to the emergency room, the providers there dismissed her symptoms and told her to go home. At each prenatal care appointment following these episodes, Annette told her midwives about the pain. They, too, dismissed her. As Annette recalled, her midwives advised her, "'You should probably just take Tums,' or 'You should get a bigger bra that provides more support for your breasts.' They were like, 'It's probably just your body doing weird things in pregnancy.' Or 'Maybe it's stress.'" They ordered no tests. They brought in no specialists.

The pain continued regularly throughout the rest of Annette's pregnancy and persisted even after she delivered her daughter. Instead of attempting to discover the cause of Annette's enduring symptoms, her midwives made different dismissive guesses about what was wrong with her. They began telling her, "Well, it's probably a stress response to the traumatic labor you had." They were wrong:

> What finally happened was that my husband took me to the ER when my daughter was six months old because I had been in such incredible pain all day and was almost delirious. Scary amount of pain. And initially, we had paged the midwives, and they told us that it sounded like stress [and that we didn't need to go the ER]. But then it went on so long, and I'm fucking peeing the bed and throwing up and stuff. So we went [to the ER]. And that's where they did the test that showed elevated enzymes levels.
>
> I ultimately ended up having emergency surgery for pancreatitis. My levels were very close to the lethal. You can die from pancreatitis if it's not treated. I'd been having these acute bouts of it, and I was showing textbook symptoms the entire time. Nobody ordered a test. Nobody asked me questions about it. Nobody followed up. It was just like I was making it up. . . . Everyone was telling me to get a better bra.

We might theorize about the work performed by Annette's abnormality along the axis of race (if white race is the unstated norm, then nonwhite people are, by definition, abnormal) as it intersects with her abnormality along the axis of body size. That is, her wayward body—deviating from established norms—might have led her providers to be unmoored. The baselines that guided them might have become useless. When the body in its entirety is understood as abnormal, then bodily phenomena that are objectively abnormal might become unrecognizable as such. Differently stated, Annette's providers might have viewed her—black, fat—through a lens of pathology. When seen through such a lens, how does one's actual, objective pathology become visible? The body *is* pathology. Pathology is everywhere. Discrete moments of pathology become impossible to see and diagnose.

* * *

The stories of Jenna, Meredith, Giselle, Harlow, Ifeoma, and Annette provide insights into class-privileged black women's strategies for achieving positive pregnancy outcomes in a country that is in the throes of a black maternal health crisis. High-income pregnant black people manipulate levers—they consciously perform their wealth and status, they choose black providers, they elect to be cared for by midwives—to attempt to liberate themselves from race-based disadvantage and receive the same quality of care that their white counterparts collectively enjoy. But these levers are imperfect. The protection from antiblackness that class privilege can provide can fail under certain circumstances, as when Giselle theorized that Dr. Tal, when confronted with an urgent medical condition, may forget that Giselle "is paying for" her healthcare. Some black providers will be incapable of fulfilling their black patient's desires around the clinical encounter, as when Dr. Anderson was unable to offer the warmth that Giselle craved. Further, some nonblack providers will provide everything that their black patients want and more, as when Meredith described in glowing terms the relationship that she had with her previous gynecologist, a white woman. Midwifery training may not liberate midwives from assumptions about body size and black race that leave them incapable of identifying actual pathology in fat people of color, as when Annette's midwives repeatedly failed to diagnose her heart condition and pancreatitis, despite the deeply concerning symptoms that she exhibited throughout her pregnancy.

Crucially, class-privileged black people who manipulate race-, class-, and training-based levers during their pregnancy are very aware of the levers' imperfections. They know that there is no magical formula that will guarantee them the experience with healthcare that they want. As the next chapter explores, high-income black people know that in making choices around healthcare, they are doing no more than dealing in probabilities. These choices are significant, however, as they are choices that are unavailable to their low-income counterparts, who frequently receive care from whomever is present that day in the obstetrics clinic at the public hospital.

The fact that class-privileged black people even have to make these types of decisions reveals that the nation has offloaded responsibility for a social, cultural, and political failure—that is, the sad state of black maternal health in the United States—onto individuals. By choosing to receive their prenatal care from a black provider, or from a midwife, or while wearing the paraphernalia of the elite colleges that they attended, or while accompanied by their white spouse, Jenna, Meredith, Giselle, Harlow, Ifeoma, and Annette are doing the best that they can to solve a fundamentally structural problem for themselves.

However, according to the political and economic philosophy of neoliberalism, this is the appropriate and preferred approach to addressing the high rates of maternal mortality and morbidity in the country today. Geographer David Harvey describes neoliberalism as "a theory of political economic practices that proposes that human well-being can best be advanced by liberating individual entrepreneurial freedoms and skills within an institutional framework characterized by strong private property rights, free markets, and free trade. The role of the state is to create and preserve an institutional framework appropriate to such practices."[22] Neoliberalism claims that governments should enable robust markets and that, beyond this, its actions should be kept to a minimum. In fact, the philosophy says that the state often acts illegitimately when it does anything other than ensure that markets are strong. Further, neoliberalism claims that the proper role of citizens is to be consumers.[23] In other words, citizens are no longer expected—and should no longer expect—to find freedom through political activity. Instead, they should expect to find freedom through consuming goods in the market.

The choices that Jenna, Meredith, Giselle, Harlow, Ifeoma, and Annette have made around their prenatal care—choices that they perceive as preserving their health and life—are evidence that the neoliberal project is alive and well in the United States today.[24] Within neoliberalism, the state has washed its hands of intervening in the processes that produce avoidable and tragic maternal deaths in the country. Instead, individuals are given the responsibility of consuming their way to better health outcomes. With every decision to receive care from a black provider, every selection of a midwife instead of an obstetrician, and every purchase of an Ivy League sweatshirt to (hopefully) broadcast deservingness, individuals are performing the unfair task that neoliberalism demands of them.

Critical theorist Saidiya Hartman is helpful here. She has described the immediate aftermath of slavery's abolition in the United States, noting that the law could have been a tool for reorganizing society into something that was appreciably different from the one that existed during the reign of chattel slavery. Instead, the law withdrew and allowed white people's aversion to black people to be the principle around which society was ordered—creating a nation that was devastatingly similar to the one that existed prior to slavery's abolition. She writes, "[T]his withdrawal of law is at the same time a declaration of value."[25] Similarly, the law has withdrawn from the processes, systems, narratives, and institutions that have resulted in black people being much less likely than their white peers to survive pregnancy and childbirth. Following Hartman, this withdrawal is a declaration of the *nonvalue* of black lives.

RACIAL RENUNCIATION AS A TECHNIQUE FOR NAVIGATING RACISM

There is another method of navigating racism and race-based disadvantage that deserves mention. This is racial renunciation. By this, I mean that some class-privileged black people have refused to think of racism as relevant to their experiences.[26] These individuals do not deny the existence of racism. Indeed, the black people I interviewed who practiced racial renunciation were as familiar with the shameful statistics around racial disparities in maternal mortality and morbidity as the black people who consciously attempted to avoid racism. In other words, black people engaging in racial renunciation were aware that, statistically speaking, they were more likely than their white counterparts to die or to be severely injured during pregnancy, childbirth, or the postpartum period. However, their strategy for managing this fact was to refuse to interpret their experiences in light of it.

I met Jody, a black woman who was pregnant with her first child, at one of her prenatal care appointments in the general obstetrics clinic on Golden Health's East Hills campus. (Golden's Black Wellbeing Clinic had not yet begun operations during Jody's pregnancy, so she did not have the option of receiving her care in the specialty clinic.) Jody was born in New Jersey and moved to California to pursue a master of science degree in human genetics at the University of California in San Francisco. She met her future husband, who is white, during her graduate studies and remained in the Bay Area after finishing her program. When we talked, she was working as a genetic counselor at a Stanford University–affiliated hospital. She explained that she had chosen to receive her prenatal care from Golden instead of where she worked because she knew that "there is so much research going on" at the hospital and that, "altruistically," she wanted to be able to contribute to it. She continued, "So I'm here in part because of altruism. But more selfishly, I'm a minority. And I know that disparities around maternal mortality are very much not ignored here." I asked her whether she felt that the care that she had received at Golden reflected the institution's commitment to addressing racial disparities in maternal outcomes:

> **Jody:** I haven't really encountered anything specifically that tells me that Golden is not ignoring those disparities. But. . . . [pause] I will admit to you that I am not always someone who [pause] goes to race when things don't feel right in medical care, to be honest. And that could be partial bias because I work in the medical field and I am a clinician. But I would say that I am peripherally aware that Golden is not ignoring those disparities—just by looking on the website and reading the emails that

come through. I am aware that there are studies that are being done and talks that are being given at the institution.

Khiara: That's super interesting. Of course, it is impossible to know in most cases whether or not race explains an outcome. So what I gather from what you just said is that you don't go to that explanation. You know that it—race as an explanation—is out there, of course. But you don't go to it. And you think that is a function of the fact that you work in the medical field?

Jody: Maybe partially. But it also goes a little deeper. I think it was how I was raised. Other people in my family—my mom, grandmother—we tend to see things similarly in that way. And there have been conversations and things growing up that, maybe, were formative.

Khiara: What kind of conversations?

Jody: I can't think of any specific examples right now. But I have vague memories of things happening and people saying, "Oh, it's because we're black." And then at home, in dialogues—in private dialogues—I would hear my family members expressing that they can't stand when people jump to that.

Khiara: Jump to race?

Jody: Yeah.

While listening to Jody, I began thinking that her decision to reject racism as an explanation for events likely helped her feel less disempowered. Being subjected to racism, whether structural or interpersonal, invariably is beyond the control of the individual so subjected. Explaining a negative experience in terms of a factor over which one has no power can be unsettling. Perhaps it may be an act of agency to refuse to embrace that factor—to conceptualize events entirely in terms of causes that are within one's ability to influence. So I asked Jody if her approach has helped. She did not answer the question directly:

> I think that we've all had encounters that are like, "Mmmmm—that doesn't seem right." [laughs] My approach is to say, "Regardless of what the reason is, if it doesn't feel right, you try to change your situation." So that's always been how I've tried to handle things.

Jody was not the only person whom I encountered during my research who avoided explaining negative experiences in terms of racism. Olivia, who was thirteen weeks pregnant with her second child when I met her at her first prenatal care appointment in the Black Wellbeing Clinic, had a similar approach. Olivia, who lived in the wealthy Mission Bay neighborhood of San Francisco, was born in Kenya and had moved to the United States as a child. She was working as a registered nurse in a cancer facility when we met. She explained that the prenatal care she received during her first pregnancy at Golden had been wonderful, so she decided to return to Golden for prenatal care for her second. Olivia explained the positive prenatal care experience at Golden during her first pregnancy entirely in terms of her midwife, Georgia, a white woman who had since retired. Olivia described her affection for Georgia:

> She was very warm and caring, and she just made it seem like everything with my pregnancy was normal—everything was progressing well—which, as a first-time mom, was the precise type of assurance that I needed. She really allayed my anxieties. But beyond that, I felt that we were simply socializing during our interactions. [laughs] I guess her personality and mine gelled together. We were the perfect fit. She had a lot of work experience in Africa, and she would tell me about her work in Uganda and Tanzania and Burundi. And we just connected around that aspect of her career. And she was, like, what's the word—holistic? So we didn't just talk "medical." We talked about my life and my family history and things like that, and she was able to bring that into my care. And of course, you know, they're busy and everything. But she made time for me. And I just appreciated her so much.

While Olivia's prenatal care appointments with Georgia exceeded her expectations, her labor and childbirth were traumatic—physically, mentally, and emotionally. Georgia, like many of the midwives who work at Golden Health, also worked in the labor and delivery department at the General, the city's public hospital. The General had a fairly new Family Birth Center that featured private birth rooms large enough to accommodate several family members and friends throughout the entire labor, as well as deep bathtubs for soaking in order to help manage labor pains. A team of midwives was present at all times to care for patients who were in labor, so a low-risk patient at the Family Birth Center never was cared for by an obstetrician simply because a midwife was unavailable. According to its promotional materials, the Family Birth Center's healthcare workers "believe in supporting women to have normal labors,"[27] and its midwives "are experts in supporting you to have a normal childbirth." It claimed that it "has the lowest cesarean birth rate of any hospital in San Francisco—15 percent for midwife patients, 19 percent for all patients."[28] Because Georgia's patients delivered their babies at the General's Family Birth Center, she and Olivia planned for Olivia to deliver her baby at the center—irrespective of whether Georgia was on duty when Olivia went into labor.

When Olivia reached forty-two weeks without going into labor, Georgia scheduled an induction of labor. Olivia recalls that Georgia told her, "Once you check into the hospital after you're induced, it will be about two days for you to start having contractions for the birth to even happen. We're going to give you Pitocin and other things to speed things up, if needed. But after about two days, you'll have your baby." As it were, things did not proceed according to Georgia's forecast. Olivia ultimately did not give birth until a full week after she checked into the hospital, and her time in the hospital was filled with anxiety about her baby's health. She repeatedly urged her midwives to enlist the help of a physician who could perform a Caesarian section. "But they weren't listening to me," recalled Olivia:

> I was just there for too long. And they kept saying "It's okay, it's fine." And I'm like, "Oh no, it's not fine." [quietly laughs]
>
> The first and second days were fine. But, you know, the third day came and went, and—still no baby. So after the third day, I started to ask for a C-section. And they would say, "Oh, no, no, no, no. It's going to be good. We're not there yet. We're not there yet."
>
> I was dilating. But not very quickly. Also, they couldn't even agree on how far I had dilated. Each person who checked my cervix would say something different. One person said five; another person said seven. And then someone else would say six. And then another person would say five. And they would go back and forth, back and forth.
>
> I was very, very worried. They were giving me Pitocin and all of these other medications. I was full of drugs. Completely full of medicine. And I was worried about how the drugs were affecting my daughter. But the whole time—there's this thing they kept saying. "Oh, the baby's happy, the baby's happy." But it just didn't seem possible to me. I couldn't wrap my head around it.

During the sixth day of Olivia's stay at the hospital, her care team performed an amniotomy—a rupture of her amniotic sac—to facilitate the progression of her labor. Olivia recalled that meconium—the baby's feces—was in her amniotic fluid, providing evidence that her baby was in distress: "I was thinking that it was an emergency. But all they did was tell me that I should get a good night's rest because I was going to deliver the next day. And I asked them, 'I'm supposed to sleep with the baby's poop inside of me?' And they just told me what they had been telling me the entire time: 'Oh no, it's fine.' But I'm thinking to myself, 'But in nursing school. . . . I could have sworn in nursing school, they said meconium is a sign that things are not fine.' But then I would second-guess myself. Because I haven't thought about meconium in years."

The next morning, a cervical exam revealed that Olivia had dilated nine centimeters, at which point her care team decided that she should start to push—even though the cervix is considered fully dilated when it is at ten centimeters: "I didn't quite get to ten. It was clear that they were worried that something bad was going to happen if the baby was not born soon." However, every time Olivia pushed, the baby's heart rate would drop precipitously: "The ICU [intensive care unit] triage team rushed to my room at least four times. Three to four times. It was terrifying. I thought my baby was dying. I kept asking them for a C-section. And they kept telling me that everything was fine." After three hours of her pushing—and several visits from the emergency unit dispatched to revive dying infants—the care team attempted a vacuum-assisted delivery, which involves applying suction and traction to the baby's head to attempt to move the baby down the birth canal. The procedure was unsuccessful. Olivia recalled that every time she pushed with the instrument inserted into her vagina, she heard a "pop" shortly thereafter—which she supposed was the sound of the suction breaking on the baby's head.

Although Olivia asked for a C-section "at least a hundred times" during her week in the hospital, she reported that they "acknowledged" every request but always gave a reason for denying it. Usually, the reason centered around the baby being "fine" or that "they weren't there yet." However, after the vacuum-assisted delivery proved unsuccessful, a provider offered a new reason for denying the C-section that Olivia so badly wanted:

After the vacuum didn't work, I asked one of the midwives for a C-section, and she said, "No, sorry." And then one of the attending physicians came in, and I asked her the same thing. And she said, "Honestly, Olivia, we don't have an operating room available right now. So we need to keep on trying to do a vaginal birth." And I was stunned. I couldn't believe that that was the reason I had to keep on trying to push—because there were no available operating rooms. That's when I was like, "Oh shit. We really have to do this." I had to stop thinking about the impossible and start doing what I could. I just knew that I had to get me and my baby out of there.

Olivia did not recall how much time passed between being told that there were no available operating rooms and delivering her daughter. She remembered being told to push whenever she felt a contraction and being unable to feel contractions due to the epidural that had been administered. She recalled looking at a monitor that was at her bedside and discerning that she should push whenever she saw a crescendo build in the displayed numbers: "I didn't tell them that I wasn't feeling contractions because at that point, I was like, 'What's the point?' They weren't listening to me anyhow. And I think they thought that because I was a nurse, I would know how the monitors worked and know that I should push when I saw a certain frequency. But I didn't. I had to figure out everything by myself in the moment." After some time, she recalled a provider "yelling" at her to push: "And then manually, I think they went in there, and they just, sort of, pulled." Her daughter, finally, had been born.

The end of Olivia's story is, mercifully, unremarkable. Both Olivia and her daughter developed fevers, and they both were given antibiotics and monitored. When their fevers subsided three days later, they were discharged from the hospital.

It is not unreasonable to believe that race and racism had something to do with the way Olivia's labor and delivery proceeded. Olivia's black race might at least partially explain her providers' refusal to listen to her over the course of her weeklong ordeal in the hospital. Moreover, there is a fascinating inconsistency in the way that Olivia's care team treated her. On one hand, team members assumed that Olivia had some specialized knowledge due to her training as a registered nurse. They believed that she would be able to interpret the tocodynamometer that measured the length and strength of her contractions and push when appropriate. On the other hand, they would not tell Olivia why they believed that the baby was "happy." What indicators supported their conclusion? While Olivia was "not there yet" and a C-section was not yet indicated, when would it be? On what evidence were they waiting? We are not irrational if we suppose that Olivia's race helps to explain how her care team both acknowledged that Olivia was a healthcare worker with some expertise in medical technologies and also infantilized her by speaking to her about "happy" babies and asserting that everything was "fine"—objective evidence to the contrary notwithstanding. As so many of my interlocutors told me, race disadvantage sometimes works to make class privilege (in this case, Olivia's training as a nurse) invisible.

Further, we might be curious about how the care team's treatment of Olivia is informed by the Family Birth Center's location inside of the General. As noted in chapter 2, the General is a "poor people's hospital"—a place that the commercially insured avoid with explicit intention and steadfast determination. For this reason, the patients who receive their healthcare from the General are overwhelmingly indigent and, as a result, disproportionately people of color. Consequently, the General itself has become racialized as an unprivileged, nonwhite site where unprivileged, nonwhite people go when they need to see the doctor. How might this fact have informed the treatment that Olivia's care team delivered to her? Had Olivia's status as a patient within the General contributed to her being racialized in a particular way—as an uneducated, low-income, nonwhite person who would not be able to understand the reasoning behind the care team's treatment decisions? Had Olivia's status as a patient in San Francisco's county hospital worked to make invisible the privilege (the education and high income) that, if recognized, might have led Olivia's care team to interact with her in a more affirming, less condescending way?

In light of the reasonableness of the conclusion that Olivia's blackness played some role in the negative birth experience that she had in the Family Birth Center, perhaps the most extraordinary aspect of Olivia's story is that *she rejected race as an explanation.* Olivia attributed the failure of her care team to listen to her pleas for a C-section to their training as midwives.

(Interestingly, Olivia was aware that obstetricians were also part of her care team: She described the person who told her that no operating rooms were available as "an attending physician.")

Because Olivia believed that her providers' status as midwives explained why her daughter's birth was harrowing, she sought to receive her prenatal care from obstetricians during her second, current pregnancy in order to try to avoid repeating that ordeal. Moreover, because Olivia disavowed that race had played a role in the frightening delivery of her daughter, she had no preferences around the race of her providers for her second pregnancy. She explained that she was currently receiving her prenatal care from the Black Wellbeing Clinic purely out of convenience. While there were few prenatal care appointments available in Golden Health's general obstetrics clinic, there were many more available in the specialty Black Wellbeing Clinic. Olivia found this out when she was initially struggling to book a prenatal care appointment and a staff member told her that she would not have any trouble getting appointments if she received her care from the Black Wellbeing Clinic. When the staff member asked if Olivia wanted to be seen in the Black Wellbeing Clinic, she told me that she replied, "Sure. It doesn't matter." I asked her why the race of her provider did not matter to her:

> Um, for me, I—maybe I have never had any traumatic experience with the nonblack providers to push me towards black providers. So I don't have a preference one way or the other. I just—for me, I think anybody's anybody. I've never had a really bad experience to make me want to choose a black provider versus someone else.

After making this assertion, Olivia then spent close to an hour recounting her self-described "traumatic" birth experience at the hands of a nearly all-white care team.

There is a deep dissonance between Olivia's self-reports of her daughter's birth and her assertion that she has "never had a really bad experience." We are wise to wonder whether Olivia is protecting herself by refusing to conclude that race helps to explain why the birth of her daughter unfolded in the way that it did. Denying that race and racism disadvantaged her might be a way to claw back some agency from structures, systems, institutions, processes, and narratives that work to shape our experiences. When racism haunts your entire neighborhood, could it be empowering to declare that your house, somewhat miraculously, remains free of ghosts?

If we find ourselves upset by the racial renunciations that Olivia, Jody, and other people of color practice, we might ask whether that uneasiness is due to the fact that powerful actors in the United States insist that this orientation to racism is correct and proper—the only orientation that sensible people could possibly have. At least since Reconstruction, actors have offered racial renunciation as a political program. Uncommitted to dismantling (or even acknowledging the existence of) structural and interpersonal racism, they have insisted that racism does not impact experiences—the overwhelming empirical evidence of the opposite being neither here nor there. They have insisted that if—*if*—racism disadvantages a person of color, that individual ought to worry about the things that they can control. They ought to make good choices. They ought to pull themselves up by their bootstraps. The fact that racial renunciation has been politically weaponized might explain any disappointment that we feel when black people, attempting to navigate racial disadvantage in their own lives, find it a useful tool for surviving the country's racial hierarchy.

* * *

As a whole, healthcare institutions have found racial disparities in health to be disconcerting, and they have been troubled by the possibility that they have been dispensing inequitable care to their patients. For this reason, many institutions, including Golden Health, have committed themselves to exploring ways to eliminate these disparities. As this chapter explores, many black patients elect to receive their healthcare from black providers as a strategy to avoid ending up on the losing end of racial disparities in maternal mortality. The next chapter discusses a provocative innovation that Golden Health embarked on in 2022 that formalizes the mechanisms by which black patients can elect to be seen by a black provider within the health system: Golden opened a specialty clinic that provides racially concordant healthcare.

6 The Racially Concordant Care Intervention (and Its Discontents)

The Women's Health Center on Golden Health's Yerba Buena campus is housed in a squat, drab concrete structure that is very unlike the glass and steel towers of Golden's East Hills campus. On one of my observation days, I sat in a spacious, somewhat worn office in the center with Dr. Helen Volante and midwife Francine Hunt as they manned the Black Wellbeing Clinic. Dr. Volante, a black woman who completed a highly selective residency at Golden a few years earlier and was currently a faculty member in Golden's OB/GYN department, popped an orange slice into her mouth and said, "I liked it! I've always been a big Rihanna fan. She didn't disappoint, in my opinion." Hunt, the only black midwife at Golden and a patient favorite, nodded her head in agreement as she scanned a computer screen showing that her first patient of the day was expected to arrive in five minutes. After finishing her review of her schedule, she said, "I was just blown away by the fact that she did the Super Bowl while pregnant! I saw so many people online criticizing her performance. I'm thinking to myself, 'You couldn't do it even without being pregnant.' And this woman is in her second trimester—standing on a stage, floating above thousands of people."

Dr. Marie Clark and Dr. Semret Iggi then entered the office, dropped their bags at separate workstations, and dove into the conversation without missing a beat. Dr. Clark, a black obstetrician whose résumé reads like a listing of elite institutions and competitive fellowships, opined, "I saw this article where the author was saying that black women are held to this impossibly high standard—where we all have to be Beyoncé. But Rihanna's not

Beyoncé! Rihanna is Rihanna. And Rihanna is exquisite in her own right." Dr. Iggi, a black maternal-fetal medicine specialist whose credentials are as impressive as those of the three other black women in the room, laughed as she threw a white coat over her blue and green polka-dot dress: "It's always 'black girl magic,' 'black girl magic,' 'black girl magic.' We can do that. Clearly, we can do that. But do we have to be magical all the time? Can't we just be human every once in a while?"

The conversation stayed for a few more minutes on Rihanna's Super Bowl performance, which had taken place a couple of days prior, but eventually shifted to other more routine matters. Dr. Clark told Dr. Volante that her 9 a.m. patient, a black woman, began prenatal care at the General, the county hospital that primarily serves San Francisco's most disadvantaged, but that the General had not sent over the patient's medical records when she transferred to Golden. Dr. Clark expressed frustration that without the medical records, she would have to order testing that the patient likely already had done. Hunt offered Dr. Volante a chocolate from a box of candies given to her by a former patient—a black woman who worked as a registered nurse at Golden. Hunt had cared for the patient during her stay at the hospital after giving birth. Dr. Iggi told Hunt that she was scheduled to see a pregnant black woman that day who had had two prior C-sections, had suffered a stillbirth, and had a history of molar pregnancies—a rare condition in which a noncancerous tumor develops in the uterus as a result of a nonviable pregnancy. "Plus she has a heart murmur," said Dr. Iggi, "and she is experiencing some housing instability. I'm going to act like I have all the time in the world when I meet with her." And so began a typical day in the Black Wellbeing Clinic.

The Black Wellbeing Clinic, which opened its doors shortly after I began conducting research at Golden, is one of the first clinics of its kind in the nation, offering what the literature calls "racially concordant care" to black women and other black people capable of pregnancy. Its website explains the clinic's mission: "We are a collective of Black Sexual and Reproductive Health providers committed to providing care to Black individuals within a reproductive justice framework. We strive to provide care that honors your authentic experience, voice, and knowledge about your body."

The Black Wellbeing Center is not the only site within Golden Health that provides racially concordant care to black patients who desire it. Golden's AFFIRM program offers black patients prenatal care in a group setting with five to seven other Golden patients who have similar due dates. AFFIRM's website explains that "Group Prenatal Care (GPC) has been shown to decrease emergency visits, promote breastfeeding, and provide higher quality of care and decrease rates of preterm birth, especially among Black participants. Despite widespread acknowledgment of GPC benefits, there is no racially responsive GPC curriculum [that] address[es] health consequences of anti-Black racism." AFFIRM aims to attend to the "inequitable outcomes in obstetrical care [that stem] from systemic and interpersonal anti-Black racism" by offering prenatal care "from an intentional angle of racial consciousness."

A program similar to AFFIRM is available across the San Francisco Bay in Oakland. BElovedBIRTH Black Centering is a racially concordant group prenatal care program for low-income, black patients who receive their care from the county's public health system. BElovedBIRTH's promotional materials explain that the program exists for the following reasons:

- We are in crisis. Every day Black mothers, birthing people and their babies are experiencing disproportionately high rates of traumatic experiences and preventable complications in pregnancy and birth. But it doesn't have to be this way. These differences in rates of birth complications are caused by racism.

We know that:

- There is nothing wrong with Black birthing people. We are not predisposed to ill health or birth complications.
- Black people are strong[,] resilient, and perfectly capable of having healthy pregnancies and births.
- The answers to this crisis are in the Black community. We are the experts in our needs, and programs to address this crisis must be led by us.

BElovedBIRTH Black Centering was created by, for, and with Black people. Our program is specially designed to address the problem of racism increasing the risk for birth complications in our Black community.[1]

Golden's Black Wellbeing Clinic, AFFIRM, and BElovedBIRTH are responses to the racial disparities in maternal mortality and morbidity that have been a feature of American society for centuries. As such, they are efforts to save black people's lives, allowing black people to receive care from black providers as a way to navigate the United States' failure to protect black people during the perinatal period. But these programs are controversial in a country in which many people insist that the way to get beyond racism is to pretend that it does not exist. It seems inevitable that these endeavors will be met with resistance. Indeed, they made uncomfortable some of the self-identified liberals who spoke with me during my fieldwork. This chapter explores the future of racially concordant care clinics in a country increasingly committed to ignoring race, racism, and racial inequality. It begins, however, with an exploration of the approaches that the medical community has taken in the past to address racial disparities in health, including implicit bias trainings; cultural competence curricula and workshops; diversity, equity, and inclusion (DEI) initiatives; and instruction in the structural competency framework.

IMPLICIT BIAS TRAININGS

As chapter 3 explores, implicit bias has been an extremely popular way for people to explain racial inequality in the United States. The medical community is no exception. Medical and nursing schools, residency and fellowship programs, and hospitals and health systems have embraced the possibility that providers' implicit biases lead them to provide inferior care to patients of color, thereby contributing to racial disparities in health. Many of these institutions have responded by encouraging—and, in some cases, requiring—their clinicians and students to attend an implicit bias training or series of trainings.

The goal of these trainings is to educate attendees about implicit bias and its possible effects on the quality of the healthcare that providers deliver to their patients. During some trainings, attendees take an implicit association test, which reveals the existence and extent of their implicit biases. More effective trainings teach attendees techniques for mitigating bias. For example, psychologists have shown that people are less likely to act on their negative implicit biases if they engage in individuation of the person in front of them—that is, if they "deliberately obtain information specific to an individual rather than rely on assumptions based on the individual's membership in a certain social group."[2] Providers who engage in individuation of their patients are less likely to conceptualize the patient as simply a single member of a larger group of others. Instead, individuation increases the likelihood that the provider will perceive the patient as belonging to the provider's group—one of "us" as opposed to one of "them." For example, if a white provider engages in individuation of a Puerto Rican patient and discovers that the patient stayed up late the night before catching up on *White Lotus*, she is less likely to perceive the patient as "Puerto Rican" and more likely to perceive the patient as a *White Lotus* enthusiast like herself. Psychologists have also demonstrated that providers are less likely to act on their negative implicit biases when they engage in "perspective-taking"—that is, when they attempt to put themselves in the patient's position and consider the situation from the patient's perspective.[3] Further, implicit biases may be dulled when an individual is exposed to counterstereotypes—that is, when they are confronted with images and stories involving persons whose lives or behaviors are inconsistent with the stereotypes that exist about the group to which the person belongs. As an example, in order to reduce the strength of an individual's unconscious association of Puerto Ricans and welfare dependency, the individual may be asked to read the biography of Justice Sonia Sotomayor, a woman born to Puerto Rican parents whose life is far from stereotypical.

The most effective trainings inform trainees that negative implicit biases may be mitigated or eliminated when people encounter individuals from outside groups under conditions of equality. It bears repeating that to diminish the strength of a negative implicit bias, the individual must engage with those belonging to an outside group as equals and not as subordinates or inferiors. The evidence indicates that there must be "shared goals and equal status between both parties. Otherwise, such interactions have the potential to strengthen previously held stereotypes."[4] For example, a nonblack provider is less likely to have negative implicit biases about black people—and, therefore, is less likely to provide inferior care to her black patients—if she has black colleagues, black supervisors, black neighbors, black in-laws, and so on. In other words, the establishment of meaningful relationships with members of an outside group may be one of the best means for eliminating negative implicit biases. This may be a radical proposition, as it suggests that society needs to reorganize itself dramatically if we want to make it impossible for negative implicit biases to harm members of marginalized groups.

While implicit bias trainings in medical schools and other healthcare settings are common, the evidence that they work to improve patient outcomes is not as overwhelming as might be expected. Many healthcare institutions have adopted implicit bias trainings as a way to ensure that providers are dispensing equal care to their patients, but the research has not established that these trainings actually improve the quality of care that providers deliver to patients about whom they may have negative implicit biases. As law professor Osamudia James summarizes it, the evidence of the ability of implicit bias trainings to "change behavior" is "limited."[5]

CULTURAL COMPETENCE WORKSHOPS AND CURRICULA

The most popular approach that medical schools and healthcare institutions have taken to address racial disparities in health is cultural competence training.[6] While definitions of cultural competence are plentiful (and while many of its principles are taught under different titles, including "cultural awareness," "cultural safety," "cultural intelligence," "cultural sensitivity," and "cultural respect"),[7] the Agency for Healthcare Research and Quality offers a starting point for an analysis of the concept, proposing that "[c]ulturally competent care is defined as care that respects diversity in the patient population and cultural factors that can affect health and health care, such as language, communication styles, beliefs, attitudes, and behaviors."[8] The cultural competence framework endeavors to reduce racial disparities in health by equipping providers with the knowledge that they need to navigate and reduce gaps in understanding that may exist during a clinical encounter involving patients with cultures different from the providers' own.

Most scholars agree that the cultural competence framework began to emerge in the 1960s, as the medical community in the United States tried to respond to the civil rights movement and the antidiscrimination legislation that Congress passed in light of the movement's demands.[9] In the 1980s, the cultural competence framework crystallized and has maintained dominance ever since. Part of its dominance may be explained by the fact that powerful organizations have vouched for it. For example, the Liaison Committee on Medical Education (LCME), which provides accreditation to schools that issue medical degrees, has declared that cultural competence should be a part of medical education. LCME has stated that accredited schools should teach a curriculum that "includes content" touching on "[t]he diverse manner in which people perceive health and illness and respond to various symptoms, diseases, and treatments" as well as "[t]he basic principles of culturally . . . competent health care."[10] Further, the Office of Minority Health, the federal agency whose charge is to improve the health of minority groups in the country, created the National Standards for Culturally and Linguistically Appropriate Services (CLAS) in Health and Health Care: "The CLAS standards specify that health care organizations should ensure that their staff receive ongoing education and training in culturally and linguistically appropriate service delivery."[11]

The principle behind the cultural competence framework is that patients may come from cultures that conceptualize health, sickness, and disease differently from the way they are conceptualized within medicine as it is practiced in the Western world. The framework says that providers should become "competent" in their patients' cultures so that they can communicate effectively with them and give them the healthcare that they need and desire. As physicians and researchers Jonathan Metzl and Helena Hansen explain, cultural competence trainings have come to assume a typical form:

> Clinical professionals learn approaches to communication, diagnosis and treatment that take into account culturally specific sources of stigma, such as the stigma of mental health diagnoses among Asian immigrants . . . Doctors train by analyzing vignettes that depict instances where "cultural" variables impact symptom presentations or attitudes about care. "Mrs. Jones is an African American woman in her mid-60s who comes late to her office visit and

refuses to take her blood pressure medication as prescribed." Or, "You see a Mexican migrant who just received health counseling for Type II diabetes eating fried tortillas in the waiting room." Meanwhile, nurses develop "linguistic competencies" that teach them culturally sensitive, non-judgmental ways to build rapport with such patients.[12]

Although the intentions that motivate the cultural competence framework are good, it ultimately is a problematic way to think about the causes of and solution to racial disparities in health. At least five critiques of the framework deserve examination.

First, the framework is an individualist account of racial disparities in health, locating the causes of racial disparities in health in a deficient encounter between the provider and patient in a clinical setting. As an individualist account, it ignores the large-scale forces—such as environmental injustices, lack of health insurance or access to quality preventative healthcare, housing insecurity, food deserts, epigenetics, stress and weathering, and healthcare segregation—that are most responsible for generating different health outcomes across racial groups.

Of course, it is possible for the cultural competence framework to coexist with awareness of the structural conditions that generate racial disparities in health. We could pay attention to the role played by culture during the clinical encounter while also paying attention to the unjust structural conditions that damage health. As one scholar has noted, "Cultural competence is not designed to draw attention away from . . . the larger factors that contribute to racial/ethnic disparities in health, such as poverty, lack of education, the environment, and poor access to care."[13] However, as one set of scholars has said, an "[u]ndue focus on culture can divert attention from those issues."[14] And this is what we have witnessed. The medical community has devoted *a lot* of energy to ensuring that providers are fluent in their patients' cultures while devoting relatively little energy to ensuring that providers are knowledgeable about the structural conditions that compromise their patients' health. As one set of researchers explain, focusing on culture "without also attending to occupational and environmental exposures, access to health care, affordability of medications, and linguistic barriers, among other factors, is to overestimate the role of individual choices in producing health, disease, and treatment outcomes."[15] Training our attention on the patient's culture might lead us to overlook the systemic processes that have the greatest responsibility for sickening marginalized people and shortening their lives. We might be fixating on the clinical encounter—which "has been shown to have only a small impact on patient outcomes and on improving population health at large"[16]—while ignoring the background conditions that do most of the work of producing higher rates of morbidity and mortality in vulnerable groups.

Second, the cultural competence framework may trade in stereotypes. The framework charges clinicians with the task of learning about a patient's culture so that the clinician can provide care that fits the patient's needs. Does this mean that if the patient is black, for example, the clinician must learn about "black culture"? As chapter 3 discusses, it may be inappropriate to assume that any individual black patient subscribes to and participates in "black culture." More important, as that chapter investigates, what is "black culture"? What are clinicians learning when they try to become proficient in "black culture"? If, as is explored in chapter 3, the clinician learns that "black culture" consists of eating fried foods, failing to exercise, and practicing Christianity, then the clinician is learning a caricature of blackness. These behaviors and beliefs do not describe the breadth and depth of the ways in which black people exist in this world. To reduce that vast collection of ways of existing to eating fried foods, failing to exercise, and practicing Christianity—and then to presume that this reduction applies to the black patient who is sitting in the exam room—is to participate in a particularly egregious form of stereotyping. Moreover, this cartoonish account of blackness may contribute to doctors' perceptions of black patients as noncompliant and as culturally incapable of adhering to medical advice. It might lead some doctors to provide a higher quality of care to their nonblack patients, who physicians would have learned do not have the same cultural obstacles to following doctors' recommendations.

Although the danger of reductionist renderings of any individual culture should have been apparent from the outset, the cultural competence literature nonetheless is filled with caricatures of individual cultures. Consider the following excerpts from this body of scholarship:

Many African Americans have either a religious orientation or a viewpoint grounded in African American social and cultural history, which may emphasize a holistic approach to health and health care. Religion is a source of enormous emotional support for African Americans. . . . Home or natural remedies are commonly known and are used by African Americans, particularly among the elderly.[17]

Three health-related traditions common in Hispanic culture include *familismo* (family involvement in medical decision making, which reduces the patient's control over the treatment and course of illness), *machismo* (gender roles that give males the power to make medical decisions for females in the family) and *fatalismo* (the belief that health and illness are preordained and, therefore, beyond control). Medical professionals [should] learn that these traditional scripts vary according to social class and level of acculturation, and [should] learn to be sensitive to these concerns as they acquire information, make a diagnosis and recommend treatment and prevention measures to Hispanic patients.[18]

[A] cultural nuance specific to the Japanese population is the removal of one's shoes upon entering a home. This is a very strict requirement among many Japanese people, requiring the use of provided slippers prior to walking on the floors of their homes. Nonadherence to this requirement is considered rude, inappropriate, and unhygienic. As another example, in certain sects of the Muslim community, women are mostly covered and can reveal only certain body parts, usually their faces (in some instances, limited to their eyes, hands, and feet), when in public in an effort to maintain modesty, respect, and privacy for the women per their religious scripture, the Koran . . . As a final example, people from Spain find stretching and yawning to be very bad manners and in poor taste. They are also very casual about keeping appointments.[19]

These examples illustrate how the cultural competence framework is uncomfortably consistent with cultural explanations of racial disparities in health—which, as chapter 3 establishes, is a flawed explanation of the increased morbidity and mortality among some groups of (usually nonwhite) people. Providers are being instructed that black, Latine, Japanese, Muslim, and Spanish cultures have the features contained in the examples above. And while the cultural competence framework instructs providers that they should be aware of these features in order to provide high-quality healthcare to patients belonging to these cultures, these same features also could be supposed to *cause* racial disparities in health. The above examples could be interpreted to mean that if African Americans are sicker than people from other groups, it is because they rely on their religion to keep them healthy or cure them of their ailments instead of adhering to their doctors' advice. If Latine people have higher rates of uncontrolled diabetes than their white counterparts, it might be because they subscribe to *fatalismo* and refuse to take their medication. If Japanese people have lower rates of some illnesses than white people, it might be due to their superior hygiene habits. And so on. As chapter 3 shows, this is a harmful and empirically unsupported way to think about why some groups live longer, healthier lives than others.

Further, there are African Americans who are not religious or whose religious faiths do not inform their approach to health and illness. There are Latine people who do not embrace *familismo*, *machismo*, and *fatalismo*. There are Japanese people who do not take off their shoes when entering their homes. There are Muslim women who do not wear niqabs or burqas. Enormous difference can be found within any given culture. However, the cultural competence framework may trade in simplified versions of any individual culture. In so doing, it may do violence to the culture it purports to describe and to the complexity that characterizes the persons who are supposed to belong to the culture.

For this reason, observers have insisted that clinicians receive instruction about the diversity within a culture when they are learning about culture during cultural competence training. They warn that when clinicians are taught crude, unsophisticated renderings of a culture, they are less likely to hear and be responsive to information that patients share that is inconsistent with what the clinician believes to be true about the patient by virtue of their culture. In those cases, the clinician will be treating a stereotype of the patient and not the actual patient. This is a recipe for the provision of inferior care—despite the intention of the cultural competence framework to improve the quality of the care delivered to patients from marginalized groups.

One physician has made this point about diversity within a culture by using black people as an example, writing, "Not only can various cultures be seen among those living in different regions, but cultures may also differ among those living in the same region. For example, in the South, the culture of certain Blacks living in Charleston, South Carolina, may differ from those in New Orleans, Louisiana, whose culture may also be different from those in Selma, Alabama."[20] For this physician, this diversity means that the goal of cultural competence trainings must not be to "teach future practitioners everything they will need to know about a minority group but instead to make them aware that different cultures exist."[21] However, if the goal of cultural competence trainings is simply to make clinicians aware that different cultures exist, then are these trainings necessary? By the time people are old enough to go to medical school, are they not aware that different cultures exist?

Perhaps this is why some who seek to redeem the cultural competence framework insist that there has to be some specificity in lessons about culture. However, these redeemers caution that any instruction on specific cultural practices or beliefs that may affect a patient's experience of health and healthcare must be coupled with instruction that teaches that culture is not a static object but rather is a fluid entity that changes over time. Trainings should instruct trainees that the way individuals express their culture will be affected by the other identities that the individual has. Further, redeemers assert that trainees should be informed that individuals' attachment to or identification with their culture varies greatly. They should be told that "black culture" will mean different things depending on the person. "Black culture" in an African American woman who is straight and cisgender, is class privileged, has no visible disabilities, and feels only a loose connection with her racial identity will likely mean different things and have different effects than "black culture" in an African American woman who is a transgender lesbian, is experiencing poverty, has a disability, and loves and values her identity as a black person. While the interventions that redeemers of the cultural competence framework propose complicate the culture concept to make it more sophisticated and *true* (culture is a complicated thing, indeed), it leaves many skeptics curious about what exactly clinicians are supposed to do with the information that has been imparted. It is fairly obvious how clinicians are supposed to use culture when it is rendered in a reductionist, simplified, caricatured way—that is, in a way that is consistent with a professional training that instructs clinicians to treat variables (such as race) as constants. But when culture is understood to be what it actually is—shifting, messy, dynamic, and undefined—then it is not clear how knowledge about it will help the provider interact with the patient during the clinical encounter. Clinicians will know that their patients are black, but they will not know what that blackness means in light of patients' other identities and experiences.

Third, because the cultural competence framework, as it is typically implemented, has not adequately theorized the concept of culture, it is not apparent what culture is supposed to encompass and what it is supposed to exclude. Sometimes culture appears to be everything, including sexuality, physical or mental ability, vocation, and pastimes. In these formulations, it is unclear what culture is *not*. Consider the story recounted by an occupational therapist about her work with a woman, Ruby, whose physical disability left her unable to leave her home.[22] The therapist wanted to help Ruby navigate the world outside her home. Ruby, however, was very satisfied with living her life inside of the four corners of her apartment. The therapist writes that it took a while before she was able to hear and respect Ruby's wishes. She attributes this disconnection to "culture," writing that "[a]lthough Ruby did not have a background different from mine ethnically, she did have a vastly different cultural experience as a homebound woman with multiple sclerosis. The subcultures I adhere to as a traveler, therapist, dancer, and academic center on constant movement and change."[23] While it is undeniable that the author's status as a "traveler, therapist, dancer, and academic" likely led her to value things differently than Ruby did, it is not clear why being a traveler, therapist, dancer, or academic are *cultural* traits. They may be. But why? What makes something "cultural"? While it is problematic to propose that culture is *only* race and ethnicity, it might also be problematic to propose that culture is everything.

Fourth, the cultural competence framework may be either insulting to those whose culture is different from their provider's, or it may exaggerate the provider's capabilities. According to the cultural competence framework, the clinician can gain a mastery of a patient's culture in a training or two.

Presuming that clinicians who take a couple of workshops will know all that is necessary to know about blackness, Mexican-ness, indigeneity, disability, or trans-ness and will be able to cross any existing cultural chasms that exist between themselves and their patients suggests that the cultures of marginalized people and groups are awfully simple or the intelligence of the provider is awfully vast.

Observers within the medical community have responded to this critique and have championed the *cultural humility* framework as superior to the cultural competence framework. According to the cultural humility framework, providers cannot become "competent" in any culture that is not their own. The framework denies that any culture is so finite—so bounded and fixed—that it can be learned. Instead, it proposes that providers will deliver high-quality care to patients from different cultures if the provider is simply curious about difference and open to self-reflection and self-critique. As one clinician has described it, "Cultural humility is a lifelong, learning-oriented approach to working with people with diverse cultural backgrounds. . . . [It embraces] an emphasis on learning rather than knowing, recognition of patient and client cultural perspectives as equally valid, and critical reflection on how systemic issues and power differences affect health care."[24] As another set of researchers put it, cultural humility "is a continuous commitment, and not an endpoint."[25]

Although the framework of cultural humility might be an improvement over cultural competence, they both attempt to use culture as the lever for improving patient care. They both may suffer from an undue focus on interpersonal interactions during the clinical encounter and may ignore the structural constraints that bear most of the responsibility for the shortened, sickened lives of marginalized people.

Fifth and finally, perhaps the most damaging critique of the cultural competence framework involves the uncertainty about its efficacy. The evidence that cultural competence trainings improve patient outcomes is not clear. Researchers have not definitively established that providers who have received instruction within the cultural competence framework provide better care than providers without such instruction. After conducting a review of the literature evaluating the effects of cultural competence trainings, one set of researchers concluded that the evidence revealed such trainings to be "both associated with *and unrelated to* positive patient outcomes."[26] In fact, these researchers found that few studies sought to examine whether cultural competence trainings actually improved the quality of the care that providers give their more vulnerable patients or reduced morbidity and mortality among these patients.[27] This led them to conclude that "the rationale supporting a cultural competence approach remains circular and rests strongly on the theoretical benefits of cultural competence, rather than on rigorous empirical evidence with respect to client outcomes."[28]

Nevertheless, cultural competence trainings remain a feature of medical education, leading some critics to wonder why it has enjoyed such prominence within medical education in the absence of proof that it generates the outcomes that it was introduced to generate. Some have concluded that institutions' professed dedication to ensuring that their faculties and students are culturally competent is just an exercise in virtue signaling. Psychologist Stephane Shepherd has written about this possibility in damning terms:

> The evident impracticability of a short-lived workshop on individual and organisational attitudes and behaviours suggests that there are broader financial, political and socio-historical objectives to running the training. A clear motive is for the organization to give the impression that diversity matters are of importance to them. While this may be genuine in some cases, cultural awareness trainings often exist symbolically as a corporate "tick-box," or perhaps even as a protection against litigation. One view is that organisations adopt diversity training mechanisms for "ceremonial" purposes, with full knowledge of the weak evidence base. This is to give the appearance of organisational legitimacy and alignment with contemporary social movements.[29]

In essence, by holding a cultural competence training every quarter or so, institutions can claim that they have an interest in racial equity and social justice while liberating themselves from the obligation to do the hard work—and make the sacrifices—that realizing racial equity and achieving social justice require.

DIVERSITY, EQUITY, AND INCLUSION INITIATIVES

Diversity, equity, and inclusion (DEI) initiatives in medical schools and healthcare institutions can take many forms—ranging from the tried-and-true training or workshop that explores a topic that might be relevant to understanding the experiences of people from disadvantaged groups[30] to a climate survey intended to measure whether and to what extent employees, students, or affiliates experience the institution as a welcoming, fair, or otherwise desirable place to work or study.[31] It deserves emphasis that many DEI initiatives are intended to address the experiences of people from disadvantaged groups *as employees or students of an institution.* That is, the focus of many DEI efforts—including the DEI offices established by health systems or the deanships and chairs of DEI created by medical schools—have focused on making these institutions more hospitable as places of employment or as schools where students learn how to be health professionals. To this end, DEI programs frequently concern themselves with hiring or recruiting more faculty, staff, students, and residents from marginalized groups[32] and ensuring that these individuals, once a part of the institution, do not confront barriers (whether structural or interpersonal) that hamper their ability to succeed within the institution.[33] While the direct goal of many of these DEI endeavors is to address the racism (or sexism, homophobia, transphobia, xenophobia, or ableism) that may make a healthcare institution a hostile place for an employee to work or a student to study, they may have the indirect effect of reducing racial disparities in health. This might happen if, for example, a health system intentionally hires more black doctors, thereby enabling it to provide racially concordant healthcare that improves health outcomes for its black patients. In the words of one set of advocates, the issues that DEI initiatives address may "not only negatively impact [an institution's] climate; they [may] also negatively impact the patients and communities that [the institution] serve[s]."[34] In this way, these initiatives may have "downstream effects on patient care."[35]

The most exciting DEI efforts have these "downstream effects." For example, one of a nursing school's DEI initiatives established a committee to identify areas in the nursing curriculum where issues related to race, gender, class, sexuality, ability, immigration status, or religion could be explored in greater depth.[36] While some might have justified this effort in terms of improving student experience (a more "inclusive" curriculum would feel less alienating to nursing students from marginalized groups and would allow them to become more engaged participants in their education),[37] it might be better justified in terms of diminishing racial disparities in health. This effect on racial disparities in health might be expected because the revised curriculum included lessons about false but common beliefs that compromise the quality of the care that vulnerable patients receive—for example, that due to a race-specific genetic variation, the kidney function of black patients is fundamentally different from that of nonblack patients, justifying "race correction" in measures of kidney health.[38] Revising the curriculum to address topics related to "social determinants of health and equity, climate change and climate justice, race, intersectionality, and race-based medicine" may certainly have a positive effect on students' sense of "belonging" to the department.[39] However, that effect might not be as important as the effect that the curriculum revision would have on the improved quality of care that students ultimately would deliver to their patients.

Unfortunately, DEI initiatives in healthcare institutions are not always effective. This is because they frequently take the form of a one-time training or workshop—a form that allows such efforts to fall victim to the critiques outlined above about the one-time training or workshop that purports to educate trainees and attendees about everything they need to know about a culture. An hour-long training about structural racism will not provide a doctor with a rich understanding of how racism shows up in the lives and compromises the health of their patients of color. Similarly, administering a climate survey and doing nothing more—or creating a new position of vice chancellor for diversity, equity, and inclusion without ensuring that the person who occupies the role has the power to implement change—will not solve a structural problem. When DEI initiatives take such forms, they are dangerous because they suggest that "one more implicit bias session, diversity executive, or DEI statement is enough; that with minimal investment, racism can be eliminated from institutions where it is as foundational as their bricks and mortar."[40] Nevertheless, this is what DEI efforts have looked like in too many institutions across the country. They have become "performative"[41]—a way to maintain the status quo while signaling an institution's commitment to social justice to the watching public.

Many institutions voluntarily terminated their DEI efforts after Donald Trump was reelected president in 2024 and his administration did its best to make such efforts politically inadvisable, if not illegal. Observers who have been critical of DEI initiatives because of their performative nature were not sad to see these programs go, understanding their disappearance as an opportunity for the development of more effective efforts to make the institutions that animate society more reflective of the nation.

INSTRUCTION IN THE STRUCTURAL COMPETENCY FRAMEWORK

In 2014, physicians Jonathan Metzl and Helena Hansen published an article that threatened the dominance that the cultural competence framework had over the ways that medical schools and healthcare institutions thought about the clinician's role in reducing racial disparities in health.[42] Their article reflected a growing sense that the cultural competence framework had proven largely unsuccessful during the three decades of its reign over medical education. Observers were dissatisfied that clinicians remained largely incapable of describing the myriad ways in which systems harm health. The cultural competence framework trained providers to look solely to the clinical encounter—specifically to communication failures between the provider and patient caused by their different cultures—as the primary site where the health of their marginalized patients was compromised. This led many clinicians to ignore the various ways the social world affects their patients' health—although scores of studies were demonstrating just that. As Metzl describes it:

> We now know that structural violence and institutional racism directly alter biologies and health outcomes. Epigenetics research demonstrates, at the level of gene methylation, how living in a resource-poor environment can impact risk factors for cardiovascular disease for generations. Meanwhile, neuroscientists demonstrate linkages between poverty, hampered brain development,

and various forms of mental illness. And economists show that low-income minority persons can lower their rates of obesity, diabetes, and major depression by moving to safer, more affluent neighborhoods.[43]

Although science had made these shocking discoveries about the relationship between structural conditions and states of unhealth, Metzl, Hansen, and like-minded thinkers were frustrated that most clinicians remained unaware of this relationship, as social structures fell outside of the cultural competence framework and medical education, more generally. Clinicians trained in accredited medical schools still largely believed that the only social factors that mattered in their patients' lives involved whether their patients smoked cigarettes, drank alcohol, or used illicit drugs. Many were eager to fault these individual shortcomings, as opposed to structural inequities, for the increased rates of sickness and death found among their patients of color.

Hansen and Metzl proposed the structural competency framework as a supplement—or an antidote[44]—to the cultural competence framework. In their words, structural competency "encourages clinical practitioners to recognize how social, economic, and political conditions produce health inequalities in the first place. Structural competency calls on health care professionals to recognize ways that institutions, neighborhood conditions, market forces, public policies, and health care delivery systems shape symptoms and diseases, and to mobilize for correction of inequalities as they manifest both in physician-patient interactions and beyond the clinic walls."[45] Moreover, structural competency responds to the critique made against the cultural competence framework regarding the idea that a clinician can know everything that needs to be known about a culture after sitting through one or two workshops. Metzl and Hansen understood that we may be exaggerating the capabilities of clinicians if we assume that they will be able to develop a fluency over something as multifaceted and complex as structure in the course of completing their medical education. They explain that structural competency "does not imply mastery of these protean forces within the context of already overbooked schedules or curricula."[46] Instead, clinicians will be structurally competent when they have developed "the humility to recognize the complexity of the structural constraints that patients and doctors operate within."[47]

The framework of structural competency recognizes that while cultural competence may help improve the interactions that providers have with patients in the exam room, clinicians also ought to have knowledge about the health-impacting conditions that exist prior to and outside of the clinical encounter. Without this knowledge, providers may continue to fixate on the individual—attributing health and sickness wholly to the individual's biological processes, behavioral choices, or cultural beliefs. According to the structural competency framework, it is dangerously shortsighted to believe that structure does not matter in the lives of patients. Structure is everywhere. It even dictates the parameters of the clinical encounter, determining how much time a provider can spend with the patient in the exam room.[48]

Metzl and Hansen's intervention challenges the prevailing idea that medicine ought to be unconcerned with the social world and should focus solely on the individual's biologic processes. Metzl and Hansen claim that if medicine, as a discipline, conceptualizes health as its object of inquiry, then the discipline should also conceptualize the systems that damage health as its object of inquiry. In their view, medicine should leverage its status as a health-preserving practice to engage in "structural level critiques and, perhaps more importantly, structural-level interventions."[49] If they are right, then a medical education is incomplete if students graduate without some level of proficiency in these health-compromising structures. A complete medical education would leave clinicians empowered to critique the systems and processes that sicken and kill their patients.

In effect, there are multiple ways for clinicians to conserve the health of a patient. For example, a provider could conserve a patient's health by diagnosing her with asthma and prescribing an inhaled corticosteroid to manage the condition, or the provider could conserve a patient's health by signing a statement objecting to the construction of a major road through the patient's neighborhood, as it is well-established that the air pollution generated by motor vehicles causes asthma and aggravates it in those who already have the condition. Both modes of involvement help the patient tremendously, and, according to the structural competency framework, there is no reason that medicine should participate in the former intervention and not the latter. As Metzl and Hansen frame it, many of the health conditions that providers treat "need to be understood as the sequellae of a host of financial, legal, governmental, and ultimately ethical decisions with which medicine must engage politically if it wishes to help its patients clinically."[50] They insist that "medicine has for too long located the clinical encounter as the primary site of politics."[51]

While the structural competency framework did not dethrone the cultural competence framework, it has been taught in some medical and nursing schools and residency programs,[52] usually as an adjunct or a subordinate to cultural competency. Additionally, structural competency has complicated the conversation that the medical and public health communities have been having around the social determinants of health (SDOH). The World Health Organization defines SDOH as "nonmedical factors that influence health outcomes."[53] These are "the conditions in which people are born, grow, work, live, and age, and the wider set of forces and systems shaping the conditions of daily life.[54] Essentially, SDOH refers to the structures that compromise, as well as conserve, health. In the early 2000s, interest in SDOH in the United States increased significantly, and the concept has become ubiquitous in the public health literature.[55] Physicians are also increasingly aware of the concept of SDOH. In fact, the standardized exam required for admission to medical school tests proficiency in SDOH.[56] However, some have begun to object to how SDOH is discussed. Writes one set of researchers, "many SDOH educational approaches in medicine focus on the lack of resources, rather than on systems and behaviors that perpetuate inequitable resource distribution."[57] In essence, SDOH has been deployed in a way that encourages people to think about structural inequities as the way things "just are." Some communities "just are" located in food deserts. Some neighborhoods "just are" situated next to highways. Some people "just are" employed in industries that "just are" toxic. Some groups "just are" unemployed and, consequently, lack health insurance. The structural competency framework insists on a more critical understanding of these phenomena by emphasizing that they are all the products of choices that have been made and policies that have been implemented. Things can be different. And structural competency maintains that the discipline of medicine can and should be at the forefront of efforts to change things.

THE RACIAL CONCORDANCE INTERVENTION

Racially concordant care recently has been introduced as a weapon in the fight against racial disparities in health. As chapter 3 explores, racial disparities in health are a function of many different factors. While patient–provider racial concordance (like implicit bias training and the cultural competency framework) is powerless to address racial disparities stemming from structural issues—namely, higher rates of poverty among black people, epigenetics, stress and weathering, and inferior quality of care provided at the level of the hospital—it (like implicit bias training and the cultural competency framework) can intervene in factors that operate at the level of the interpersonal. Specifically, black racially concordant care aims to improve black patients' health outcomes in three ways: by eliminating the opportunity for nonblack providers' biases to corrupt the quality of care that they give their black patients,[58] by increasing the likelihood that black patients will feel that they can trust their healthcare provider, and by improving the quality of the communication between patient and provider.

Research shows that antiblack implicit biases are pervasive in the United States—even among black people.[59] Because of the ways in which society has been organized and resources have been distributed, no one is immune from associating black people with negative characteristics. Research also shows, however, that black people—including black healthcare providers—are less likely than their nonblack counterparts to have antiblack implicit biases.[60] To the extent that provider implicit bias is a driver of increased mortality and morbidity among black people, racially concordant care helps to produce racial equity in outcomes by narrowing that pathway for inequity.

Studies have shown that, with respect to using provider–patient race concordance to increase patient trust and strengthen the channels of provider–patient communication, black patients are more likely to report that they trust black providers.[61] When there is trust, patients are more likely to follow their providers' advice and adhere to treatment regimens. Further, patients who trust their providers are more willing to share information—a "critical component of clinical care."[62] Further still, the improved communication made possible by racially concordant care is reciprocal. It flows from patient to provider as well as from provider to patient. As one set of researchers explains, "Physicians may communicate differently in medical encounters with racially, ethnically, or culturally concordant patients . . . Studies have found that . . . race-concordant visits lasted longer and include more affective communication by physicians."[63]

Even so, enhanced patient trust and increased levels of satisfaction with communication during racially concordant clinical encounters may be less meaningful if they do not lead to better clinical outcomes. So the million-dollar question is: Does being cared for by a black physician improve the black patient's health? Most studies have answered the question with a resounding "Maybe." Researchers who have conducted reviews of studies investigating whether racially concordant care improves clinical outcomes for black patients have concluded that the findings are decidedly mixed. One set of researchers surveyed the existing literature and determined that "[t]here is limited evidence that race concordance is associated with better health outcomes."[64] The theme uniting these studies is the inconclusiveness of the findings, with some studies showing improved outcomes for black patients with racially concordant care, and others showing none.[65] Some observers have proposed that the research has come back with mixed results because the efficacy of race concordance may be context-dependent.[66] It may be that race concordance matters in oncology but not in obstetrics; it might be meaningful in the emergency room but meaningless in the dialysis clinic.

However, some recent research provides evidence that race concordance in the clinical encounter does improve black patients' health outcomes—at least in the primary care physician's office. Researchers studying the effect of race concordance on clinical outcomes conducted an experiment in which they offered over a thousand black men in Oakland, California, a free health screening.[67] The study participants were shown pictures of the physician who would care for them that day and were asked whether they wanted additional cardiovascular screening services—a body mass index (BMI) measurement, a blood pressure measurement, a diabetes screening, and a cholesterol screening. The study participants then met with their physicians. Half were assigned to see a black physician, and the other half were assigned to see a nonblack physician. Among participants who initially declined additional cardiovascular screening services, those assigned to black physicians were more likely than those assigned to nonblack physicians to change their minds after talking with their physicians and to consent to those screenings. Essentially, *black physicians were more effective than nonblack physicians at convincing their black patients during the visit of the importance of such screenings.* Moreover, this effect was even more pronounced for the diabetes and cholesterol screenings—both of which involve a blood draw, unlike the BMI and blood pressure measurement. For these more invasive tests, which "carry more risk and thus likely require more trust in the person providing the service, only subjects assigned to black doctors responded[,] increasing their take-up of diabetes and cholesterol screenings by 20 and 26 percentage points . . . , respectively."[68]

The cardiovascular screenings offered in the study are well established to be lifesaving. They empower individuals with the knowledge they need to make changes in diet or lifestyle or to begin taking medication for hypertension, diabetes, or high cholesterol. The researchers estimated that if racially concordant care improves the uptake of these preventative screenings at the levels demonstrated in the study, and if such care were available to all black patients in the United States, then "black doctors would reduce mortality from cardiovascular disease by 16 deaths per 100,000, accounting for 19 percent of the black-white gap in cardiovascular mortality."[69] This would "add up to an 8 percent decline in the black–white male life expectancy gap."[70]

In a similar vein, economists Michael Frakes and Jonathan Gruber recently conducted a study that showed that black patients who received their care from black providers at military hospitals were more likely to adhere to treatment regimens for diabetes, high blood pressure, high cholesterol, and clogged arteries. They found that racially concordant care resulted in a "33% relative decline in mortality" for these conditions, leading them to conclude that "increased patient concordance could have a meaningful impact on the large racial mortality disparity in the U.S."[71]

Another recent study provides devastating support for the claim that racially concordant care improves black patients' clinical outcomes. This study investigated the effects of racial concordance on black newborns who had been hospitalized in the state of Florida between 1992 and 2015.[72] The researchers found that extremely sick, hospitalized black newborns were more likely to survive if black physicians cared for them: "Black infants experience inferior health outcomes regardless of who is treating them. However, clinical penalties for Black newborns treated by Black physicians are halved compared with penalties Black newborns experience when cared for by White physicians."[73] Further, the benefits of racially concordant care—indeed, its ability to save lives—were available to black babies without regard to socioeconomic status. Racially concordant care halved the mortality penalty for babies born to persons with Medicaid insurance as well to babies born to persons with commercial insurance.

Interestingly, the data showed that white newborns experienced no advantage or disadvantage under the care of black physicians. White babies' outcomes were the same with racially concordant and racially dissimilar care. Even more interestingly, while the data showed that racially concordant care reduces racial disparities in infant mortality, it did not provide evidence that racial concordance reduces racial disparities in *maternal* mortality. A recently postpartum black person was as likely to survive under the care of a black physician as under the care of a white physician. In this way, the study suggests that racially concordant care might be demanded in neonatology while not entirely necessary in obstetrics and gynecology.

One of the most gripping things about this study is that it demonstrates that the benefits of racially concordant care for the patients involved were not a function of the quality of patient–provider communication or the willingness of the patient to trust the provider's expertise and to adhere to prescribed treatment regimens. The patients were hospitalized *babies*, incapable of communication. Moreover, being hospitalized, the babies' care was unmediated by a third party—a parent or guardian—who could choose whether to follow the doctor's advice. In this way, the study provides evidence that if racially dissimilar care negatively affects black patients' clinical outcomes, it is not always due to something that the patient does. In some cases, the negative outcomes would be wholly attributable to the inferior care that nonblack providers deliver to their black patients.

So the evidence is mounting that racially concordant care can reduce rates of morbidity and mortality among black people.[74] However, even if institutions agreed to facilitate racially concordant care for black patients to increase their chances of having a positive health outcome—through racially concordant care clinics or other mechanisms that formalize the means by which a black patient can select a black provider—universal race concordance for black patients would be impossible to achieve for many years. And this is simply because black people are underrepresented among physicians, nurses, and other professionals who provide clinical care. While black people presently comprise 13 percent of the population in the United States, they constitute less than 6 percent of physicians[75] and about 11 percent of registered nurses.[76] Only 23 percent of black people have a black physician.[77] Moreover, black people's underrepresentation in medicine is worsening[78]—allowing us to predict that the percentage of black patients with black providers will decrease as black people's underrepresentation in medicine increases.[79]

Observers once proposed that institutions should respond to black people's underrepresentation in medicine by working to increase the number of black students who apply to, are accepted to, and graduate from medical school.[80] However, the legal and political landscape has shifted such that it is no longer clear that such efforts are permitted under federal law. In 2023, the United States Supreme Court decided *Students for Fair Admissions, Inc. v. Harvard* (*SFFA*), ruling that the race-based affirmative action programs instituted by Harvard College and the University of North Carolina violated the United States Constitution and Title VI of the Civil Rights Act, which prohibits educational institutions that receive federal funds from discriminating on the basis of race. While the Court refrained from holding that race-based affirmative action is always impermissible, the decision required institutions that implement race-conscious admissions programs to provide data about the benefits generated by their programs that will be impossible for most institutions to produce. The effect of *SFFA* is to prohibit all colleges and universities in the country—including medical schools—from administering race-based affirmative action programs.

As a technical matter, *SFFA* applies only to the college and university admissions process, when institutions determine which students will be accepted into an incoming class. However, the logic of the decision is much broader. The undeniable thrust of the opinion is that whatever racial inequities exist in the nation today should be addressed—if they are addressed at all—through colorblind courses of action. This is a decidedly political position—a position that the Constitution itself does not demand—that critical scholars of race have challenged and rejected for at least half a century.

SFFA leaves efforts to increase the number of black people in medicine and nursing on shaky legal ground. First, the decision effectively prohibits medical and nursing schools from increasing the number of black (and Latine and Native) students in their incoming classes by considering race during the admissions process. Second, *SFFA* suggests the illegality of race-conscious efforts to create pipelines to careers in medicine and nursing for black elementary, high school, and college students—especially if those efforts target black, Latine, and Native students to the exclusion of white and Asian students. Additionally, the legality of race-based efforts to increase the number of black people in medicine is a different question from their political plausibility. The United States has entered an era where interest in addressing inequities along the lines of race, class, sex, sexuality, gender identity, and ability is derided as "woke." Even if race-conscious efforts to address the underrepresentation of black people in medicine and nursing were legal, many institutions may find them politically inadvisable. As such, racially concordant healthcare will likely remain only a pipe dream for most black people.

CRITIQUES OF THE FORMALIZATION OF RACIALLY CONCORDANT CARE

Some of the critiques that have been levied against the pursuit of race concordance in clinical care come from the unusual suspects—from critics who stand at the ready to label any race-conscious effort that addresses existing racial inequality as "reverse discrimination" against white people. However, other criticism comes from places that are more unexpected—from people who would self-identify as liberals with progressive politics. The balance of the chapter looks at these critiques from the left.

Racially Concordant Care Essentializes Identity

Some observers worry that institutionalizing racially concordant care—whether through specialty clinics like the Black Wellbeing Clinic at Golden Health or through formalized methods that allow patients to select same-race providers when receiving care within a healthcare institution—will essentialize identity. They fear that that institutionalized racially concordant care will be interpreted as saying that race is the only aspect of a person that matters. They are concerned that the pursuit of patient–provider race concordance will reduce the complexity of individuals to a single facet of themselves.

Psychiatrist and researcher Helen-Maria Lekas has articulated this anxiety, writing that when healthcare institutions allow patients to select providers on the basis of race, such programs "risk reifying an assumption that matched Black people will share certain innate understandings of one another, be it of socioeconomic status, language, preferences for clinical care, and so on."[81] She argues that "even a matching program that is based on careful thinking can appear to erase the internal diversity of Black people."[82]

But Lekas's critique may misidentify the assumptions about race that motivate efforts like the Black Wellbeing Clinic, and it may fail to take into account how patients and providers who elect to participate in such efforts conceptualize the enterprise. Programs that facilitate race concordance in clinical care need not be motivated by the idea that an individual's race is the only thing that matters. Rather, such programs often are motivated by the idea that an individual's race is *one of many things* that matter. Further, when patients opt into receiving care in such a program, we can assume that they believe that race is one of their innumerable attributes that matter to them during the clinical encounter. The same is true for the provider who opts into providing care in such a program. The literature calls this racial identity salience and racial identity centrality:

> Racial identity salience explores how much [a person] considers race an important aspect of their self-concept at a particular moment in time. It is dependent on the context of the situation. . . . Racial identity centrality, on the other hand, measures how important race is to a person's perception of themselves. It is concerned with the extent to which a person normally defines themselves in relationship to their race.[83]

The concept of racial identity centrality proposes that for some individuals, their race is significant to them and for others, their race is insignificant. A program that facilitates racially concordant care should be taken to assume only that racial identity is essential to *some* black people, not *all* black people. Further, the concept of racial identity salience proposes that in some contexts, an individual's race will be highly meaningful, and, in other contexts, it will be meaningless. A program that facilitates racially concordant care should be taken to assume only that racial identity is relevant to some black people *during clinical healthcare encounters.*

When racial identity is central to people or when it is salient to them during the clinical encounter, it seems unkind not to allow them to seek care that is mindful of that aspect of their identity. Moreover, it seems unkind *and* absurd to prevent patients from receiving racially concordant care because a third party believes that a program that facilitates such care in a healthcare institution "erase[s] the internal diversity of Black people."[84] People misunderstand things all the time. And some people will probably misunderstand a program that formalizes the acquisition of racially concordant care in a physician group, hospital, or health system. Some people will mistake it as declaring that race is the only facet of a person that is relevant during the clinical encounter and that it always matters to members of the racial group. But those people will be wrong. Programs that allow patients to receive racially concordant healthcare simply assert that race matters to some patients when they are navigating healthcare systems.

Further, the patients who spoke with me at Golden Health's Black Wellbeing Clinic did not believe that a provider's blackness guaranteed that the patient–provider relationship would be a good one. Instead, most patients electing to receive care through the Black Wellbeing Clinic thought that a provider's blackness did no more than increase the likelihood that they would have a positive experience. Again, no black patient with whom I talked assumed that black providers possessed no differences from them in terms of background, worldview, socioeconomic status, or nationality that might produce challenges during the clinical encounter. Indeed, no black patient that I interviewed believed that provider blackness was a trait that would invariably generate certain experiences and produce certain outcomes—a belief that would be consistent with a problematic conceptualization of race as something that, when shared, promised "certain innate understandings" of the other person.[85] All of the patients talked about race as a lever that, if manipulated, might—or might not—work to their advantage on the way to childbirth.

The experience of Isra, a thirty-four-year-old graphic designer who was pregnant with her first child when I met her at the Black Wellbeing Clinic, exemplifies this. Isra, who was raised in Chicago, had moved to the Bay Area after living in New York City for a decade. She had become accustomed to thinking of doctors' visits as unpleasant occasions because, like so many women in the United States, her body had been criticized frequently during her childhood, adolescence, and young adulthood:

> We had a family doctor when I was growing up. I believe he was Indian. Every time I think of my interactions with him, there was always a lot of focus on my weight. And so I was super conscious about it as a young kid. I was always active—always played sports. I always ate well. But I went through puberty super early. I was much taller than everybody else. I got all the things before everybody. [laughs] And nobody ever really made me feel like that was okay.

Isra moved to Manhattan in her twenties to pursue a career in fashion, and her experience of going to the doctor in New York City was similar to many New Yorkers' experiences of healthcare. She explained, laughingly, "I had spent ten years in New York just doing ZocDoc. Whoever had an opening, I would jump on the train, and then come back to work. So I was kind of hopping around."

Isra eventually relocated to the Bay Area after accepting a job at Google, and she decided to take advantage of the medical care offered on Google's campus as an employee benefit. She received care from a black woman physician there, Dr. Elliott—the first black provider that Isra had had in her life:

> It was such a great experience. I never knew that I needed that. . . . At my first appointment with her, we started talking—about my weight, my activity level, my diet. And it was the first time that a doctor was like, "Yeah, you're perfectly healthy. You're okay." And I was stunned. Nobody had ever said that before. It had always been, "You're not doing this," or "You should be doing

that." And Dr. Elliott was just like, "You're doing great. You're healthy. There's nothing wrong with you." I just broke down crying. I didn't realize how many years I had been waiting to hear somebody tell me that.

Isra did not attribute her positive experience with Dr. Elliott to the physician's blackness. Instead, she attributed it to the fact that Dr. Elliott "talked to [her] like [she] was a person." Isra asked, "Is that because she was black? No. I think that's just who she was." Isra's experience with Dr. Elliott led her to alter her expectations around healthcare. So when Isra became pregnant, she decided to seek out care that was more than just fine. She sought care that actually felt good.

Isra's affirming experience with Dr. Elliott is helpful for thinking about the critique that programs that facilitate racially concordant care essentialize identity. For Isra, Dr. Elliott was wonderful because that is "just who she was"—not because she was black. Nevertheless, Isra decided to receive her prenatal care from Golden's Black Wellbeing Clinic because she felt that having a black provider would increase the likelihood of being related to in a way that would nourish her.

Black patients who sought care from black providers in the Black Wellbeing Clinic—of whom Isra is representative—were under no illusions that racially concordant care would ensure that they would have a positive clinical encounter. They did not think that having a black midwife or obstetrician meant that they would experience no miscommunications, slights, or pregnancy complications. Instead, the patients who spoke with me talked in terms of likelihoods and probabilities. They believed that the *odds* of having a provider who understood their needs would increase if the provider was black. They believed that there was a *greater chance* that a black provider would be attentive to and empathize with their concerns. They believed that a black physician would be *more likely* to advocate on their behalf in the labor and delivery room. That is, black patients choosing racially concordant care were trading in statistics. They understood that there were no guarantees. They sought racially concordant care to improve their prospects of achieving the outcomes that they most valued—a safe (if not fun) pregnancy, a respectful (if not empowering) labor and childbirth, and, above all, a healthy baby.

Racially Concordant Care Offloads Responsibility for Eliminating Racial Disparities in Health onto Black Providers

A more compelling critique of racially concordant care for black patients is that it burdens black providers with the task of reducing racial disparities in health. While black physicians, nurses, and other health professionals do the work of protecting black patients from the racism that is embedded within medicine and our healthcare institutions, nonblack providers can continue with business as usual—never having to confront the role that they have played in black people's poorer health outcomes.[86]

It is important to observe that many black providers welcome the "burden" of caring for black patients as a way to protect them from racism. This is certainly true of the black providers who worked in Golden Health's Black Wellbeing Clinic. They all were there because they were aware of what anthropologist Dána-Ain Davis calls "obstetric racism"—a form of "gender-based violence" that "emerges specifically in reproductive care and places Black women and their infants at risk."[87] The black providers at the Black Wellbeing Clinic offered themselves as shields against obstetric racism and foot soldiers in the struggle to decrease the rates of mortality and morbidity among black birthing people in the United States. Other studies have confirmed what I observed firsthand at Golden's Black Wellbeing Clinic. A study of black women pursuing careers in midwifery found that participants conceptualized themselves and the services that they eventually would provide to pregnant patients of color "as critical resistance to the influences of racism and other oppressive forces on individual care and within health systems. . . . [T]hey saw their pursuit of midwifery as one way to mitigate the pain and suffering in their community in a more immediate way."[88]

Not all black healthcare providers welcome the burden of caring for black patients, however. This is demonstrated by a conflict that occurred in Golden's labor and delivery department during my fieldwork. With the best of intentions, the white nurse manager started assigning admitted black patients to the black nurses as a matter of course. This affronted some of the black nurses—in part because they had to care for black patients in addition to nonblack patients. Caring for black patients required additional labor from them that their nonblack nurse counterparts did not have to expend. However, other black nurses were displeased with this arrangement not because it required them to work harder than nonblack nurses but rather because they did not want others to think of them in terms of their racial identities when they were not thinking of themselves that way. When talking with me about the conflict, Dr. Clark mused, "Black people deal with racism in different ways. And some of the black nurses are dealing with it by refusing to think about their race while they're at work. Can we blame them? Of course not. Racism is awful. And black people are not all the same. We have to respect that difference as they deal with the awfulness of racism." (Chapter 5 ends with a look at black people who deal with the awfulness of racism by declining to conceptualize race and racism as significant—a phenomenon that I call racial renunciation.)

It is probably not surprising that some people's sense of justice is offended when the individuals and the communities that have been harmed are charged with the duty of fixing the harm. As Lekas puts it, "Assigning the task of rectifying our racist, sexist, classist, and heteronormative health care system solely to Black physicians is unfair."[89] Indeed, it strikes many people as unfair that institutions have turned to black providers to deliver racially concordant care to black patients as the solution to the racial disparities in health that the institutions helped perpetuate.

We might draw an analogy to the way that doulas—unregulated, medically untrained, oftentimes poorly compensated birth workers who support and advocate for the pregnant person during labor and delivery—have been seen as the answer to black people's poor maternal health outcomes in the United States. Feminist scholar Jennifer Nash has brilliantly critiqued this positioning of doula care. There is compelling evidence demonstrating that doula-supported pregnant persons have better health outcomes than those who do not have doula support during labor and delivery: "Various analyses and theoretical models investigating improved outcomes associated with doula-supported births have concluded that women with doula care have lower odds of unindicated cesarean births and preterm births."[90] Moreover, those with doula care are more likely to initiate breastfeeding,[91] which can improve infant health outcomes. In response to this evidence, many states have turned to doulas as the way to address the black maternal health crisis in the United States by, for example, covering the cost of doula care under state Medicaid programs. Nash writes:

> The state has increasingly latched on to doulas . . . as the solution to the problem of Black maternal and infant death. Yet the outsourcing of care to nonmedical staff (and to those who explicitly reject medicalization . . .) can seem a troubling solution to a problem that unfolds in medicalized spaces and implicates institutionalized medicine. Put differently, if doulas are the bodies mobilized by the state to save Black women's lives, what does it mean that they are not required to be licensed or credentialed, that many are minimally trained? . . . We [should] ask how the state's embrace of doulas' fugitive and paraprofessional practices might actually stand as evidence of the state's deep divestment in Black maternal health.[92]

Unlike doulas, the black physicians and nurses who care for black patients in racially concordant dyads are licensed, credentialed, and well trained. Nevertheless, we might ask an analogue of the question that Nash poses: What does it mean when institutions turn to black providers as the solution to the inequitable care that black patients have received from those who are supposed to help safeguard their health? What does it mean for society to leave in place all of the toxic systems that have compromised the health of people of color while looking to black providers as the preferred way to save black lives? *How is the embrace of racially concordant care as the solution to racial disparities in health actually evidence of the nation's deep divestment in black health?*

In order to defend racially concordant care as a means to address racial disparities in health—as more than a way for nonblack actors, the state, and society to offload responsibility for fixing inequities in the healthcare system—it has to be just one prong in a multipronged effort to combat these disparities. If black people are sicker and die earlier than their white counterparts because of structural issues, then we have to tackle those structural problems *in addition* to offering black patients the option of racially concordant care.

Further, if racial disparities in health result, in part, from deficiencies in the interactions between patient and provider during the clinical encounter, then we need to address those deficiencies alongside offering racially concordant care to black patients. As chapter 3 explains, antiblack implicit biases might lead nonblack clinicians to offer inferior care to their black patients. Additionally, black patients may mistrust healthcare actors and institutions and consequently refuse to share clinically relevant information about themselves or follow treatment regimens and the advice of their providers. If these defects in the clinical encounter contribute to racial disparities in health, then they should be addressed in conjunction with pursuing the racially concordant care intervention. If providers' antiblack implicit biases contaminate the quality of the care that they give their black patients, then, as chapter 3 proposes, the most effective, just solution would be to reorganize society so that it would be irrational for individuals to associate black people with negative qualities and behaviors. If black patient mistrust is making it difficult for their healers to heal them, then we have to make healthcare actors and institutions trustworthy. In short, black providers cannot be left holding the bag. The actors and institutions that created the harm must also be fully engaged in undoing the damage that antiblackness has wrought.

Racially Concordant Care Produces Segregated Spaces

About three months before Golden Health opened the Black Wellbeing Clinic, Nancy—the kind and competent manager of the obstetrics clinic at Golden's East Hills campus—asked me to meet with her in her sunny office to discuss a recent incident involving two employees who often seemed to be in conflict. (This incident began when one employee, a white woman, saw the other employee, a black woman, disinfecting her own workstation and said that she wanted the black woman to "come and clean my house." The black employee filed a formal complaint.) After Nancy and I discussed the episode, we began talking about a number of other things. Eventually, our conversation landed on the topic of the new Black Wellbeing Clinic, which was generating a lot of interest at Golden. I told Nancy, who was racially ambiguous, that I was excited about the clinic and that Golden was going to be at the forefront of the movement for institutionalized racially concordant care. I was surprised when Nancy did not share my enthusiasm: "I don't know how to feel about it! If you take all the black providers and black staff and black patients and put them all in one place, what does that do to the other places? If we go this route, we are creating segregated spaces. And we all know the good things that come from diversity. I'm just worried about what we are going to lose when we separate black people from everyone else."

Nancy was not the only one at Golden—a proudly progressive institution in a historically liberal city in a vividly blue state—who expressed concerns about the new clinic. After the Black Wellbeing Clinic opened and was seeing patients, I spoke to Charlotte, the manager of the obstetrics clinic at Golden's Yerba Buena campus, where the Black Wellbeing Clinic was housed. Charlotte, an affable white woman, was always a blur, constantly moving, putting out proverbial fires. One morning as I was talking to the intake worker at the front desk, Charlotte hurried by. She paused to tell me that she was thrilled that I was able to see the Black Wellbeing Clinic in action. She then lowered her voice and said, "Some people might say, 'When you're creating this separate clinic, what are you doing to the general clinic? You're segregating everyone.'" She continued, a little louder, "But that's not a reason not to do it. Because what we have been doing hasn't been working for black patients." Clearly, Charlotte had spoken with people who, like Nancy, were worried about the effect that the Black Wellbeing Clinic would have on the racial demographics of other spaces in Golden's health system.

The concern that racially concordant care clinics create segregated spaces is quite intriguing because the unease is *not* that such clinics are both ineffective and create segregated spaces. Rather, the unease is that such clinics, simply, create segregated spaces—separating black people from everyone else. In this way, the critique assumes the efficacy of racially concordant care. It seems to acknowledge that black patients have better experiences and improved health outcomes when black providers care for them. But it remains interested in the clinic's effect on *everyone else*—all the nonblack people who will miss out on interactions with black people. It may be worth making plain how these critiques of racially concordant care clinics are striking the balance. On the one hand, these clinics might decrease the rates of black morbidity and mortality. On the other hand, these clinics might deprive nonblack people of the opportunity to interact with black people. Some critics seem willing to elevate nonblack people's ability to intermingle with black people over black people's health and lives. The prioritization is revealing.

Nancy's comment about "all the good things that come from diversity" invite us to put the critique that race concordance clinics create segregated spaces into conversation with the debate over race-based affirmative action. Since the Supreme Court's 1978 decision in *Regents of the University of California v. Bakke*, proponents have defended race-conscious admissions programs that seek to increase the numbers of nonwhite students in the incoming classes of colleges and universities by arguing that such efforts pursue the goal of diversity. Prior to *Bakke*, however, proponents used the language of remedy to defend these programs. These supporters argued that they were a way to remedy the effects of past and present societal discrimination against historically marginalized racial groups.[93] Indeed, remedy was the language used by the activists involved in the civil rights movement in the 1950s and 1960s when they demanded that institutions implement race-based affirmative action programs.[94] They observed that the United States had constructed a racial caste system that deprived black people of social, political, and economic power and that needed to be dismantled. Further, they demanded the implementation of programs that could move black people into the arenas of social life from which they had been formally excluded and, in so doing, help repair the injuries that had been inflicted on them. At its inception, that is what race-based affirmative action was imagined to be—a means to remedy a harm and, as such, a way to pursue racial justice.

In *Bakke*, the Court struck down the race-based affirmative action program at the medical school at University of California, Davis, and ordered the admission of a white applicant who claimed that his rights under federal law were violated when the school designated sixteen out of one hundred seats in the incoming class for black, Latine, Asian, and Native students.[95] Justice Powell wrote an opinion whose reasoning eventually became the law of the land twenty-five years later, when a majority of the Court endorsed it in the 2003 case of *Grutter v. Bollinger*. Justice Powell argued that race-based affirmative action programs were unconstitutional when schools implemented them as a remedy for historical societal discrimination. Rejecting the rationale for such programs that had been embraced by the civil rights activists who had risked their lives to make the country fulfill the commitments contained in its own founding documents, Justice Powell argued that "societal discrimination" was "an amorphous concept of injury that may be ageless in its reach into the past."[96] If schools administered such programs, Justice Powell argued that they should pursue them from a platform that, to him, was more concrete. He found that platform in diversity. He concluded that race-based affirmative action programs were permissible when schools implemented them in order to pursue the educational benefits that flow from student body diversity. In this way, Justice Powell altered the official terms of the debate about affirmative action We could no longer talk about such programs as efforts to address racism or racial inequality. We could not claim—at least not in any official capacity—that these programs were attempts to achieve some modicum of racial justice in a nation that was finally coming to terms with its centuries-long history of formal racial disenfranchisement and dispossession. Instead, we could only declare that such programs should be permitted because without them, student bodies would not be diverse, and diversity is good for students.

On the whole, critical scholars of race found the diversity rationale to be deeply unsatisfying—even though they believed that racial diversity in a classroom produces educational benefits and that diversity is good for students.[97] Critics objected that the diversity rationale shifted the focus from students of color and their inherited disadvantages to white students who would benefit from the students of color who would be present in classrooms by virtue of race-based affirmative action programs.[98] Consider that in making the case for the importance of student body diversity, the *Grutter* majority opinion claimed that "classroom discussion is livelier, more spirited, and simply more enlightening and interesting" when the students have "the greatest possible variety of backgrounds."[99] If we look closely, we will see that this framing centers white students. Without race-based affirmative action, white students would be present in the classroom and having these discussions—among themselves and with those subgroups of Asian students who excel when evaluated solely with traditional indicia of merit, like standardized test scores, grades, and extracurricular activities. However, with the admission of black, Latine, and Native students, the discussions that white students would have in the classrooms in which they would already be present will be "livelier, more spirited, and simply more enlightening and interesting." In this way, race-based affirmative action figures as good for white people.

And this is why critical scholars of race have found the diversity rationale as a justification for race-consciousness in admissions to be maddening. When race-based affirmative action was defended in terms of the benefits that would accrue to racially disadvantaged students who would now have access to educational opportunities that would otherwise be unavailable to them, a majority of Supreme Court justices was unwilling to sanction it. However, when race-based affirmative action was defended in terms of the benefits that would accrue to white people, a majority of justices, at least for a period of time, was willing to deem it constitutional.

Hence it is fascinating that Nancy that would be ambivalent about a clinic that offers black patients racially concordant care because of a concern that it will create segregated spaces and deny the hospital "all the good things that come from diversity." We have to ask, "Who benefits from diversity? Who reaps all these good things that diversity engenders?" If racially concordant care improves black patients' outcomes and helps to save black lives (which some recent studies show), then it becomes hard to say that, in this context, diversity benefits black patients. Instead, diversity appears to benefit nonblack people—the nonblack patients in the waiting room with the black patient, the nonblack medical assistants who take the black patient's vitals before they meet with their provider, the nonblack physicians, nurses, or midwives who provide the black patient's care that day—who get to interact with black people. As in the affirmative action context, black people's needs are decentered, and the experiences of nonblack people are prioritized. Indeed, the higher rates of morbidity and mortality that black people endure when cared for in racially dissimilar clinical encounters becomes a price that some people are willing to pay for the benefits of diversity.

Analogizing racially concordant care to race-based affirmative action is instructive for another reason. Like race-based affirmative action, healthcare facilities that offer institutionalized racially concordant care may be on uncertain legal ground. As explained above, the Court's decision in *Students for Fair Admissions* (*SFFA*) announced the Court's preference for interpreting the Constitution to mandate colorblindness from institutions. While the decision did not officially reverse *Grutter*'s holding that a school's pursuit of the educational benefits that flow from student body diversity may save its race-conscious admissions program from unconstitutionality, the evidence that it required schools to produce to establish the legality of their affirmative action programs will make it impossible for most schools to administer such programs. As Justice Thomas announced in his concurring opinion in *SFFA*, the majority opinion "makes clear that *Grutter* is, for all intents and purposes, overruled."[100]

The meaning of *SFFA* with respect to hospitals and health systems that offer racially concordant care clinics is unclear. On the one hand, the case could mean nothing. Because the Court's decision, as a technical matter, applies solely to college and university admissions programs, it may not constrain other institutions, like hospitals or health systems, that engage in race-conscious efforts to produce a social good—like improved health outcomes among patients of color.

On the other hand, *SFFA* could be quite meaningful to hospitals and health systems that offer racially concordant care clinics. A majority of current Supreme Court justices believes that the Constitution requires actors and institutions to be colorblind. This logic—and political commitment—makes racially concordant care clinics vulnerable to legal challenge. Vulnerable is the health system that cares for a nonblack patient who believes that the existence of such a clinic makes it more difficult for her to secure an appointment. Vulnerable is the health system that employs a nonblack provider or staff person who feels that their inability to work in such a clinic constitutes reverse discrimination. Vulnerable is the health system that employs a black provider or staff person who feels that any additional labor that is shunted their way is a function of such a clinic's existence and, therefore, a form of racial discrimination against them. Vulnerable is the health system that becomes the target of a "watchdog" organization that is convinced, or sincerely hopes, that such a clinic runs afoul of existing law.[101] The health system may find itself in court, defending itself and its innovation against the tide of colorblindness that is flooding the federal judiciary and the country.

* * *

If institutionalized racially concordant care becomes a legal impossibility, healthcare providers would likely return to implicit bias trainings, cultural competence workshops, and DEI initiatives as the preferred methods for addressing racial disparities in health. For all of the reasons explored in this book, these interventions have been problematic and unsatisfactory. Indeed, many critical thinkers of race have found them to be boring, at best. That said, a simple return to past uninspired techniques for addressing racial disparities in health may be impossible.

After the brutal murder of George Floyd by the police in May 2020, protesters took to the street in numbers that recalled the world-shattering days of the civil rights movement of the mid-twentieth century, and the nation began to undergo what optimists at the time called a "racial reckoning." However, the protests provoked an angry racial backlash, which was initially executed under the banner of a war against "critical race theory." Within months of the protests, conservative politicians, pundits, and laypersons adopted and distorted the term "critical race theory", which for forty years prior to that summer had referred to a body of literature that analyzed the relationship between law and persisting racial inequality in the post–civil rights era. Like the word "woke," which was coopted and weaponized soon thereafter, conservatives used the term "critical race theory" to describe any talk about race that they did not like. Importantly, the architects of the racial backlash that began in 2020 identified efforts like employer-led implicit bias trainings as examples of the "critical race theory" that was damaging American society and preventing racial progress.[102] The campaigns eventually turned to eliminating so-called critical race theory from the curriculum in K–12 schools. Over time, DEI programs were swept up into the maelstrom of the racial backlash, as politically conservative actors attempted to make it illegal for institutions to express any concern about individuals from historically or currently marginalized groups who found themselves within the institutions' walls.[103] One member of Congress—a medical doctor, no less—sought to deny federal funding to medical schools that undertook DEI efforts.[104]

The racial regression that the United States has been undergoing since the nation's "racial reckoning" in 2020 imperils not only the more assertive efforts (like racially concordant care clinics) that we might pursue to save black lives but also the more cautious efforts that have been pursued for decades. As proof, the Medical Board of California has been sued by challengers who seek to eliminate the requirement that physicians receive one hour of implicit bias training.[105] These are bewildering times. As one set of researchers summarized it, "Calls to action for trainings that promote the delivery of equitable care are as urgent as ever. However, they will fall short if the sociopolitical climate continues to devalue racial/ethnic diversity and if policies that penalize institutions for engaging in academic activities to address systemic racism, promote equity, and embrace antiracism are allowed to stand."[106] In these dim lights, the future looks bleak.

Conclusion: If We Really Cared—How to Solve the Black Maternal Health Crisis

The solution to the tragic, embarrassing state of black maternal health in the United States is not to leave it to individuals to buy their way to a healthy pregnancy and a safe childbirth and postpartum period. When the government in a country as wealthy and powerful as the United States sees its citizens and residents dying wholly preventable deaths and does little more than wish them good luck in finding and purchasing the goods and services in the market that may help them survive, it abdicates its responsibilities and loses legitimacy.

If we are looking for solutions to the black maternal health crisis in the United States, we will quickly notice that the delivery of healthcare in this country is, to put it plainly, odd. It is peculiar that healthcare in the United States is a profit-making, billion-dollar industry. It is strange that some people—like CEOs of health systems and high-level executives at health insurance companies—accumulate massive amounts of wealth from the delivery of something that many reasonable people around the world believe to be a human right. The profit motive that underlies healthcare in the United States leads the actors animating the system to make decisions that are not health-affirming. Performing a Caesarian section is more lucrative than waiting for a labor to progress without pharmaceutical or surgical intervention. Providing lifesaving medical care to a preterm infant in the neonatal intensive care unit is more profitable than sending a healthy baby home with its parents. Ensuring that its patient population consists primarily of commercially insured patients is more financially rewarding for a health system than focusing on providing healthcare to vulnerable (that is, uninsured and

Medicaid-insured) people. When these types of profit-maximizing decisions are made in a country that has never come to terms with its horrific racial past, black people will suffer from these health-compromising choices more frequently than their nonblack counterparts. To eradicate racial disparities in maternal mortality and morbidity, we might begin by eliminating the profit motive that undergirds the provision of healthcare in the United States. Doing so would make pregnancy safer for *all* people in the country today.

Our pursuit of an answer to the long-standing black maternal health crisis will also likely lead us to notice that the nation's two-tier healthcare system is similarly odd. It is, again, peculiar that in a country that purports to value equality (indeed, the Fourteenth Amendment of the Constitution states that people under its jurisdiction are entitled to "equal protection of the laws"), some hospitals cater to people with jobs that offer health insurance as a benefit and other hospitals are left to care for everyone else. Further, it is commonly understood that the healthcare dispensed on the lower, public tier is inferior to that dispensed on the upper, private tier. To eradicate racial disparities in maternal mortality and morbidity, we should create a system where income or wealth does not determine where people go when they need to see a doctor. As it stands, the inequality that lies at the foundation of the United States' healthcare system functions to reaffirm racial inequality.

To eliminate racial disparities in maternal mortality and morbidity, we, of course, need to take racism seriously. Racism is killing black people. It does this not only when a black man is murdered by police in broad daylight or when hundreds of thousands of black people are warehoused in the nation's prisons and jails. Racism kills when it causes epigenetic changes in fetuses that are not yet born. It kills when these epigenetic changes are transmitted to the next generation, creating a heritable trait out of the damage that racism inflicts. Further, racism kills when it is experienced as chronic stress that causes body systems to deteriorate prematurely. To make the perinatal period as safe for black people as it is for their nonblack peers, we should make it so that black people do not feel like they are entering a hostile environment when they go to work, drive their cars, shop at the grocery store, walk their dogs, turn on the TV, go online, or simply wake up in the morning while black in the United States.

And then there is the interpersonal. The inferior care that black people have received from the professionals who are charged with protecting their health contributes to racial disparities in maternal health outcomes. But this contributor will not be eliminated by compelling providers to take an implicit association test at some point in their medical or nursing education or by making health professionals sit through a workshop on "black culture." It will be eliminated when providers are no longer incorrectly taught that black people are genetically distinct from nonblack people or that they have kidneys, lungs, brains, hearts, and nerve endings that are biologically different from those that their nonblack counterparts possess.[1] And crucially, this contributor will be eliminated when society is reorganized in a way that makes it irrational to associate black people—consciously or unconsciously—with negative characteristics. We could create a country where black race does not correlate with poverty, welfare dependence, criminality, sickness, or early death. In such a world, we likely would not have to worry about antiblack implicit and explicit biases corrupting the quality of the care that providers deliver to their black patients. If we made different policy choices, we would see different things.

Finally, to the extent that black patients' mistrust of healthcare providers and institutions contributes to racial disparities in maternal mortality and morbidity, the solution is not to attempt to persuade black people to place their trust in their doctors and nurses. Instead, the solution is to recognize that medical distrust is a rational response to institutions and professionals who demonstrate again and again that they are not to be trusted. The solution is to make these institutions and providers worthy of black people's trust.

* * *

It might seem fanciful to lay out such a grand program in a country that, at this political moment, seems hellbent on undoing the racial progress that has been achieved over the last few decades. Even so, all things—including racial backlashes—must end. When this current political era of racial retrenchment finally comes to a close, we will first count the bodies of those who needlessly died. And then we must begin again the work of creating a country that is worthy of the people who never gave up hope.

Acknowledgments

I have been dreaming about this book for well over a decade. The fact that it now exists is proof that dreams really do come true.

This book would not have been possible without all of the people at Golden Health who helped me get permission to conduct my research at the institution. I truly regret that the necessity for anonymity prevents me from thanking them by name. Thanks are owed as well to the physicians, nurses, midwives, medical assistants, ultrasound technicians, lactation consultants, clinic managers, call center agents, and front desk workers who let me hang out with them and observe them. A very special thank-you to that one nurse who helped me recruit the majority of the patients that I interviewed on the East Hills campus. Most of all, I am endlessly thankful for the pregnant and recently postpartum folks who shared their stories with me. I am grateful for their generosity, vulnerability, and honesty.

Because of this book's long gestation period (pun intended), I have had the opportunity to present the ideas contained in this work as well as portions of the manuscript dozens of times—including at conferences, faculty workshops, and speaking engagements at Cleveland State University College of Law, Cornell Law School, Durham University, Emory University, Princeton University, San Francisco State University, Tulane University, UCLA School of Law, UC Law at San Francisco, the University of Edinburgh, the University of Illinois at Chicago, the University of Kentucky, the University of Leeds, the University of Maryland, the University of Michigan Law School, the University of Washington, Washington University in St. Louis,

Yale Law School, and Yale Medical School. I am thankful for all of the people in these varied audiences who offered insights, affirmations, critiques, and challenges.

I owe a debt of gratitude to Yuvraj Joshi, Osagie Obasogie, and Marc Spindelman for their invaluable feedback on several chapters of the book. Thanks also to the anonymous reviewers who offered such helpful critiques of the manuscript.

I feel so lucky to work at UC Berkeley School of Law. My colleagues are truly extraordinary. I thank them for inspiring me and for always being willing to engage with my ideas and to improve the quality of my scholarship. I am especially thankful for Erwin Chemerinsky, who has been such a wonderful boss and steadfast supporter.

I am indebted to the brilliant, diligent folks in the Berkeley Law Library who supported my research for this book—particularly Douglas Avila, Ramona Collins, Edna Lee Lewis, Dean Rowan, and I-Wei Wang. I am grateful for the army of research assistants who helped me bring this book to the world: Arni Daroy, Juliette Draper, Kennedy Edwards, Taylor Fox, Clemencia Garcia-Kasimirowski, Natalie Daniella Giron, Ortal Isaac, Simone Lieban Levine, Jacob Antonio Lusk, Hayley MacMillen, Roberto Prates, Samira Seraji, Alyssa Young, Everett Zhao, Ianna Zhu, and Amelia Zoernig. I am also thankful for my students, who are so very unsatisfied with the status quo. I thank them for insisting upon changing the world and for giving me reason for optimism.

Thanks to Matthew Browne, my original editor at the MIT Press, for his enthusiasm about this project. Thanks to Janice Audet and everyone at the MIT Press for bringing the book across the finish line. I am indebted to Jenny Stephens, my literary agent, for blowing my mind by suggesting that I write a book that speaks to audiences outside of the academy.

I am grateful for my private world. Thanks are owed to Dr. Leanh Nguyen for being the most insightful person I know. Thanks to my friends for loving me—flaws and all. I am thankful for my extended family for their unconditional love. I thank my parents-in-law, Mams and Paps, for making me a part of their cozy, little family—and for bringing Nelson and then Babs into my life. Thanks as well to my brother and sister, Khari Bridges and Algeria Bridges, for being a constant, comforting presence throughout my entire life—from the days of our childhood, when we put together (top-tier, high-quality) shows for our parents, to today, when things get loud and rambunctious at Family Game Night. I am also grateful for my brother-in-law, Dave McLeod, for making Family Game Night louder than it otherwise would be. I owe a special debt of gratitude to my Uncle J, Dr. James Bridges, for kicking down doors and being so proud of me when I follow him through them. And words fail when I try to describe my appreciation for my parents, Clive R. Bridges and Deborah A. Bridges. My father is the kindest, sweetest, funniest person I know, and I am so incredibly fortunate to be his Baby Bear. My mother taught me how to be audacious, fearless, and confident. (She also taught me that it's okay to laugh *hard* at your own jokes.) Thank you, Mama and Daddy, for loving me perfectly.

Finally, thank you to Gert Reynaert. I could not have done any of this without you. When you met me that night at the Beehive, did you think that we would build the adventure-filled, laughter-filled, love-filled life that we have? Thank you for being my ride-or-die, *mijn hartendief, mijn honing konijn*. You're my favorite person in the world.

Notes

INTRODUCTION

1. The names of institutions and individuals are pseudonyms unless otherwise noted.
2. Khiara M. Bridges, *Reproducing Race: An Ethnography of Pregnancy as a Site of Racialization* (University of California Press, 2011).
3. Elizabeth A. Howell, "Reducing Disparities in Severe Maternal Morbidity and Mortality," *Clinical Obstetrics and Gynecology* 61, no. 2 (2018): 387–399, https://doi.org/10.1097/GRF.0000000000000349.
4. Kate Kennedy-Moulton et al., "Maternal and Infant Health Inequality: New Evidence from Linked Administrative Data," Working Paper No. 30693 (National Bureau of Economic Research, September 2023), https://doi.org/10.3386/w30693; Latoya Hill et al., "Racial Disparities in Maternal and Infant Health: Current Status and Efforts to Address Them," KFF (October 25, 2024), https://www.kff.org/racial-equity-and-health-policy/issue-brief/racial-disparities-in-maternal-and-infant-health-current-status-and-efforts-to-address-them/.
5. Kennedy-Moulton et al., "Maternal and Infant Health Inequality," 5.
6. Munira Z. Gunja et al., "U.S. Health Care from a Global Perspective, 2022: Accelerating Spending, Worsening Outcomes," The Commonwealth Fund, January 31, 2023, https://www.commonwealthfund.org/publications/issue-briefs/2023/jan/us-health-care-global-perspective-2022.
7. Robert H. Shmerling, "Is Our Healthcare System Broken?," *Harvard Health Publishing*, July 13, 2021, https://www.health.harvard.edu/blog/is-our-healthcare-system-broken-202107132542#:~:text=Despite%20spending%20far%20more%20on,relatively%20low%20in%20the%20US.
8. Munira Z. Gunja et al., "Insights into the U.S. Maternal Mortality Crisis: An International Comparison," The Commonwealth Fund, June 4, 2024, https://www.commonwealthfund.org/publications/issue-briefs/2024/jun/insights-us-maternal-mortality-crisis-international-comparison.

9. John A. Ozimek and Sarah J. Kilpatrick, "Maternal Mortality in the Twenty-First Century," *Obstetrics and Gynecology Clinics of North America* 45, no. 2 (2018): 176, https://doi.org/10.1016/j.ogc.2018.01.004.

10. Ozmiek and Kilpatrick, "Maternal Mortality," 176.

11. Gunja et al., "Insights into the U.S. Maternal Mortality Crisis."

12. Black people are not the only nonwhite people who die more frequently from pregnancy-related causes than white people. The maternal mortality rates of Native and Native Hawaiian/Pacific Islander people are also higher than the maternal mortality rates of white people. United States Centers for Disease Control and Prevention, "Pregnancy Mortality Surveillance System," accessed August 31, 2024, https://www.cdc.gov/maternal-mortality/php/pregnancy-mortality-surveillance/index.html.

13. Energy and Commerce Committee Democrats, Hearing on "Better Data and Better Outcomes: Reducing Maternal Mortality in the U.S.," Subcommittee on Health (September 27, 2018), https://democrats-energycommerce.house.gov/committee-activity/hearings/hearing-on-better-data-and-better-outcomes-reducing-maternal-mortality. Similarly, one set of researchers observes that "non-Hispanic Black mothers and their infants in the *highest* income families fare worse than the *poorest* non-Hispanic white mothers and infants, and in some cases the difference in outcomes between these groups is quite large." Kennedy-Moulton et al., "Maternal and Infant Health Inequality," 16.

14. Energy and Commerce Committee Democrats, "Better Data and Better Outcomes."

15. Dána-Ain Davis, *Reproductive Injustice: Racism, Pregnancy, and Premature Birth* (New York University Press, 2019), 202.

16. Emily E. Petersen et al., "Racial/Ethnic Disparities in Pregnancy-Related Deaths—United States, 2007–2016," *Mobility and Mortality Weekly Report* 68, no. 35 (2019): 763, https://www.cdc.gov/mmwr/volumes/68/wr/pdfs/mm6835a3-H.pdf.

17. Petersen et al., "Racial/Ethnic Disparities," 763.

18. Kennedy-Moulton et al., "Maternal and Infant Health Inequality."

19. Kennedy-Moulton et al., "Maternal and Infant Health Inequality." Reporting on the NBER study, the *New York Times* explains that the infant mortality rate among the poorest black people is 653 deaths per 100,000 births, and the infant mortality rate among the poorest white people is 350 deaths per 100,000 births. Thus, poor black babies are 1.87 times as likely as poor white babies to die. Claire Cain Miller et al., "Childbirth Is Deadlier for Black Families, Even When They're Rich, Expansive Study Finds," *New York Times*, February 12, 2023, https://www.nytimes.com/interactive/2023/02/12/upshot/child-maternal-mortality-rich-poor.html.

20. Kennedy-Moulton et al., "Maternal and Infant Health Inequality." Reporting on the NBER study, the *New York Times* states that the infant mortality rate among the wealthiest black people is 437 deaths per 100,000 births, and the infant mortality rate among the wealthiest

white people is 173 deaths per 100,000 births. Thus, wealthy black babies are 2.53 times as likely as wealthy white babies to die. Miller et al., "Childbirth Is Deadlier."

21. In order to preserve the confidentiality of the identities of the remarkable people who shared their personal stories with me for this book, I have occasionally altered some insignificant details about their lives. For example, a study participant who was born in New Jersey might be described as being from Connecticut.

22. During a Foley bulb induction, a provider inserts a balloon-like catheter into the cervix and fills the catheter with a solution that causes it to expand, which encourages the cervix to dilate. Valencia Higuera, "What to Expect from a Foley Bulb Induction," *Healthline*, December 10, 2018, https://www.healthline.com/health/pregnancy/foley-bulb-induction.

23. The gravity of a vaginal tear is ranked in terms of degrees. Third-degree tears are fairly severe and extend into the muscle that surrounds the anus. Complications from third-degree tears include fecal incontinence and painful vaginal intercourse. Fourth-degree tears are the most severe, usually requiring repair in an operating room as opposed to the delivery room. Mayo Clinic, "Vaginal Tears in Childbirth," accessed August 31, 2024, https://www.mayoclinic.org/healthy-lifestyle/labor-and-delivery/in-depth/vaginal-tears/art-20546855.

24. Long overdue is an in-depth, qualitative study of the experiences that trans men and nonbinary people who were assigned female at birth have with obstetricians and gynecologists. We might safely assume that unless these individuals receive their care from providers and at practices that are attuned to the needs of gender-expansive people, the violence of nonrecognition and cisnormativity during the clinical encounter will make their encounters with obstetricians and gynecologists different from—and likely worse than—their cisgender counterparts' encounters.

25. Dána-Ain Davis, "Obstetric Racism: The Racial Politics of Pregnancy, Labor, and Birthing," *Medical Anthropology* 38, no. 7 (2019): 561–562, https://doi.org/10.1080/01459740.2018.1549389. Davis explains that obstetric racism

> includes critical lapses in diagnosis; being neglectful, dismissive, or disrespectful; causing pain; and engaging in medical abuse through coercion to perform procedures or performing procedures without consent. Informing women's interpretations of those encounters is a fluency of historically constituted racism, segregation and policing. Obstetric racism emerges specifically in reproductive care and places Black women and their infants at risk.

CHAPTER 1

1. Zuckerberg San Francisco General Hospital and Trauma Center, *FY 2021–2022 Annual Report*, uploaded May 2024, 9, https://www.zuckerbergsanfranciscogeneral.org/wp-content/uploads/2024/05/ZSFG-FY-Annual-Report-2021-2022.pdf.

2. Barbara J. Flagg, "'Was Blind, But Now I See': White Race Consciousness and the Requirement of Discriminatory Intent," *Michigan Law Review* 91, no. 5 (1993): 953, https://doi.org/10.2307/1289678.

3. United States Census Bureau, "Black Individuals Had Record Low Official Poverty Rate in 2022," September 12, 2023, https://www.census.gov/library/stories/2023/09/black-poverty-rate.html.

4. Karyn R. Lacy, *Blue-Chip Black: Race, Class, and Status in the New Black Middle Class* (University of California Press, 2007), 73.

5. At the time of Trump's declaration, 27 percent of black youth were unemployed, half the figure that he cited. Scott Detrow, "Trump Says African-American Communities in 'Worst Shape' Ever; Data Disagree," NPR, September 21, 2016, https://www.npr.org/2016/09/21/494883725/trump-says-african-americans-are-in-their-worst-shape-ever-the-data-disagrees.

6. Alana Semuels, "No, Most Black People Don't Live in Poverty—or Inner Cities," *The Atlantic*, October 12, 2016, https://www.theatlantic.com/business/archive/2016/10/trump-african-american-inner-city/503744/.

7. Yamiche Alcindor, "Ben Carson Is Confirmed as HUD Secretary," *New York Times*, March 2, 2017, https://www.nytimes.com/2017/03/02/us/politics/ben-carson-housing-urban-development.html.

8. The conflation of black race with poverty may cause or correlate with another problematic conflation—white race and wealth. This conflation obscures the reality that many white people are indigent.

9. Douglas S. Massey and Nancy A. Denton, *American Apartheid: Segregation and the Making of the Underclass* (Harvard University Press, 1998), 152–153.

10. In keeping with the definitions used by the American Community Survey, I define poverty as an annual income of less than $35,000 per year for a family of four. Social Explorer, "ACS 2021 (5-Year Estimates), U.S. Census Bureau: San Francisco City, California—Household Income in the Past 12 Months (in 2021 Inflation-Adjusted Dollars)," accessed February 16, 2023, https://www.socialexplorer.com/tables/ACS2021_5yr/R13302533.

11. Native people are the only racial group in San Francisco with poverty rates that outstrip those of black people in the city. Some 45 percent of Native San Francisco residents live in poverty. Social Explorer, "ACS 2021."

12. The Pew Research Center defines an upper-income household as a family of three earning more than $145,500 per year. Richard Fry, "Are You in the American Middle Class? Find Out with Our Income Calculator," *Pew Research Center*, September 16, 2024, https://www.pewresearch.org/short-reads/2020/07/23/are-you-in-the-american-middle-class/. However, this definition of class privilege imperfectly applies to San Francisco: "By 2018, the median asking rental price for a two-bedroom apartment in San Francisco was $4,300. Renters would need to earn $83 per hour—over $170,000 annually—to afford this rent." UC Berkeley's Urban Displacement Project and the California Housing Partnership, "Rising Costs and Re-Segregation in the San Francisco Bay Area," accessed August 2021, 2–3, https://www.urbandisplacement.org/wp-content/uploads/2021/08/bay_area_re-segregation_rising

_housing_costs_report_2019.pdf. A family of four in San Francisco with an annual household income of $145,500 would be scraping by, unable to enjoy the comforts associated with the upper middle class.

13. The percentages for Asian, Latine, and Native San Francisco residents are 37.3 percent, 28.7 percent, and 11.7 percent, respectively. Social Explorer, "ACS 2021."

14. The percentages of white, Asian, Latine, and Native residents of San Francisco are 43.4 percent, 34.4 percent, 15.4 percent, and 0.5 percent, respectively. United States Census Bureau, "Quick Facts: San Francisco City, California—Race and Hispanic Origin," https://www.census.gov/quickfacts/fact/table/sanfranciscocitycalifornia/PST045222.

15. Stephen Menedian and Samir Gambhir, "Racial Segregation in the San Francisco Bay Area, Part 2," Othering & Belonging Institute, February 7, 2019, https://belonging.berkeley.edu/racial-segregation-san-francisco-bay-area-part-2.

16. UC Berkeley's Urban Displacement Project and the California Housing Partnership, "Rising Costs and Re-Segregation in the San Francisco Bay Area."

17. Eli Moore et al., *Roots, Race, and Place: A History of Racially Exclusionary Housing in the San Francisco Bay Area* (Haas Institute for a Fair and Inclusive Society Public Education Report, 2019), 8.

18. Savannah Shange, *Progressive Dystopia: Abolition, Antiblackness, and Schooling in San Francisco* (Duke University Press, 2019), 24.

19. "Harvey Milk Becomes the First Openly Gay Person Elected to Public Office in California," *History*, published August 28, 2019, https://www.history.com/this-day-in-history/harvey-milk-first-openly-gay-person-elected-in-california.

20. Sarah Gibbens, "A Brief History of How Plastic Straws Took Over the World," *National Geographic*, January 2, 2019, https://www.nationalgeographic.com/environment/article/news-plastic-drinking-straw-history-ban; David Gorn, "San Francisco Plastic Bag Ban Interests Other Cities," NPR, March 27, 2008, https://www.npr.org/2008/03/27/89135360/san-francisco-plastic-bag-ban-interests-other-cities; Dion Lim and Ken Miguel, "San Francisco Bans Some Commonly Used Plastic Items," *ABC7 News*, July 1, 2019, https://abc7news.com/san-francisco-plastic-ban-plastics-straw/5368614/.

21. Nadine Jelsing, "How a 1934 Waterfront Strike Was a Major Turning Point for West Coast Labor," *Oregon Public Broadcasting*, July 11, 2022, https://www.opb.org/article/2022/07/11/1934-west-coast-ilwu-longshore-big-strike-labor-victory/.

22. Ahimsa Porter Sumchai, "Reflections . . . On the Unspeakable History of Animal Cruelty at the Hunters Point Naval Shipyard," *Medium*, August 25, 2021, https://ahimsaportersumchaimd.medium.com/reflections-efc3cc6156ac.

23. Moore et al., *Roots, Race, and Place*, 16.

24. Moore et al., *Roots, Race, and Place*, 16.

25. Moore et al., *Roots, Race, and Place*, 17.

26. Moore et al., *Roots, Race, and Place*, 23.
27. Christopher Chou, "Land Use and the Chinatown Problem," *UCLA Asian Pacific American Law Journal* 19 (2014): 49–50, https://doi.org/10.5070/P3191024222.
28. Chou, "Land Use and the Chinatown Problem," 50.
29. Moore et al., *Roots, Race, and Place*, 29.
30. *Yick Wo v. Hopkins*, 118 U.S. 356 (1886).
31. *Yick Wo*, 118 U.S. at 359.
32. Moore et al., *Roots, Race, and Place*, 30.
33. *Yick Wo*, 118 U.S. at 374.
34. *Yick Wo*, 118 U.S. at 373–374.
35. Moore et al., *Roots, Race, and Place*, 19.
36. Moore et al., *Roots, Race, and Place*, 20.
37. Committee on African American Parity of the Human Rights Commission of San Francisco, *The Unfinished Agenda: The Economic Status of African Americans in San Francisco 1964–1990* (Polaris Research and Development, 1993), 2–3.
38. Committee on African American Parity of the Human Rights Commission of San Francisco, *The Unfinished Agenda*, 4.
39. Richard Rothstein, *The Color of Law: A Forgotten History of How Our Government Segregated America* (Liveright, 2017), 5.
40. Committee on African American Parity of the Human Rights Commission of San Francisco, *The Unfinished Agenda*, 4.
41. United States Department of the Interior, "National Register of Historic Places Multiple Property Documentation Form for African Americans in California, 1850–1974," https://ohp.parks.ca.gov/pages/1067/files/CA_Multiple%20Counties_African%20Americans%20in%20CA%20MPDF_DRAFT.pdf.
42. Marilynn S. Johnson, *The Second Gold Rush: Oakland and the East Bay in World War II* (University of California Press, 1993), 55.
43. Committee on African American Parity of the Human Rights Commission of San Francisco, *The Unfinished Agenda*, 5.
44. Committee on African American Parity of the Human Rights Commission of San Francisco, *The Unfinished Agenda*, 4.
45. Shange, *Progressive Dystopia*, 39–40.
46. Walter Thompson, "How Urban Renewal Destroyed the Fillmore in Order to Save It," *Hoodline*, January 3, 2016, https://hoodline.com/2016/01/how-urban-renewal-destroyed-the-fillmore-in-order-to-save-it/.
47. Thompson, "How Urban Renewal Destroyed the Fillmore."

48. Bianca Taylor, "Why San Francisco's Fillmore District Is No Longer the 'Harlem of the West,'" KQED, June 25, 2010, https://www.kqed.org/news/11825401/how-urban-renewal-decimated-the-fillmore-district-and-took-jazz-with-it.

49. Adam Brinklow, "San Francisco Has Done Everything to the Bayview Except Fix Problems," *Curbed SF*, February 18, 2020, https://sf.curbed.com/2020/2/18/21142590/bayview-black-population-sfmta-transit-report.

50. Committee on African American Parity of the Human Rights Commission of San Francisco, *The Unfinished Agenda*, 6.

51. Thompson, "How Urban Renewal Destroyed the Fillmore."

52. Thompson, "How Urban Renewal Destroyed the Fillmore."

53. Thompson, "How Urban Renewal Destroyed the Fillmore."

54. Thompson, "How Urban Renewal Destroyed the Fillmore."

55. Elsa Devienne, "The Right to the Beach? Urban Renewal, Public Space Policing and the Definition of a Beach Public in Postwar Los Angeles, 1940s–1960s," *Revue française d'études américaines* 148, no. 3 (2016): 31, 34, https://doi.org/10.3917/rfea.148.0031.

56. Elie Mystal, "Let's Talk About the Taking of Black Land," *The Nation*, March 7/14, 2022, https://www.thenation.com/article/society/black-land-seneca-village/; Ann Pfau et al., "Using Urban Renewal Records to Advance Reparative Justice," *Russell Sage Foundation Journal of the Social Sciences* 10, no. 2 (2024): 113–131, https://doi.org/10.7758/RSF.2024.10.2.05.

57. While the targets of urban renewal were usually neighborhoods of color, white neighborhoods occasionally were objects of these projects. For example, Boston's West End was an Italian American enclave when it was declared a slum and targeted for renewal. Leland T. Saito, *Building Downtown Los Angeles: The Politics of Race and Place in Urban America* (Stanford University Press, 2022), 23–57.

58. Alisa Chang et al., "Beneath the Santa Monica Freeway Lies the Erasure of Sugar Hill," NPR, May 4, 2021, https://www.npr.org/2021/05/04/993605428/beneath-the-santa-monica-freeway-lies-the-erasure-of-sugar-hill.

59. Devienne, "The Right to the Beach," 31, 34.

60. Christina Jackson and Nikki Jones, "Remember the Fillmore: The Lingering History of Urban Renewal in Black San Francisco," in *Black California Dreamin': The Crises of California's African American Communities*, ed. C. Woods (University of California, Santa Barbara Center for Black Studies Research, 2012), 62, https://escholarship.org/uc/item/63g6128j.

61. Thompson, "How Urban Renewal Destroyed the Fillmore."

62. Thompson, "How Urban Renewal Destroyed the Fillmore."

63. Thompson, "How Urban Renewal Destroyed the Fillmore."

64. Thompson, "How Urban Renewal Destroyed the Fillmore."

65. Thompson, "How Urban Renewal Destroyed the Fillmore."
66. Thompson, "How Urban Renewal Destroyed the Fillmore."
67. Moore et al., *Roots, Race, and Place*, 46.
68. Moore et al., *Roots, Race, and Place*, 46.
69. Jessica Lin, "Lincoln Square Renewal Project (New York, 1955–1969)," *ArcGIS StoryMaps*, December 16, 2020, https://storymaps.arcgis.com/stories/d6c942630bee454bae0c7b459a081f07.
70. Lin, "Lincoln Square Renewal Project."
71. Lilia Fernández, *Brown in the Windy City: Mexicans and Puerto Ricans in Postwar Chicago* (University of Chicago Press, 2012), 92, 96.
72. Fernández, *Brown in the Windy City*, 92.
73. Fernández, *Brown in the Windy City*, 92–93.
74. Fernández, *Brown in the Windy City*, 99.
75. Francesca Russello Ammon, "Commemoration Amid Criticism: The Mixed Legacy of Urban Renewal in Southwest Washington, D.C.," *Journal of Planning and History* 8, no. 3 (2009): 178, https://doi.org/10.1177/1538513209340630.
76. Russello Ammon, "Commemoration Amid Criticism," 178.
77. Russello Ammon, "Commemoration Amid Criticism," 188.
78. Russello Ammon, "Commemoration Amid Criticism," 199.
79. Quinlyn R. Spellmeyer, "Southwest DC: A Cycle of Urban Renewal and 'Revitalization,'" *ArcGIS StoryMaps*, December 16, 2020, https://storymaps.arcgis.com/stories/f43a96703b3e4d098b7c242d680e3498.
80. Russello Ammon, "Commemoration Amid Criticism," 202.
81. Russello Ammon, "Commemoration Amid Criticism," 202.
82. Milan Dluhy et al., "Creating a Positive Future for a Minority Community: Transportation and Urban Renewal Politics in Miami," *Journal of Urban Affairs* 24, no. 1 (2002): 75–95, https://doi.org/10.1111/1467-9906.00115.
83. N. D. B. Connolly, "Colored, Caribbean, and Condemned: Miami's Overtown District and the Cultural Expense of Progress, 1940–1970," *Caribbean Studies* 34, no. 1 (2006): 24, https://www.redalyc.org/pdf/392/39211247001.pdf.
84. Richard F. Weingroff, "Federal-Aid Highway Act of 1956: Creating the Interstate System," *Public Roads* 60, no. 1 (1996), https://highways.dot.gov/public-roads/summer-1996/federal-aid-highway-act-1956-creating-interstate-system-sidebars.
85. Connolly, "Colored, Caribbean, and Condemned," 33.
86. Connolly, "Colored, Caribbean, and Condemned," 37.

87. Connolly, "Colored, Caribbean, and Condemned," 38.

88. Connolly, "Colored, Caribbean, and Condemned," 38.

89. Chang et al., "Beneath the Santa Monica Freeway."

90. Chang et al., "Beneath the Santa Monica Freeway."

91. Chang et al., "Beneath the Santa Monica Freeway."

92. Chang et al., "Beneath the Santa Monica Freeway."

93. Chang et al., "Beneath the Santa Monica Freeway."

94. Jackson and Jones, "Remember the Fillmore."

95. Thompson, "How Urban Renewal Destroyed the Fillmore."

96. Shange, *Progressive Dystopia*, 24.

97. Shange, *Progressive Dystopia*, 39.

98. Thomas Fuller, "The Loneliness of Being Black in San Francisco," *New York Times*, July 20, 2016, https://www.nytimes.com/2016/07/21/us/black-exodus-from-san-francisco.html.

99. As sociologists Megan Tobias Neely, Patrick Sheehan, and Christine Williams explain, "[T]he tech industry across the United States is more white, more Asian (a category that includes Asian Americans and Asian immigrants), and more male than the private sector generally." Megan Tobias Neely et al., "Social Inequality in High Tech: How Gender, Race, and Ethnicity Structure the World's Most Powerful Industry," *Annual Review of Sociology* 49 (2023): 319, https://dx.doi.org/10.1146/annurev-soc-031021-034202.

100. Redfin, "Cole Valley, CA Housing Market," accessed August 30, 2024, https://www.redfin.com/neighborhood/548/CA/San-Francisco/Cole-Valley/housing-market.

101. Debra Kamin, "Cole Valley, San Francisco: Where High Prices Meet Low Inventory," *New York Times*, December 31, 2019, https://www.nytimes.com/2019/12/31/realestate/cole-valley-san-francisco-where-high-prices-meet-low-inventory.html.

102. Vanessa Racehorse and Anna Hohag, "Achieving Climate Justice through Land Back: An Overview of Tribal Dispossession, Land Return Efforts, and Practical Mechanisms for #LandBack," *Colorado Environmental Law Journal* 34, no. 2 (2023): 183, https://ssrn.com/abstract=4575288.

103. Emily E. Petersen et al., "Racial/Ethnic Disparities in Pregnancy-Related Deaths—United States, 2007–2016." *Morbidity and Mortality Weekly Report* 68, no. 35 (2019): 762–763, http://dx.doi.org/10.15585/mmwr.mm6835a3.

104. Kate Kennedy-Moulton et al., "Maternal and Infant Health Inequality: New Evidence from Linked Administrative Data," Working Paper No. 30693 (National Bureau of Economic Research, September 2023), 19–20, https://doi.org/10.3386/w30693.

105. Raj Chetty et al., "Race and Economic Opportunity in the United States: An Intergenerational Perspective," Working Paper No. 24441 (National Bureau of Economic Research, December 2019), https://doi.org/10.3386/w24441.

106. Robin Pearce, *The Sick Side of Town: How Place Shapes Disparities in Health* (Haas Institute for a Fair and Inclusive Society, 2018), 10, https://belonging.berkeley.edu/sites/default/files/haasinstitute_thesicksideoftown_healthdisparitiesweb.pdf?file=1&force=1.

107. William A. Smith et al., "Challenging Racial Battle Fatigue on Historically White Campuses: A Critical Race Examination of Race-Related Stress," in *Faculty of Color: Teaching in Predominately White Colleges and Universities*, ed. Christine A. Stanley (Anker Publishing, 2007); Marlo Vernon et al., "Maternal Mortality," in *Black Health in the South*, ed. Steven S. Coughlin et al. (Johns Hopkins University Press, 2023), 387.

108. Pearce, *The Sick Side of Town*, 10.

CHAPTER 2

1. I have not used a pseudonym for Zuckerberg San Francisco General Hospital and Trauma Center.

2. Medicaid, "Medicaid," accessed August 15, 2024, https://www.medicaid.gov/medicaid/index.html.

3. Medicaid, "Medicaid."

4. California Department of Health Care Services, "Medi-Cal Resources," accessed August 15, 2024, https://www.dhcs.ca.gov/services/medi-cal/Pages/default.aspx.

5. United States Department of Health and Human Services, "Who's Eligible for Medicare?," last modified December 8, 2022, https://www.hhs.gov/answers/medicare-and-medicaid/who-is-eligible-for-medicare/index.html.

6. Zuckerberg San Francisco General Hospital and Trauma Center, *FY 2022–2023 Annual Report* (2023), 9, https://www.sf.gov/sites/default/files/2023-10/05%20ZSFG%20FY%20Annual%20Report%202022-2023.pdf.

7. Zuckerberg San Francisco General Hospital, *FY 2022–2023 Annual Report*, 9.

8. Zuckerberg San Francisco General Hospital, *FY 2022–2023 Annual Report*, 9. Some 33 percent of the General's inpatients and 23 percent of its outpatients were Medicare-insured in 2022–2023. A significant portion of the General's Medicare-insured population, like the General's Medi-Cal-insured and uninsured patients, can be assumed to be indigent.

9. Zuckerberg San Francisco General Hospital, *FY 2022–2023 Annual Report*, 9.

10. Shawna Chen et al., "How San Francisco's Racial Demographics Have Changed since 2000," *Axios San Francisco*, July 6, 2023, https://www.axios.com/local/san-francisco/2023/07/06/san-francisco-demographic-trends; Jinyun Tsai, "One in Three Homes in This San Francisco Neighborhood Lives below the Poverty Line," *San Francisco Standard*, December 8, 2022, https://sfstandard.com/2022/12/08/san-francisco-neighborhood-new-census-data-maps/; Zuckerberg San Francisco General Hospital, *FY 2022–2023 Annual Report*, 8.

11. Tsai, "One in Three Homes"; Zuckerberg San Francisco General Hospital, *FY 2022–2023 Annual Report*, 8.

12. California Department of Health Care Access and Information, "Hospital Profile," accessed August 17, 2024, [url redacted].
13. California Department of Health Care Access and Information, "Hospital Profile."
14. Uché Blackstock, "'At the Private Hospital, the Disrespect Was Just More Subtle': A Tale of America's Two Healthcare Systems," *The Guardian*, January 23, 2024, https://www.theguardian.com/wellness/2024/jan/23/us-hospital-segregation-racism-public-private; Rachel Wilkinson et al., "Leveraging Clerkship Experiences to Address Segregated Care: A Survey-Based Approach to Student-Led Advocacy," *Teaching and Learning in Medicine* 35, no. 4 (2022): 381, https://doi.org/10.1080/10401334.2022.2088538.
15. Wilkinson et al., "Leveraging Clerkship Experiences," 381.
16. Khiara M. Bridges, *Reproducing Race: An Ethnography of Pregnancy as a Site of Racialization* (University of California Press, 2011), 31–32, https://doi.org/10.1525/california/9780520268944.001.0001; Wilkinson et al., "Leveraging Clerkship Experiences," 381.
17. Wilkinson et al., "Leveraging Clerkship Experiences," 381.
18. Julia Craven, "How Do Black Patients and White Patients Get Different Doctors in the Same Hospitals?," *Slate*, May 26, 2021, https://slate.com/technology/2021/05/hospital-segregation-study.html.
19. Carlos Barrientos, "25 Popular San Francisco Neighborhoods: Where to Live in San Francisco in 2025," Redfin, April 22, 2024, https://www.redfin.com/blog/san-francisco-ca-neighborhoods/.
20. California Department of Health Care Access and Information, "Hospital Profile: [name redacted]," accessed August 17, 2024, [url redacted]; California Department of Health Care Access and Information, "Hospital Profile: [name redacted]," accessed August 17, 2024, [url redacted].
21. California Department of Health Care Access and Information, "Hospital Profile: [name redacted] Hospital–San Francisco," accessed August 17, 2024, [url redacted].
22. Katherine Tam, "Expanded Partnership at [redacted] to Advance Care for Publicly Insured Pregnant Patients," *Science of Caring*, January 25, 2023, [url redacted].
23. Jamie Godwin et al., "Understanding Mergers between Hospitals and Health Systems in Different Markets," KFF, August 23, 2023, https://www.kff.org/health-costs/issue-brief/understanding-mergers-between-hospitals-and-health-systems-in-different-markets/.
24. Godwin et al., "Understanding Mergers."
25. Godwin et al., "Understanding Mergers."
26. Godwin et al., "Understanding Mergers"; Hoag Levins, "Hospital Consolidation Continues to Boost Costs, Narrow Access, and Impact Care Quality," University of Pennsylvania Leonard Davis Institute of Health Economics, January 19, 2023, https://ldi.upenn.edu/our-work/research-updates/hospital-consolidation-continues-to-boost-costs-narrow-access-and-impact-care-quality/.

27. Godwin et al., "Understanding Mergers."
28. Michael Cohen et al., *The Prices That Commercial Health Insurers and Medicare Pay for Hospitals' and Physicians' Services* (Congressional Budget Office, January 2022), https://www.cbo.gov/system/files/2022-01/57422-medical-prices.pdf.
29. [name redacted] Health, "How [redacted] Hospital–Brooklyn Became One of the Safest Hospitals in the Country," [name redacted] Health, November 2, 2022, [url redacted].
30. [name redacted] Health, "How [redacted] Hospital."
31. [name redacted], "The Value of an Integrated Healthcare Network" (2020), [url redacted].
32. [name redacted], "Our 340B Story," accessed August 17, 2024, [url redacted].
33. This data is on file with author.
34. Victoria Colliver, "For-Profit Hospitals Give Back as Much as Nonprofits, Study Finds," *SFGate*, August 4, 2015, https://www.sfgate.com/health/article/For-profit-hospitals-give-back-as-much-as-6422790.php; Bradley Herring et al., "Comparing the Value of Nonprofit Hospitals' Tax Exemption to Their Community Benefits," *Inquiry* 55 (2018).
35. Colliver, "For-Profit Hospitals Give Back."
36. Colliver, "For-Profit Hospitals Give Back."
37. Joseph D. Bruch and David Bellamy, "Charity Care: Do Nonprofit Hospitals Give More than For-Profit Hospitals?," *Journal of General Internal Medicine* 36, no. 10 (2020), https://doi.org/10.1007/s11606-020-06147-9.
38. Jessica Silver-Greenberg and Katie Thomas, "They Were Entitled to Free Care. Hospitals Hounded Them to Pay," *New York Times*, last updated December 15, 2022, https://www.nytimes.com/2022/09/24/business/nonprofit-hospitals-poor-patients.html.
39. Silver-Greenberg and Thomas, "They Were Entitled to Free Care."
40. Douglas McCarthy and Kimberly Mueller, "The New York City Health and Hospitals Corporation: Transforming a Public Safety Net Delivery System to Achieve Higher Performance," The Commonwealth Fund, October 2008, https://www.commonwealthfund.org/sites/default/files/documents/___media_files_publications_fund_report_2008_oct_the_new_york_city_health_and_hospitals_corporation__transforming_a_public_safety_net_delivery_system_mccarthy_nychlthospitalscorpcasestudy_1154_pdf.pdf.
41. Zuckerberg San Francisco General Hospital and Trauma Center, "Home," accessed August 17, 2024, https://www.zuckerbergsanfranciscogeneral.org/.
42. [name redacted], "Team Lily / Patient Information," [url redacted].
43. Canopy Health, "Canopy Health, San Francisco Health Network Announce Collaboration That Will Expand Hospital-Based Midwifery Access in San Francisco," last modified August 5, 2019, https://www.canopyhealth.com/canopy-health-san-francisco-health-network-announce-collaboration-that-will-expand-hospital-based-midwifery-access-in-san-francisco/.

44. Canopy Health, "Canopy Health, San Francisco Health Network."
45. Sarah Kliff, "Prices at Zuckerberg Hospital's Emergency Room Are Higher than Anywhere Else in San Francisco," *Vox*, January 22, 2019, https://www.vox.com/2019/1/22/18183534/zuckerberg-san-francisco-general-hospital-er-prices; Andrew Whalen, "Zuckerberg Hospital ER Doesn't Take Private Insurance, Sticking San Francisco Patients with Huge Bills," *Newsweek*, January 7, 2019, https://www.newsweek.com/zuckerberg-hospital-er-private-insurance-medicare-medicaid-mark-facebook-san-1282274.
46. Jenny Gold and Sarah Kliff, "A Baby Was Treated with a Nap and a Bottle of Formula. His Parents Received an $18,000 Bill," *Vox*, July 20, 2018, https://www.vox.com/2018/6/28/17506232/emergency-room-bill-fees-health-insurance-baby; Sarah Kliff, "Hit by a City Bus—and Hit with a $27,660 City Hospital Bill," *Vox*, February 19, 2019, https://www.vox.com/2019/2/19/18213948/zuckerberg-hospital-emergency-room-bill-bus-accident; Sarah Kliff, "A $20,243 Bike Crash: Zuckerberg Hospital's Aggressive Tactics Leave Patients with Big Bills," *Vox*, January 24, 2019, https://www.vox.com/policy-and-politics/2019/1/7/18137967/er-bills-zuckerberg-san-francisco-general-hospital.
47. California Department of Health Care Services, "Information on the Presumptive Eligibility for Pregnant Women," accessed February 11, 2025, https://www.dhcs.ca.gov/services/medi-cal/eligibility/Pages/PE_Info_women.aspx.
48. Mariana Alexander et al., *A New Approach to Funding New York City Health + Hospitals* (Citizens Budget Commission, December 2019), 1, https://cbcny.org/sites/default/files/media/files/CBCREPORT_Health%2BHospitals_12162019_1.pdf.
49. Alexander et al., "A New Approach to Funding," 1.
50. Bridges, *Reproducing Race*, 25.
51. Denise Clay-Murray, "The HBCU Endowment Gap: Why Black Colleges Lag So Far behind PWIs," *BET*, October 7, 2022, https://www.bet.com/article/3d5ktm/black-colleges-endowment-gap.
52. Michael L. Lomax, "Why HBCUs Still Matter," United Negro College Fund, https://uncf.org/the-latest/why-hbcus-still-matter#:~:text=While%20Black%20and%20White%20students,STEM%20degrees%20come%20from%20HBCUs.
53. Jonathan Gruber and Benjamin D. Sommers, "Fiscal Federalism and the Budget Impacts of the Affordable Care Act's Medicaid Expansion," Working Paper No. 26862 (National Bureau of Economic Research, March 2020), https://doi.org/10.3386/w26862. This is not meant to suggest that there are no or few restraints on the federal budget. When Medicare reimbursement rates increase, the government has to find the money to pay those higher rates. That money typically comes from higher federal taxes or other politically unpopular policy choices—a fact that works to keep Medicare reimbursement rates from increasing greatly over time. Cohen et al., *The Prices That Commercial Health Insurers and Medicare Pay*.
54. Sean McElwee, "One Big Reason Congress Ignores the Poor: They Don't Vote," *Vox*, September 24, 2015. https://www.vox.com/2015/9/24/9388045/2014-voter-turnout-redistribution.

55. Cindy Mann and Adam Striar, "How Differences in Medicaid, Medicare, and Commercial Health Insurance Payment Rates Impact Access, Health Equity, and Cost," The Commonwealth Fund, August 17, 2022, https://www.commonwealthfund.org/blog/2022/how-differences-medicaid-medicare-and-commercial-health-insurance-payment-rates-impact. As the Congressional Budget Office explains, "Hospitals and physicians groups may have market power because they have a dominant share of the market in an area or because an insurer sees them as essential to its network of providers." Cohen et al., *The Prices That Commercial Health Insurers and Medicare Pay*.

56. Because commercial insurance reimbursement rates are a function of the negotiating power that commercial insurance companies have with providers, they vary greatly across the country. Mann and Striar, "Differences in Medicaid." Further, some types of providers are able to demand higher reimbursement rates from commercial insurers than others. For example, obstetrics and gynecology, family medicine, and a handful of other specialties "had the lowest commercial markups relative to Medicare prices" at around 110 percent; "[r]adiology and neurosurgery received commercial payment rates of 180 and 220 percent of Medicare rates"; "emergency department and critical care specialties received commercial payment rates of 250 percent of Medicare rates"; and "[a]nesthesia received the highest markup of 330 percent of Medicare rates." Stacey McMorrow et al., "Commercial Health Insurance Markups over Medicare Prices for Physician Services Vary Widely by Specialty" (Urban Institute, 2021), 2, https://www.urban.org/sites/default/files/publication/104945/commercial-health-insurance-markups-over-medicare-prices-for-physician-services-vary-widely-by-specialty_0.pdf. Consequently, there is no easy answer to the question of how much more commercial insurance companies pay providers relative to Medicare.

57. This certainly holds true in the context of maternity care. Different sets of researchers have conducted studies to estimate the disparity in reimbursement rates between commercial insurance and Medicaid with respect to maternity care. Some studies conclude that commercial insurance rates for maternity care are twice Medicaid rates; others conclude that commercial insurance rates for maternity care are five times Medicaid rates. Melora Simon, "Medi-Cal Explained: Paying for Maternity Services" (California Health Care Foundation, September 2020), https://www.chcf.org/wp-content/uploads/2020/09/MediCalExplainedPayingMaternityServices.pdf; Truven Health Analytics, *The Cost of Having a Baby in the United States* (January 2013), 6, https://nationalpartnership.org/wp-content/uploads/2023/02/the-cost-of-having-a-baby-in-the-us.pdf.

58. University of California Health, "Our Commitment to Medi-Cal," accessed August 19, 2024, https://health.universityofcalifornia.edu/about-us/our-commitment-medi-cal.

59. To offset some of the losses that come with caring for Medi-Cal patients, California's Department of Health Care Services (DHCS) gives supplemental payments to hospitals with significant numbers of uninsured and Medi-Cal-insured patients. Medicaid and CHIP Payment and Access Commission (MACPAC), "Medicaid Hospital Payment: A Comparison across States and to Medicare," updated April 2017, https://www.macpac.gov/publication/medicaid-hospital-payment-a-comparison-across-states-and-to-medicare/.

60. [name redacted], "About [redacted] at [redacted]: Partners in Health," accessed August 19, 2024, [url redacted].

61. [name redacted], "About [redacted] at [redacted]."

62. [name redacted], "Training Sites," accessed August 19, 2024, [url redacted].

63. Ellen S. Lazarus, "What Do Women Want? Issues of Choice, Control, and Class in Pregnancy and Childbirth," *Medical Anthropology Quarterly* 8, no. 1 (1994): 40, https://doi.org/10.1525/maq.1994.8.1.02a00030.

64. Lazarus, "What Do Women Want?," 40.

65. Lazarus, "What Do Women Want?," 40.

66. Mann and Striar, "How Differences in Medicaid."

67. Mann and Striar, "How Differences in Medicaid."

68. Bridges, *Reproducing Race*, 51.

69. Bridges, *Reproducing Race*, 51.

70. Bridges, *Reproducing Race*, 51.

71. MyChart is a web portal that gives patients online access to their medical records and enables patients to make appointments, communicate with their providers, receive the results of laboratory tests, and accomplish other healthcare-related tasks. MyChart, "Home," accessed August 19, 2024, https://www.mychart.org/.

72. Crilhien R. Francisco, *Report on the Fiscal 2024 Preliminary Plan and the Fiscal 2023 Mayor's Management Report for the New York City Health + Hospitals* (New York City Council Finance Division, 2023), https://council.nyc.gov/budget/wp-content/uploads/sites/54/2023/03/HH.pdf.

73. American Hospital Association, "Metropolitan Anchor Hospital (MAH) Case Study," June 2022, https://aha.org/case-studies/2022-11-22-nyc-health-hospitals-new-york.

74. McCarthy and Mueller, "The New York City Health and Hospitals Corporation."

75. McCarthy and Mueller, "The New York City Health and Hospitals Corporation."

76. American Hospital Association, "Metropolitan Anchor Hospital (MAH) Case Study."

77. New York State designates a hospital as a "safety net" institution when it is either publicly owned or approximately one third of its patients are Medicaid-insured, are uninsured, or qualify for both Medicare and Medicaid. New York State Department of Health, "Safety Net Definition," revised February 2016, https://www.health.ny.gov/health_care/medicaid/redesign/dsrip/safety_net_definition.htm.

78. Alexander et al., "A New Approach to Funding," 1.

79. Alexander et al., "A New Approach to Funding," 1.

80. [name redacted], *In the Community 2023: Our Commitment to Nursing Excellence* (2023), [url redacted].

81. [name redacted], *In the Community 2023: Our Commitment to Nursing Excellence.*
82. Sarah Kliff and Jessica Silver-Greenberg, "'Major Trustee, Please Prioritize': How [redacted]'s E.R. Favors the Rich," *New York Times*, December 22, 2022, [url redacted].
83. Kliff and Silver-Greenberg, "Major Trustee, Please Prioritize.'"
84. [name redacted] Health, "How [redacted] Hospital."
85. [name redacted] Health, "How [redacted] Hospital."
86. DHCS describes federally qualified health centers as "primary care clinics that receive federal funds to provide healthcare services to underserved communities." California Department of Health Care Services, "Federally Qualified Health Centers and Rural Health Clinics," https://www.dhcs.ca.gov/services/medi-cal/Pages/FQHC_RHC.aspx.
87. [name redacted] Health, "Family Health Centers at [redacted]," [url redacted].
88. [name redacted] Health, "How [redacted] Hospital."

CHAPTER 3

1. Jonathan Custodio, "This Bronxite Died Weeks after an Emergency C-Section: Her Family Wants Answers, and Changes," *The City*, September 24, 2023, https://www.thecity.nyc/2023/09/24/bronxcare-maternal-mortality-elaina-boone-death/.
2. Custodio, "This Bronxite Died Weeks after an Emergency C-Section."
3. Irth (@irthapp), "Rest in Peace Elaina Boone," TikTok, September 15, 2023, https://www.tiktok.com/@irthapp/video/7279295156648414510.
4. Irth (@irthapp), "Rest in Peace Elaina Boone."
5. American Anthropological Association, "AAA Statement on Race," https://americananthro.org/about/policies/statement-on-race/; Ashley Montagu, *Statement on Race: An Extended Discussion in Plain Language of the UNESCO Statement by Experts on Race Problems* (Schuman, 1951), 15; Dorothy Roberts, *Fatal Invention: How Science, Politics, and Big Business Re-Create Race in the Twenty-First Century* (New Press, 2011), 49.
6. American Anthropological Association, "AAA Statement on Race."
7. Christopher W. Kuzawa and Elizabeth Sweet, "Epigenetics and the Embodiment of Race: Developmental Origins of US Racial Disparities in Cardiovascular Health," *American Journal of Human Biology* 21, no. 1 (January 2009): 3, https://doi.org/10.1002/ajhb.20822.
8. Kuzawa and Sweet, "Epigenetics and the Embodiment of Race," 2.
9. Kuzawa and Sweet, "Epigenetics and the Embodiment of Race," 11.
10. Yadav Sapkota et al., "Genetic Variants Associated with Therapy-Related Cardiomyopathy among Childhood Cancer Survivors of African Ancestry," *Cancer Research* 81, no. 9 (2021): 2556–2565, https://doi.org/10.1158/0008-5472.CAN-20-2675.
11. Sapkota et al., "Genetic Variants," 2556.

12. Sapkota et al., "Genetic Variants," 2560.
13. Dolores Acevedo-Garcia et al., "The Differential Effect of Foreign-Born Status on Low Birth Weight by Race/Ethnicity and Education," *Pediatrics* 115, no. 1 (2005): e20–e30, https://doi.org/10.1542/peds.2004-1306; Howard Cabral et al., "Foreign-Born and US-Born Black Women: Differences in Health Behaviors and Birth Outcomes," *American Journal of Public Health* 80, no. 1 (1990): 71, https://doi.org/10.2105/AJPH.80.1.70; Fatu Forna et al., "Pregnancy Outcomes in Foreign-Born and US-Born Women," *International Journal of Gynecology and Obstetrics* 83, no. 3 (2003): 257–265, https://doi.org/10.1016/S0020-7292(03)00307-2; Gopal K. Singh and Stella M. Yu, "Adverse Pregnancy Outcomes: Differences Between US- and Foreign-Born Women in Major US Racial and Ethnic Groups," *American Journal of Public Health* 86, no. 6 (1996): 842, https://doi.org/10.2105/AJPH.86.6.837.
14. James W. Collins Jr. et al., "Differing Intergenerational Birth Weights among the Descendants of US-Born and Foreign-Born Whites and African Americans in Illinois," *American Journal of Epidemiology* 155, no. 3 (2002): 214, https://doi.org/10.1093/aje/155.3.210.
15. Kuzawa and Sweet, "Epigenetics and the Embodiment of Race," 8–9.
16. Kuzawa and Sweet, "Epigenetics and the Embodiment of Race," 9.
17. Dorothy E. Roberts, "What's Wrong with Race-Based Medicine? Genes, Drugs, and Health Disparities," *Minnesota Journal of Law, Science & Technology* 12, no. 1 (2011): 15, https://scholarship.law.umn.edu/mjlst/vol12/iss1/3.
18. Khiara Bridges and Douglas White, "COVID-19 Is Not an Equalizer: Early Data Shows African Americans Are Dying at Higher Rates," interview by Lizzie O'Leary, *The Takeaway*, WNYC Studios and WGBH, April 6, 2020, https://www.wnycstudios.org/podcasts/takeaway/segments/covid19-black-people-dying-at-higher-rates.
19. Jonathan M. Metzl et al., "Using a Structural Competency Framework to Teach Structural Racism in Pre-health Education," *Social Science and Medicine* 199 (2018): 189–201, https://doi.org/10.1016/j.socscimed.2017.06.029.
20. Metzl et al., "Using a Structural Competency Framework," 197.
21. Metzl et al., "Using a Structural Competency Framework," 197.
22. Metzl et al., "Using a Structural Competency Framework," 197.
23. Julie Beaulac et al., "A Systematic Review of Food Deserts, 1966–2007," *Preventing Chronic Disease* 6, no. 3 (2009): 1, http://www.cdc.gov/pcd/issues/2009/jul/08_0163.htm.
24. William Dressler et al., "Race and Ethnicity in Public Health Research: Models to Explain Health Disparities," *Annual Review of Anthropology* 34, no. 1 (October 2005): 238, https://doi.org/10.1146/annurev.anthro.34.081804.120505.
25. Michael Marmot and Richard Wilkinson, eds., *Social Determinants of Health*, 2nd ed. (Oxford University Press, 2005).
26. KFF, "Poverty Rate by Race/Ethnicity," accessed August 14, 2024, https://www.kff.org/other/state-indicator/poverty-rate-by-raceethnicity/.

27. KFF, "Poverty Rate by Race/Ethnicity."
28. Marlo Vernon et al., "Maternal Mortality," in *Black Health in the South*, ed. Steven S. Coughlin et al. (Johns Hopkins University Press, 2023), 387.
29. Vernon et al., "Maternal Mortality," 394.
30. Shriya Joshi et al., "Epigenetic Determinants of Racial Disparity in Breast Cancer: Looking beyond Genetic Alterations," *Cancers* 14, no. 8 (2022): 1905, https://doi.org/10.3390/cancers14081903.
31. Kuzawa and Sweet, "Epigenetics and the Embodiment of Race," 5.
32. Kuzawa and Sweet, "Epigenetics and the Embodiment of Race," 6.
33. Chantel L. Martin et al., "Understanding Health Inequalities through the Lens of Social Epigenetics," *Annual Review of Public Health* 43 (2022): 241, https://doi.org/10.1146/annurev-publhealth-052020-105613.
34. Kuzawa and Sweet, "Epigenetics and the Embodiment of Race," 7.
35. Riya R. Kanherkar et al., "Epigenetics across the Human Lifespan," *Frontiers in Cell and Developmental Biology* 2 (2014): 9, https://doi.org/10.3389/fcell.2014.00049.
36. Susanne R. De Rooij et al., "Lessons Learned from 25 Years of Research into Long Term Consequences of Prenatal Exposure to the Dutch Famine 1944–45: The Dutch Famine Birth Cohort," *International Journal of Environmental Health Research* 32, no. 7 (2022): 1432–1436, https://doi.org/10.1080/09603123.2021.1888894; Elmar W. Tobi et al., "DNA Methylation Signatures Link Prenatal Famine Exposure to Growth and Metabolism," *Nature Communications* 5 (2014): 1–13, https://doi.org/10.1038/ncomms6592.
37. De Rooij et al., "Lessons Learned," 1436–1437; Tobi et al., "DNA Methylation," 8.
38. De Rooij et al., "Lessons Learned," 1433–1436; M. V. E. Veenendaal et al., "Transgenerational Effects of Prenatal Exposure to the 1944–45 Dutch Famine," *BJOG: An International Journal of Obstetrics & Gynaecology* 120, no. 5 (2013); 548–554, https://doi.org/10.1111/1471-0528.12136.
39. Arline T. Geronimus, "The Effects of Race, Residence, and Prenatal Care on the Relationship of Maternal Age to Neonatal Mortality," *American Journal of Public Health* 79, no. 12 (1986): 1416–1421, https://doi.org/10.2105/ajph.76.12.1416.
40. Geronimus, "The Effects of Race, Residence, and Prenatal Care," 1417.
41. Arline T. Geronimus, *Weathering: The Extraordinary Stress of Ordinary Life in an Unjust Society* (Little, Brown Spark, 2023).
42. Arline T. Geronimus, "Making the Case That Discrimination Is Bad for Your Health," interview by Gene Demby, *Code Switch*, NPR, January 14, 2018, https://www.npr.org/sections/codeswitch/2018/01/14/577664626/making-the-case-that-discrimination-is-bad-for-your-health.
43. Vernon et al., "Maternal Mortality," 394.

44. Geronimus, "Making the Case."

45. McEwen and Stellar defined allostatic load "as the cost of chronic exposure to fluctuating or heightened neural or neuroendocrine response resulting from repeated or chronic environmental challenge that an individual reacts to as being particularly stressful." Bruce S. McEwen and Eliot Stellar, "Stress and the Individual: Mechanisms Leading to Disease," *Archives of internal Medicine* 153, no. 18 (1993): 2093, https://doi.org/10.1001/archinte.1993.00410180039004.

46. Arline T. Geronimus et al., "'Weathering' and Age Patterns of Allostatic Load Scores among Blacks and Whites in the United States," *American Journal of Public Health* 96, no. 5 (2006): 826–833, https://doi.org/10.2105/AJPH.2004.060749.

47. Elizabeth A. Howell, "Reducing Disparities in Severe Maternal Morbidity and Mortality," *Clinical Obstetrics and Gynecology* 61, no. 2 (2018): 391, https://doi.org/10.1097/GRF.0000000000000349.

48. Elizabeth A. Howell et al., "Black–White Differences in Severe Maternal Morbidity and Site of Care," *American Journal of Obstetrics and Gynecology* 214, no. 1 (2016): 122.e1, https://doi.org/10.1016/j.ajog.2015.08.019.

49. Howell et al., "Black–White Differences," 122.e3.

50. Howell et al., "Black–White Differences," 122.e5.

51. Elizabeth A. Howell et al., "Site of Delivery Contribution to Black–White Severe Maternal Morbidity Disparity," *American Journal of Obstetrics and Gynecology* 215, no. 2 (2016): 146, https://doi.org/10.1016/j.ajog.2016.05.007.

52. Brittney T. Anderson, "Access to Quality, Culturally Appropriate Health Care," in *Black Health in the South*, ed. Steven S. Coughlin et al. (Johns Hopkins University Press, 2023), 33.

53. Anderson, "Access to Quality, Culturally Appropriate Health Care," 33.

54. Kartik K. Ganju et al., "The Role of Decision Support Systems in Attenuating Racial Biases in Healthcare Delivery," *Fox School of Business Research Paper* (2019): 5, https://doi.org/10.2139/ssrn.3465839; Frank M. McClellan et al., "It Takes a Village: Reforming Law to Promote Health Literacy and Reduce Orthopedic Health Disparities," *Journal of Health and Biomedical Law* 8, no. 3 (2013): 338, https://doi.org/10.2139/ssrn.2275424.

55. David A. Paul et al., "Racial Differences in Prenatal Care of Mothers Delivering Very Low Birth Weight Infants," *Journal of Perinatology* 26 (2006): 74, https://doi.org/10.1038/sj.jp.7211428.

56. Paul et al., "Racial Differences in Prenatal Care," 74.

57. Paul et al., "Racial Differences in Prenatal Care," 74.

58. Paul et al., "Racial Differences in Prenatal Care," 74.

59. Heba M. Eltoukhi et al., "The Health Disparities of Uterine Fibroid Tumors for African American Women: A Public Health Issue," *American Journal of Obstetrics and Gynecology* 210, no. 3 (2014): 195–197, https://doi.org/10.1016/j.ajog.2013.08.008.

60. Paul et al., "Racial Differences in Prenatal Care," 74.

61. Reed Mszar et al., "Racial/Ethnic Disparities in Screening for and Awareness of High Cholesterol among Pregnant Women Receiving Prenatal Care," *Journal of the American Heart Association* 10, no. 1 (2021): 8, https://doi.org/10.1161/JAHA.120.017415; Lakshmi S. Tummala et al., "Management Considerations for Lipid Disorders during Pregnancy," *Current Treatment Options in Cardiovascular Medicine* 23, no. 50 (May 2021): 2, https://doi.org/10.1007/s11936-021-00926-1.

62. Michael D. Kogan et al., "Racial Disparities in Reported Prenatal Care Advice from Health Care Providers," *American Journal of Public Health* 84, no. 1 (1994): 86, https://doi.org/10.2105/AJPH.84.1.82.

63. Maya A. Wright et al., "Changing Trends in Black–White Racial Differences in Surgical Menopause: A Population-Based Study," *American Journal of Obstetrics and Gynecology* 225, no. 5 (2021): 502.e1–502.e13, https://doi.org/10.1016/j.ajog.2021.05.045.

64. Allison S. Bryant et al., "Racial/Ethnic Disparities in Obstetric Outcomes and Care: Prevalence and Determinants," *American Journal of Obstetrics and Gynecology* 202, no. 4 (2010): 338, https://doi.org/10.1016/j.ajog.2009.10.864.

65. Elise G. Valdes, "Examining Cesarean Delivery Rates by Race: A Population-Based Analysis Using the Robson Ten-Group Classification System," *Journal of Racial and Ethnic Health Disparities* 8, no. 4 (2021): 844, 846, https://doi.org/10.1007/s40615-020-00842-3.

66. Colleen Campbell, "Medical Violence, Obstetric Racism, and the Limits of Informed Consent for Black Women," *Michigan Journal of Race and Law* 26, special issue (2021): 62, https://doi.org/10.36643/mjrl.26.sp.medical.

67. Campbell, "Medical Violence," 62–63.

68. Osamudia James, "The 'Innocence' of Bias," *Michigan Law Review* 119, no. 6 (2021): 1346, https://doi.org/10.36644/mlr.119.6.innocence.

69. Ivy W. Maina et al., "A Decade of Studying Implicit Racial/Ethnic Bias in Healthcare Providers Using the Implicit Association Test," *Social Science and Medicine* 199 (2018): 224, https://doi.org/10.1016/j.socscimed.2017.05.009.

70. Maina et al., " A Decade of Studying Implicit Racial/Ethnic Bias," 222–223.

71. Maina et al., " A Decade of Studying Implicit Racial/Ethnic Bias," 226.

72. Samreen Vora et al., "Recommendations and Guidelines for the Use of Simulation to Address Structural Racism and Implicit Bias," *Simulation in Healthcare: The Journal of the Society for Simulation in Healthcare* 16, no. 4 (2021): 275, https://doi.org/10.1097/SIH.0000000000000591.

73. Patricia G. Devine and Tory L. Ash, "Diversity Training Goals, Limitations, and Promise: A Review of the Multidisciplinary Literature," *Annual Review of Psychology* 73 (January 2022): 404, https://doi.org/10.1146/annurev-psych-060221-122215; Starbucks, "Starbucks to

Close All Stores Nationwide for Racial-Bias Education on May 29," accessed December 11, 2024, https://stories.starbucks.com/press/2018/starbucks-to-close-stores-nationwide-for-racial-bias-education-may-29/.

74. L. Song Richardson and Phillip A. Goff, "Implicit Racial Bias in Public Defender Triage," *Yale Law Journal* 122, no. 8 (2013): 2629, https://www.jstor.org/stable/23528687.

75. Celeste S. Royce et al., "The Time Is Now: Addressing Implicit Bias in Obstetrics and Gynecology Education," *American Journal of Obstetrics and Gynecology* 228, no. 4 (2023): 378, https://doi.org/10.1016/j.ajog.2022.12.016.

76. Khiara M. Bridges, *Critical Race Theory: A Primer* (West Academic Publishing, 2018).

77. Sirry Alang et al., "Police Brutality and Mistrust in Medical Institutions," *Journal of Racial and Ethnic Health Disparities* 7, no. 4 (2020): 761, https://doi.org/10.1007/s40615-020-00706-w; Marcella Alsan et al., "Does Diversity Matter for Health? Experimental Evidence from Oakland," *American Economic Review* 109, no. 12 (2019): 4072–4073, https://doi.org/10.1257/aer.20181446; Adolfo G. Cuevas and Kerth O'Brien, "Racial Centrality May Be Linked to Mistrust in Healthcare Institutions for African Americans," *Journal of Health Psychology* 24, no. 14 (2019): 2022, https://doi.org/10.1177/1359105317715092; Lillie D. Williamson, "Beyond Personal Experiences: Examining Mediated Vicarious Experiences as an Antecedent of Medical Mistrust," *Health Communication* 37, no. 9 (2022): 1061–1074, https://doi.org/10.1080/10410236.2020.1868744.

78. Allan M. Brandt, "Racism and Research: The Case of the Tuskegee Syphilis Study," *Hastings Center Report* 8, no. 6 (1978): 21, https://doi.org/10.2307/3561468.

79. Brandt, "Racism and Research," 21, 24.

80. Brandt, "Racism and Research," 27.

81. Brandt, "Racism and Research," 21, 25–27.

82. Brandt, "Racism and Research," 21.

83. Hetty Chang, "Combating Vaccine Hesitancy among Black Americans after Mistrust Caused by Unethical Study," NBC Los Angeles, September 11, 2021, https://www.nbclosangeles.com/news/local/combating-vaccine-hesitancy-among-black-americans-after-mistrust-caused-by-unethical-study/2690303/.

84. Chang, "Combating Vaccine Hesitancy."

85. Ruha Benjamin, "Cultura Obscura: Race, Power, and 'Culture Talk' in the Health Sciences," *American Journal of Law and Medicine* 43, no. 2–3 (2017): 234, https://doi.org/10.1177/0098858817723661.

86. Simar Singh Bajaj and Fatima Cody Stanford, "Beyond Tuskegee: Vaccine Distrust and Everyday Racism," *New England Journal of Medicine* 384, no. 5 (2021): e12(1), https://doi.org/10.1056/NEJMpv2035827.

87. Benjamin, "Cultura Obscura," 234.

CHAPTER 4

1. "CDC on Infant and Maternal Mortality in the United States: 1900–99," *Population and Development Review* 25, no. 4 (December 1, 1999): 824. https://www.jstor.org/stable/172510.

2. Helena Andrews-Dyer, "This Isn't Another Horror Story About Black Motherhood," *Washington Post*, September 4, 2019, https://www.washingtonpost.com/graphics/2019/lifestyle/black-motherhood/.

3. Jessica Grose, "Black Maternal Mortality Is Still a Crisis," *New York Times*, June 22, 2022, https://www.nytimes.com/2022/06/22/opinion/black-maternal-mortality.html.

4. Erica L. Green, "'I Don't Want to Die': Fighting Maternal Mortality among Black Women," *New York Times*, January 18, 2023, https://www.nytimes.com/2023/01/18/us/doula-black-women.html.

5. Claire Cain Miller et al., "Childbirth Is Deadlier for Black Families Even When They're Rich, Expansive Study Finds," *New York Times*, February 12, 2023, https://www.nytimes.com/interactive/2023/02/12/upshot/child-maternal-mortality-rich-poor.html.

6. Anna Malaika Tubbs, "'I Knew How Dangerous Things Could Become': The Perils of Childbirth as a Black Woman," *The Guardian*, June 26, 2021, https://www.theguardian.com/lifeandstyle/2021/jun/26/i-knew-how-dangerous-things-could-become-perils-of-childbirth-as-a-black-woman.

7. Brianna Scott et al., "The Rates of Death for Pregnant Black Women Have Doubled the Last 20 Years," NPR, July 7, 2023, https://www.npr.org/2023/07/07/1186531829/the-rates-of-death-for-pregnant-black-women-have-doubled-the-last-20-years.

8. Nina Martin and Renee Montagne, "Nothing Protects Black Women from Dying in Pregnancy and Childbirth," *ProPublica*, December 7, 2017, https://www.propublica.org/article/nothing-protects-black-women-from-dying-in-pregnancy-and-childbirth.

9. Tianna Madison, "I Survived the Black Maternal Health Crisis. My Friend Didn't," *Newsweek*, June 26, 2023, https://www.newsweek.com/black-maternity-crisis-tori-bowie-1808651.

10. Cierra Bryant and Brooke Muya, "We Must Treat the Black Maternal Health Crisis with the Urgency It Deserves," *Newsweek*, July 7, 2023, https://www.newsweek.com/we-must-treat-black-maternal-health-crisis-urgency-it-deserves-opinion-1811127.

11. Minvonne Burke, "She Was a Black Pediatrician But Still Died after Giving Birth to Her 1st Child," *Today*, November 6, 2022, https://www.today.com/health/she-was-black-pediatrician-still-died-after-giving-birth-her-t198011.

12. Maia Niguel Hoskin, "Black Women Are Dying during Childbirth and No One Seems to Care," *Forbes*, February 20, 2023, https://www.forbes.com/sites/maiahoskin/2023/02/20/black-mothers-report-feeling-ignored-or-dismissed-by-health-care-providers-as-maternal-health-disparities-persist/?sh=2737e681d857.

13. Ann M. Simmons, "The Quiet Crisis among African Americans: Pregnancy and Childbirth Are Killing Women at Inexplicable Rates," *Los Angeles Times*, October 26, 2017, https://www

.latimes.com/world/global-development/la-na-texas-black-maternal-mortality-2017-html story.html.

14. Katie Kindelan et al., "US Olympian Dies from Pregnancy Complication That Disproportionately Impacts Black Women," ABC News, June 13, 2023, https://abcnews.go.com/GMA/Wellness/us-olympian-dies-pregnancy-complication-disproportionately-impacts-black/story?id=100045363.

15. Lyndon Haviland, "Regardless of Income, Black Women Face Death to Give Birth in America," *The Hill*, March 1, 2023, https://thehill.com/opinion/healthcare/3879248-regardless-of-income-black-women-face-death-to-give-birth-in-america/.

16. Rachel Jones, "Maternal Mortality Is Shockingly High in the U.S.—Especially If You're Black," *National Geographic*, June 22, 2023, https://www.nationalgeographic.com/premium/article/maternal-mortality-usa-health-motherhood.

17. Anushay Hossain, "We Should All Be Talking About America's Black Maternal Health Crisis," *Harper's Bazaar*, November 5, 2021, https://www.harpersbazaar.com/culture/features/a38094736/americas-black-maternal-health-crisis/.

18. Denetra Walker and Kelli Boling, "Black Maternal Mortality in the Media: How Journalists Cover a Deadly Racial Disparity," *Journalism* 24, no. 7 (2023): 1538, https://doi.org/10.1177/14648849211063361.

19. Walker and Boling, "Black Maternal Mortality in the Media," 1538.

20. Nina Martin and Renee Montagne, "Lost Mothers: Maternal Mortality in the U.S.," NPR, 2017, https://www.npr.org/series/543928389/lost-mothers.

21. Nina Martin and Renee Montagne, "Black Mothers Keep Dying after Giving Birth. Shalon Irving's Story Explains Why," NPR, December 7, 2017, https://www.npr.org/2017/12/07/568948782/black-mothers-keep-dying-after-giving-birth-shalon-irvings-story-explains-why.

22. Martin and Montagne, "Black Mothers Keep Dying after Giving Birth."

23. Rob Haskell, "Serena Williams on Motherhood, Marriage, and Making Her Comeback," *Vogue*, January 10, 2018, https://www.vogue.com/article/serena-williams-vogue-cover-interview-february-2018; Walker and Boling, "Black Maternal Mortality in the Media," 1538.

24. Haskell, "Serena Williams on Motherhood."

25. Haskell, "Serena Williams on Motherhood."

26. Haskell, "Serena Williams on Motherhood."

27. Linda Villarosa, "Why America's Black Mothers and Babies Are in a Life-or-Death Crisis," *New York Times*, April 11, 2018, https://www.nytimes.com/2018/04/11/magazine/black-mothers-babies-death-maternal-mortality.html.

28. Jennifer C. Nash, *Birthing Black Mothers* (Duke University Press, 2021), 3, https://doi.org/10.2307/j.ctv1s04wng.

29. *Homecoming: A Film by Beyoncé*, directed by Beyoncé Knowles-Carter, aired April 17, 2019, on Netflix, https://www.netflix.com/title/81013626.

30. Derecka Purnell, "If Even Beyoncé Had a Rough Pregnancy, What Hope Do Other Black Women Have?," *The Guardian*, April 23, 2019, https://www.theguardian.com/commentisfree/2019/apr/23/beyonce-pregnancy-black-women.

31. Alissa Chang et al., hosts, *Summer of Racial Reckoning*, podcast, season 1, episode 1, "The Match Lit," NPR, August 16, 2020, https://www.npr.org/2020/08/16/902179773/summer-of-racial-reckoning-the-match-lit.

32. Michelle S. Phelps and Amber M. Hamilton, "Visualizing Injustice or Reifying Racism? Images in the Digital Media Coverage of the Killing of Michael Brown," *Sociology of Race and Ethnicity* 8, no. 1 (2021): 161, https://doi.org/10.1177/23326492211015696.

33. Nash, *Birthing Black Mothers*, 22.

34. Haile Eshe Cole, "Reproduction on Display: Black Maternal Mortality and the Newest Case for National Action," *Journal of the Motherhood Initiative for Research and Community Involvement* 9, no. 2 (2018): 89, 92 https://jarm.journals.yorku.ca/index.php/jarm/article/view/40511; Jacqueline Golsby, *A Spectacular Secret: Lynching in American Life and Literature* (University of Chicago Press, 2006); Amy Louise Wood, *Lynching and Spectacle: Witnessing Racial Violence in America, 1890–1940* (University of North Carolina Press, 2009).

35. Walker and Bolling, "Black Maternal Mortality in the Media," 1539–1540.

36. Cole, "Reproduction on Display," 90.

37. David Pilgrim, "The Mammy Caricature," Jim Crow Museum, October 2000, last modified 2024, https://jimcrowmuseum.ferris.edu/mammies/homepage.htm.

38. Daniel Patrick Moynihan, *The Negro Family: The Case for National Action* (United States Department of Labor, 1965), 29–45, https://web.stanford.edu/~mrosenfe/Moynihan's%20The%20Negro%20Family.pdf.

39. Gene Demby, "The Truth behind the Lies of the Original 'Welfare Queen,'" NPR, December 20, 2013, https://www.npr.org/sections/codeswitch/2013/12/20/255819681/the-truth-behind-the-lies-of-the-original-welfare-queen.

40. Charles Krauthammer, "Children of Cocaine," *Washington Post*, July 30, 1989.

41. Cole, "Reproduction on Display," 95.

42. Nash, *Birthing Black Mothers*, 4.

43. Nash, *Birthing Black Mothers*, 175.

44. Nash, *Birthing Black Mothers*, 4.

45. Walker and Boling, "Black Maternal Mortality in the Media," 1544.

46. Walker and Boling, "Black Maternal Mortality in the Media," 1548.

47. Martha Minow, *Saving the News: Why the Constitution Calls for Government Action to Preserve Freedom of Speech* (Oxford University Press, 2021), 16.

48. Safiya Umoja Noble, "Teaching Trayvon: Race, Media, and the Politics of Spectacle," *Black Scholar* 44. no. 1 (2014): 25, https://www.jstor.org/stable/10.5816/blackscholar.44.1.0012.

49. Wesley Lowery, "A Test of the News: Objectivity, Democracy, and the American Mosaic," *Columbia Journalism Review*, April 25, 2023, https://www.cjr.org/analysis/a-test-of-the-news-wesley-lowery-objectivity.php.

50. Jesse Holcomb et al., "The Revenue Picture for American Journalism and How It Is Changing," Pew Research Center, March 26, 2014, 2, https://www.pewresearch.org/wp-content/uploads/sites/8/2014/03/Revnue-Picture-for-American-Journalism.pdf.

51. Technically, cable providers pay cable fees to cable channels for the right to offer the channel in the packages that customers can purchase from the provider. Providers ultimately "pass along those fees to consumers in the form of their monthly bills." Holcomb et al., "The Revenue Picture for American Journalism," 10.

52. Holcomb et al., "The Revenue Picture for American Journalism," 6.

53. Holcomb et al., "The Revenue Picture for American Journalism," 2.

54. Thomas E. Patterson, "Time and News: The Media's Limitations as an Instrument of Democracy," *International Political Science Review* 19, no. 1 (1998): 56.

55. Frances Robles, "The Citizen's Arrest Law Cited in Arbery's Killing Dates Back to the Civil War," *New York Times*, May 13, 2020, https://www.nytimes.com/article/ahmaud-arbery-citizen-arrest-law-georgia.html.

56. Tonia Sutherland, "Making a Killing: On Race, Ritual, and (Re)Membering in Digital Culture," *Preservation, Digital Technology & Culture* 46, no. 1 (2017): 20, https://doi.org/10.1515/pdtc-2017-0025.

57. Sutherland, "Making a Killing," 38; see also Noble, "Teaching Trayvon," 23.

58. Noble observes that punditry comprises a "whole industry" wherein people "make a living off of commenting," and she notes that there likely will be "Pulitzer Prize–winning journalism that will come out of black horror." Safiya Umoja Noble, "Media Coverage and the Political Economy of Black Death," interview by Jared Ball, *¡MWiL!*, July 14, 2016, video, 19:43, https://imixwhatilike.org/2016/07/14/media-coverage-and-the-political-economy-of-black-death/.

59. Minow, *Saving the News*, 20.

60. However, Minow notes that the democratic crisis that the first Trump presidency posed to the nation resulted in a rash of new subscribers for the *New York Times* and *Washington Post*, which "brought those top papers to record numbers and sustaining revenues." The vast majority of newspapers, however, have not been as fortunate. Minow, *Saving the News*, 14.

61. Minow, *Saving the News*, 18.

62. Zachary Hagen-Smith, "Salience Bias: The 24-Hour News Cycle Is a Market Failure," *Berkeley Economic Review*, April 25, 2022, https://econreview.studentorg.berkeley.edu/salience-bias-the-24-hour-news-cycle-is-a-market-failure/.

63. Howard Rosenberg and Charles S. Feldman, *No Time to Think: The Menace of Media Speed and the 24-Hour News Cycle* (Bloomsbury Publishing, 2009), 52–53.

64. The ideological commitments of Fox News make it unlikely that the TV channel has ever provided significant coverage of black maternal deaths. Moreover, if Fox News were to cover the phenomenon, it might be expected to frame the deaths as products of black insufficiency as opposed to structural inequality.

65. Saidiya Hartman, *Scenes of Subjection: Terror, Slavery, and Self-Making in Nineteenth-Century America* (W. W. Norton, 1997), 243.

66. Hartman, *Scenes of Subjection*, 21.

67. Noble, "Media Coverage and the Political Economy of Black Death."

68. Hartman, *Scenes of Subjection*, 22.

69. Alisha Ebrahimji, "Some Say Sharing Videos of Police Brutality against Black People Is Just 'Trauma Porn,'" CNN, August 25, 2020, https://www.cnn.com/2020/08/25/us/police-brutality-videos-trauma-porn-trnd/index.html. Some have also described "videos showing violent black death" as "death porn or perverse entertainment." Kia Gregory, "How Videos of Police Brutality Traumatize African Americans and Undermine the Search for Justice," *New Republic*, February 13, 2019, https://newrepublic.com/article/153103/videos-police-brutality-traumatize-african-americans-undermine-search-justice.

70. Gregory, "How Videos of Police Brutality Traumatize African Americans."

71. Phelps and Hamilton, "Visualizing Injustice or Reifying Racism?," 162.

72. Equal Justice Initiative, "Bloody Sunday: Civil Rights Activists Brutally Attacked in Selma," accessed February 11, 2025, https://calendar.eji.org/racial-injustice/mar/7#:~:text=On%20March%207%2C%201965%2C%20state,the%20state%20capitol%20in%20Montgomery; Library of Congress, "Today in History—March 7: First March from Selma," accessed August 1, 2024, https://www.loc.gov/item/today-in-history/march-07/.

73. Library of Congress, "First March from Selma."

74. Rasul A. Mowatt, "Black Lives as Snuff: The Silent Complicity in Viewing Black Death," *Biography* 41, no. 4 (September 2018): 781, https://doi.org/10.1353/bio.2018.0079.

75. Villarosa, "Why America's Black Mothers and Babies Are in a Life-or-Death Crisis."

76. Cole, "Reproduction on Display," 92.

77. Mowatt, "Black Lives as Snuff," 778.

78. Debra Walker King, *African Americans and the Culture of Pain* (University of Virginia Press, 2008), 13.

79. Mowatt, "Black Lives as Snuff," 787.

80. Nash, *Birthing Black Mothers*, 4–6.

81. Nash, *Birthing Black Mothers*, 7.

82. Nash, *Birthing Black Mothers*, 177.
83. Andrews-Dyer, "This Isn't Another Horror Story About Black Motherhood."
84. Andrews-Dyer, "This Isn't Another Horror Story About Black Motherhood."
85. Nash, *Birthing Black Mothers*, 3, 21, 56. See also Leith Mullings and Alaka Wali, *Stress and Resilience: The Social Context of Reproduction in Central Harlem* (Springer Nature, 2001).
86. As of January 17, 2025, forty-nine states and the District of Columbia provide Medicaid coverage for up to twelve months postpartum. KFF, "Medicaid Postpartum Coverage Extension Tracker," last modified January 17, 2025, https://www.kff.org/medicaid/issue-brief/medicaid-postpartum-coverage-extension-tracker/.
87. Tanesha Mondestin, "State Momentum on Medicaid Doula Coverage, Rate Increases," Center for Children & Families at the Georgetown University McCourt School of Public Policy, April 11, 2024, https://ccf.georgetown.edu/2024/04/11/state-momentum-on-medicaid-doula-coverage-rate-increases/.
88. California Maternal Quality Care Collaborative, "Who We Are," accessed August 1, 2024, https://www.cmqcc.org/who-we-are.
89. California Maternal Quality Care Collaborative, "Toolkits," accessed August 1, 2024, https://www.cmqcc.org/resources-tool-kits/toolkits.
90. California Maternal Quality Care Collaborative, "Toolkits."
91. California Maternal Quality Care Collaborative, "California Hospital Membership," accessed January 24, 2025, https://www.cmqcc.org/about-cmqcc/member-hospitals/california-hospital-membership.
92. Rachel Frazin, "Warren Unveils Plan to Reward Hospitals That Make Childbirth Safer for Black Women," *The Hill*, April 25, 2019, https://thehill.com/homenews/campaign/440629-warren-unveils-plan-to-reward-hospitals-that-make-childbirth-safer-for/.
93. Andrews-Dyer, "This Isn't Another Horror Story About Black Motherhood."
94. Samantha Vincenty, "Kamala Harris Is Fighting to Protect Black Mothers from Medical Bias," *Oprah Daily*, August 13, 2020, https://www.oprahdaily.com/entertainment/a33577853/kamala-harris-black-maternal-health-care-crisis/. The Momnibus Act, which never made it out of congressional committees, consisted of "nine bills aimed at combating maternal health disparities through investment in community-based programs and other efforts to rectify social determinants of health." Edwin Rios, "'Birthing While Black' Is a National Crisis for the US. Here's What Black Lawmakers Want to Do about It," *The Guardian*, April 19, 2022, https://www.theguardian.com/us-news/2022/apr/19/black-mothers-birth-maternal-mortality.
95. "Fact Sheet: Vice President Kamala Harris Announces Call to Action to Reduce Maternal Mortality and Morbidity," The White House, December 7, 2021, https://web.archive.org/web/20250116071958/https://www.whitehouse.gov/briefing-room/statements-releases/2021/12/07/fact-sheet-vice-president-kamala-harris-announces-call-to-action-to-reduce-maternal-mortality-and-morbidity/.

96. The White House, "Fact Sheet."

97. Joan E. Greve, "Senate Passes $739 Bn Healthcare and Climate Bill after Months of Wrangling," *The Guardian*, August 7, 2022, https://www.theguardian.com/us-news/2022/aug/07/inflation-reduction-act-senate-democrats-pass.

98. Nash, *Birthing Black Mothers*, 15. In 2018, Congress passed the Preventing Maternal Deaths Act, which allocates $60 million to states over five years to fund maternal mortality review commissions to investigate every pregnancy-related death in the jurisdiction and compile data on these events. The Preventing Maternal Deaths Act is an exasperating piece of legislation. For a critique of the act, see Khiara M. Bridges, "Racial Disparities in Maternal Mortality," *New York University Law Review* 95, no. 5 (2020): 1229–1318.

99. Safiya Umoja Noble, "Critical Surveillance Literacy in Social Media: Interrogating Black Death and Dying Online," *Black Camera* 9, no. 2 (2018): 149, https://doi.org/10.2979/blackcamera.9.2.10.

100. Michelle A. Williams, "The Cost of Bearing Witness: Watching and Sharing Videos of Police Brutality Online," *BMJ*, March 16, 2023, https://doi.org/10.1136/bmj.p616.

101. Nash, *Birthing Black Mothers*, 4.

102. Nash, *Birthing Black Mothers*, 5.

103. Khiara M. Bridges, *Reproducing Race: An Ethnography of Pregnancy as a Site of Racialization* (University of California Press, 2011), 12.

CHAPTER 5

1. Sociologist Karyn Lacy makes a similar observation in her investigation of class-privileged black people, writing that the "middle-class blacks" that she studied "actively correct[ed] the misapprehensions of white strangers"—who tended to "equate race with class and then reflexively consign[ed] all blacks to the lowest class level"—by signaling their class privilege through their clothing, speech, and "mannerisms." Karyn R. Lacy, *Blue-Chip Black: Race, Class, and Status in the New Black Middle Class* (University of California Press, 2007), 73.

2. Journalist Linda Villarosa's recounts engaging in the same tactic in her powerful exposition on racial disparities in health, *Under the Skin*. Linda Villarosa, *Under the Skin: The Hidden Toll of Racism on American Lives and on the Health of Our Nation* (Vintage, 2023), 18.

3. Most black patients who choose racially concordant care are aware that a provider's black race imperfectly predicts the characteristics that the patient hopes a provider will have. Chapter 6 elaborates on this point.

4. Future studies might explore the similarities and differences between the comfort that black patients hope to experience in racially concordant clinical encounters and the comfort that leads many cisgender women to choose cisgender women as providers for obstetrical and gynecological care. Does a cisgender woman's desire for sex and gender concordance in reproductive healthcare similarly stem from the expectation that providers who were assigned female at birth will have shared experiences with them? Do cisgender women similarly believe

that they share a common foundation with providers who are also cisgender women and that this common foundation will lead to the provision of quality healthcare? Or are the two situations completely different?

5. Annette Burfoot and Derya Güngör, "The Medicalization of Pregnancy and Birth," in *Women and Reproductive Technologies: The Socio-Economic Development of Technologies Changing the World* (Routledge, 2022), 35.

6. Kristin K. Barker, "A Ship upon a Stormy Sea: The Medicalization of Pregnancy," *Social Science and Medicine* 47, no. 8 (1998): 1068, https://doi.org/10.1016/S0277-9536(98)00155-5.

7. Burfoot and Güngör, "The Medicalization of Pregnancy and Birth," 26.

8. Robbie E. Davis-Floyd, "The Technocratic Body: American Childbirth as Cultural Expression," *Social Science and Medicine* 38, no. 8 (1994): 1137, https://doi.org/10.1016/0277-9536(94)90228-3.

9. Davis-Floyd, "The Technocratic Body," 1138.

10. Davis-Floyd, "The Technocratic Body," 1127.

11. Iris Marion Young, "Pregnant Embodiment: Subjectivity and Alienation," *Journal of Medicine and Philosophy: A Forum for Bioethics and Philosophy of Medicine* 9, no. 1 (1984): 57–58, https://doi.org/10.1093/jmp/9.1.45. Many people assume that rates of maternal and infant mortality and morbidity started falling when medicine began managing pregnancy and childbirth. However, the data do not support this conclusion. One researcher observes that while there was a dramatic reduction in maternal and infant mortality rates in the United Kingdom between 1900 and 1920, "biomedicine made little direct contribution. . . . Standards of living for poorer sections of society increased substantially during the war years; if pregnant women were able to avail themselves of a better diet, clearly both they and their unborn infants would benefit, which is the most probable explanation for falling mortality rates." Heather A. Cahill, "Male Appropriation and Medicalization of Childbirth: An Historical Analysis," *Journal of Advanced Nursing* 33, no. 3 (2001): 336.

12. Sarah Jane Brubaker, "Denied, Embracing, and Resisting Medicalization: African American Teen Mothers' Perceptions of Formal Pregnancy and Childbirth Care," *Gender & Society* 21, no. 4 (2007): 532, https://doi.org/10.1177/0891243207304972.

13. Gertrude Jacinta Fraser, *African American Midwifery in the South: Dialogues of Birth, Race, and Memory* (Harvard University Press, 1998), 178.

14. Fraser, *African American Midwifery in the South*, 178.

15. Khiara M. Bridges, *Reproducing Race: An Ethnography of Pregnancy as a Site of Racialization* (University of California Press, 2011).

16. Ellen S. Lazarus, "What Do Women Want? Issues of Choice, Control, and Class in Pregnancy and Childbirth," *Medical Anthropology Quarterly* 8, no. 1 (1994): 30, https://doi.org/10.1525/maq.1994.8.1.02a00030.

17. Lazarus, "What Do Women Want?," 39.

18. Annette's experience is consistent with reports from the literature. As sociologist Julia Chinyere Oparah and coauthors write, "In black communities, alternative ideas of beauty and different body ideals exist, leading to a greater acceptance and celebration of roundness and curves, and an appreciation for 'thick' women." Julia Chinyere Oparah et al., *Battling over Birth: Black Women and the Maternal Health Crisis* (Praeclarus Press, 2017), 34.

19. Annette's experience has scholarly affirmation. See Joy Arlene Renee Cox, *Fat Girls in Black Bodies: Creating Communities of Our Own* (North Atlantic Books, 2020); Da'Shaun L. Harrison, *Belly of the Beast: The Politics of Anti-Fatness as Anti-Blackness* (North Atlantic Books, 2021); Sabrina Strings, *Fearing the Black Body: The Racial Origins of Fat Phobia* (New York University Press, 2018).

20. Dominique Tobbell and Patricia D'Antonio, "The History of Racism in Nursing: A Review of Existing Scholarship" (National Commission to Address Racism in Nursing, 2022), 13, https://www.nursingworld.org/globalassets/practiceandpolicy/workforce/commission-to-address-racism/1thehistoryofracisminnursing.pdf.

21. American Midwifery Certification Board, *2023 Demographic Report* (2024), 1, https://www.amcbmidwife.org/docs/default-source/default-document-library/demographic-report-2023.pdf?sfvrsn=432df54b_0.

22. David Harvey, *A Brief History of Neoliberalism* (Oxford University Press, 2005), 2.

23. Niklas Olsen, *The Sovereign Consumer: A New Intellectual History of Neoliberalism* (Palgrave MacMillan, 2019).

24. The rise of far-right, white Christian nationalism in the United States suggests the country might be turning toward fascism more than neoliberalism. Nevertheless, it is possible that fascism can exist within neoliberalism.

25. Saidiya Hartman, *Scenes of Subjection: Terror, Slavery, and Self-Making in Nineteenth-Century America* (W. W. Norton, 1997), 171.

26. This is akin to what anthropologist Dána-Ain Davis observed among the nonblack healthcare professionals that she interviewed for her research on premature births among black people. She noted that even though many interviewees knew that higher rates of premature births persist across income levels, they typically insisted on talking about the issue as a problem of class, not race. Davis uses the term "racial refusal" to describe this tendency. Dána-Ain Davis, *Reproductive Injustice: Racism, Pregnancy, and Premature Birth* (New York University Press, 2019), 88. The racial renunciations that I observed are different from Davis's racial refusals insofar as racial renunciations were made by black patients—as opposed to nonblack providers and other interested third parties. Moreover, while racial refusals represent a disinclination to engage with race and racism out of discomfort or due to a political commitment that racism is not meaningful in a post–civil rights era, racial renunciations represent a disinclination to engage with race and racism as a way to survive racism.

27. [name redacted], "Midwifery at [redacted]," accessed August 8, 2024, [url redacted].

28. [name redacted], "Midwifery at [redacted]."

CHAPTER 6

1. Alameda Health System, "Black Centering Is a New Kind of Care Made for You and Your Baby," accessed July 31, 2024, https://www.alamedahealthsystem.org/family-birthing-center/black-centering/.

2. Ivy W. Maina et al., "A Decade of Studying Implicit Racial/Ethnic Bias in Healthcare Providers Using the Implicit Association Test," *Social Science and Medicine* 199 (2018): 227, https://doi.org/10.1016/j.socscimed.2017.05.009.

3. See Monica B. Vela et al., "Eliminating Explicit and Implicit Biases in Health Care: Evidence and Research Needs," *Annual Review of Public Health* 43 (2022): 482, https://doi.org/10.1146/annurev-publhealth-052620-103528.

4. Sonya T. Gleicher et al., "Confronting Implicit Bias toward Patients: A Scoping Review of Post-graduate Physician Curricula," *BMC Medical Education* 22, no. 1 (2022): 7, https://doi.org/10.1186/s12909-022-03720-0.

5. Osamudia James, "The 'Innocence' of Bias," *Michigan Law Review* 119, no. 6 (2021): 1359.

6. Crystal Jongen et al., *Cultural Competence in Health: A Review of the Evidence* (Springer, 2018), 5; Sunil Kripalani et al., "A Prescription for Cultural Competence in Medical Education," *Journal of General Internal Medicine* 21, no. 10 (2006): 1116, https://doi.org/10.1111/j.1525-1497.2006.00557.x.

7. Stephane Shepherd, "Cultural Awareness Workshops: Limitations and Practical Consequences," *BMC Medical Education* 19, no. 1 (2019): 1, https://doi.org/10.1186/s12909-018-1450-5; Elizabeth Vella et al., "Does Cultural Competence Training for Health Professionals Impact Culturally and Linguistically Diverse Patient Outcomes? A Systematic Review of the Literature," *Nurse Education Today* 118, no. 1 (2022): 2, https://doi.org/10.1016/j.nedt.2022.105500.

8. Agency for Healthcare Research and Quality, "Improving Cultural Competence to Reduce Health Disparities for Priority Populations," Effective Health Care Program, archived July 8, 2014, https://effectivehealthcare.ahrq.gov/products/cultural-competence/research-protocol.

9. Shepherd, "Cultural Awareness," 1.

10. Liaison Committee on Medical Education, "Functions and Structure of a Medical School: Standards for Accreditation of Medical Education Programs Leading to the MD Degree" (2023), 11.

11. Jeff Stone and Gordon B. Moskowitz, "Non-Conscious Bias in Medical Decision Making: What Can Be Done to Reduce It?," *Medical Education* 45, no. 8 (2011): 771, https://doi.org/10.1111/j.1365-2923.2011.04026.x.

12. Jonathan M. Metzl and Helena Hansen, "Structural Competency: Theorizing a New Medical Engagement with Stigma and Inequality," *Social Science and Medicine* 103, no. 126 (2014): 126, https://doi.org/10.1016/j.socscimed.2013.06.032.

13. Joseph R. Betancourt, "Cultural Competence and Medical Education: Many Names, Many Perspectives, One Goal," *Academic Medicine* 81, no. 6 (2006): 500, https://doi.org/10.1097/01.ACM.0000225211.77088.cb.

14. Jeffrey T. Berger and Dana Ribeiro Miller, "Health Disparities, Systemic Racism, and Failures of Cultural Competence," *American Journal of Bioethics* 21, no. 4 (2021): 7, https://doi.org/10.1080/15265161.2021.1915411.

15. Scott D. Stonington et al., "Case Studies in Social Medicine: Attending to Structural Forces in Clinical Practice," *New England Journal of Medicine* 379, no. 20 (2018): 1959, https://doi.org/10.1056/NEJMms1814262.

16. Shepherd, "Cultural Awareness Workshops," 7.

17. Arnold R. Eiser and Glenn Ellis, "Cultural Competence and the African American Experience with Health Care: The Case for Specific Content in Cross-Cultural Education," *Academic Medicine* 82, no. 2 (2007): 177–178, https://doi.org/10.1097/ACM.0b013e31802d92ea.

18. Stone and Moskowitz, "Non-Conscious Bias," 771.

19. Patti Renee Rose, *Health Equity Diversity, and Inclusion: Context, Controversies, and Solutions* (Jones & Bartlett Learning, 2021), 429.

20. Brittney T. Anderson, "Access to Quality, Culturally Appropriate Health Care," in *Black Health in the South*, ed. Steven S. Coughlin et al. (Johns Hopkins University Press, 2023), 35.

21. Anderson, "Access to Quality, Culturally Appropriate Health Care," 35.

22. Joy Agner, "Moving from Cultural Competence to Cultural Humility in Occupational Therapy: A Paradigm Shift," *American Journal of Occupational Therapy* 74, no. 4 (2020): 3, https://doi.org/10.5014/ajot.2020.038067.

23. Agner, "Moving from Cultural Competence," 3.

24. Agner, "Moving from Cultural Competence," 1.

25. Imbi Drame et al., "Strategies for Incorporating Health Disparities and Cultural Competency Training into the Pharmacy Curriculum and Co-Curriculum," *American Journal of Pharmaceutical Education* 86, no. 3 (2022): 201, https://doi.org/10.5688/ajpe8631.

26. Patricia G. Devine and Tory L. Ash, "Diversity Training Goals, Limitations, and Promise: A Review of the Multidisciplinary Literature," *Annual Review of Psychology* 73, no. 1 (2022): 414, https://doi.org/10.1146/annurev-psych-060221-122215.

27. Devine and Ash, "Diversity Training," 414.

28. Devine and Ash, "Diversity Training," 414.

29. Shepherd, "Cultural Awareness Workshops," 6.

30. Tennyson S. Jellins et al., "Diversity, Equity, and Inclusion (DEI) in Medical Education: DEI at the Bedside," *Journal of the Neurological Sciences* 459 (2024): 2, https://doi.org/10.1016/j.jns.2024.122946.

31. Kyle A. Bersted et al., "A Path toward Equity and Inclusion: Establishing a DEI Committee in a Department of Pediatrics," *Journal of Clinical Psychology in Medical Settings* 30 (2023): 342–345, https://doi.org/10.1007/s10880-022-09929-x.
32. Bersted et al., "A Path toward Equity and Inclusion," 342–355.
33. Loretta Brancaccio-Taras et al., "The PULSE Diversity Equity and Inclusion (DEI) Rubric: A Tool to Help Assess Departmental DEI Efforts," *Journal of Microbiology and Biology Education* 23, no. 3 (2022): 1–8, https://doi.org/10.1128/jmbe.00057-22; Sonja R. Solomon et al., "Diversity Is Not Enough: Advancing a Framework for Antiracism in Medical Education," *Academic Medicine* 96, no. 11 (2021): 1513–1517, https://doi.org/10.1097/acm.0000000000004251.
34. Bersted et al., "A Path toward Equity and Inclusion," 352.
35. Simar S. Bajaj et al., "Medicine's DEI Backlash Offers an Opportunity to Refocus on Evidence-Based Approaches," *Nature Medicine* 30 (2024): 3040, https://doi.org/10.1038/s41591-024-03236-8.
36. Rachel Cox et al., "A Guide to Application of Diversity, Equity, and Inclusion (DEI) Principles for Prelicensure Nursing Education," *Journal of Professional Nursing* 46 (2023): 146–154, https://doi.org/10.1016/j.profnurs.2023.03.002.
37. Brancaccio-Taras et al., "The PULSE Diversity Equity and Inclusion (DEI) Rubric," 5.
38. Nwamaka D. Eneanya et al., "Reconsidering the Consequence of Using Race to Estimate Kidney Function," *JAMA* 322, no. 2 (2019): 113–114, https://doi.org/10.1001/jama.2019.5774.
39. Cox et al., "A Guide to Application of Diversity," 146–154.
40. Bajaj et al., "Medicine's DEI Backlash," 3040–3041.
41. Bajaj et al., "Medicine's DEI Backlash," 3040–3041.
42. Metzl and Hansen, "Structural Competency: Theorizing a New Medical Engagement," 126–133.
43. Jonathan M. Metzl, "Structural Competency," *American Quarterly* 64, no. 2 (2012): 214, http://www.jstor.org/stable/23273514.
44. Stonington et al., "Case Studies," 1959.
45. Jonathan M. Metzl and Helena Hansen, "Structural Competency and Psychiatry," *JAMA Psychiatry* 75, no. 2 (2018): 115, https://doi.org/10.1001/jamapsychiatry.2017.3891.
46. Metzl and Hansen, "Structural Competency: Theorizing a New Medical Engagement," 128.
47. Metzl and Hansen, "Structural Competency: Theorizing a New Medical Engagement," 128.
48. Metzl and Hansen, "Structural Competency: Theorizing a New Medical Engagement," 128.

49. Metzl and Hansen, "Structural Competency: Theorizing a New Medical Engagement," 215.

50. Metzl and Hansen, "Structural Competency: Theorizing a New Medical Engagement," 126.

51. Metzl and Hansen, "Structural Competency: Theorizing a New Medical Engagement," 132.

52. Jonathan M. Metzl et al., "Responding to the COVID-19 Pandemic: The Need for a Structurally Competent Health Care System," *JAMA* 324, no. 3 (2020): 231, https://doi.org/10.1001/jama.2020.9289.

53. World Health Organization, "Social Determinants of Health," accessed August 2, 2024, https://www.who.int/health-topics/social-determinants-of-health#tab=tab_1.

54. World Health Organization, "Social Determinants of Health."

55. Paula Braveman et al., "The Social Determinants of Health: Coming of Age," *Annual Review of Public Health* 32, no. 1 (2011): 382, https://doi.org/10.1146/annurev-publhealth-031210-101218.

56. Jonathan M. Metzl et al., "Using a Structural Competency Framework to Teach Structural Racism in Pre-Health Education," *Social Science and Medicine* 199, no. 1 (2018): 191, https://doi.org/10.1016/j.socscimed.2017.06.029.

57. Jennifer Edgoose et al., "Teaching About Racism in Medical Education: A Mixed-Method Analysis of a Train-the-Trainer Faculty Development Workshop," *Family Medicine* 53, no. 1 (2021): 24, https://doi.org/10.22454/FamMed.2021.408300.

58. Nia Johnson, "From a Reckoning to Racial Concordance: A Strategy to Protect Black Mothers, Children, and Infants," *Hastings Center Report* 52, no. 2 (2022): S32–S34, https://doi.org/10.1002/hast.1366.

59. Maina et al., "A Decade of Studying," 222.

60. Maina et al., "A Decade of Studying," 222.

61. Marcella Alsan et al., "Does Diversity Matter for Health? Experimental Evidence from Oakland," *American Economic Review* 109, no. 12 (2019): 4073, https://doi.org/10.1257/aer.20181446; Anderson, "Access to Quality, Culturally Appropriate Health Care," 31–50; Ann Neville Miller et al., "The Relationship of Ethnic, Racial, and Cultural Concordance to Physician–Patient Communication: A Mixed-Methods Systematic Review Protocol," *Health Communication* 38, no. 11 (2022): 2370–2376, https://doi.org/10.1080/10410236.2022.2070449.

62. Alsan et al., "Does Diversity Matter for Health?," 4073.

63. Miller et al., "The Relationship of Ethnic," 2370; Megan Johnson Shen et al., "The Effects of Race and Racial Concordance on Patient–Physician Communication: A Systematic Review of the Literature," *Journal of Racial and Ethnic Health Disparities* 5, no. 1 (2018): 136, https://doi.org/10.1007/s40615-017-0350-4.

64. Lisa A. Cooper and Neil R. Powe, "Disparities in Patient Experiences, Health Care Processes, and Outcomes: The Role of Patient–Provider Racial, Ethnic, and Language Concordance,"

The Commonwealth Fund, July 1, 2004, https://www.commonwealthfund.org/publications/fund-reports/2004/jul/disparities-patient-experiences-health-care-processes-and.

65. Claire E. Ashton-James et al., "Understanding the Contribution of Racially and Ethnically Discordant Interactions to Pain Disparities: Proximal Mechanisms and Potential Solutions," *Pain* 164, no. 2 (2023): 224. https://doi.org/10.1097/j.pain.0000000000002698; Sonia V. Otte, "Improved Patient Experience and Outcomes: Is Patient–Provider Concordance Key?," *Journal of Patient* 9 (2022): 1, https://doi.org/10.1177/23743735221103033; Cindy Zhao et al., "Race, Gender, and Language Concordance in the Care of Surgical Patients: A Systematic Review," *Surgery* 166, no. 5 (2019): 786, https://doi.org/10.1016/j.surg.2019.06.012.

66. Ashton-James et al., "Understanding the Contribution," 224.

67. Alsan et al., "Does Diversity Matter for Health?," 4071.

68. Alsan et al., "Does Diversity Matter for Health?," 4075.

69. Alsan et al., "Does Diversity Matter for Health?," 4077.

70. Alsan et al., "Does Diversity Matter for Health?," 4107.

71. Michael D. Frakes and Jonathan Gruber, "Racial Concordance and the Quality of Medical Care: Evidence from the Military," Working Paper No. 30767, National Bureau of Economic Research (December 2022), 30, http://www.nber.org/papers/w30767.

72. Brad R. Greenwood et al., "Physician–Patient Racial Concordance and Disparities in Birthing Mortality for Newborns," *Proceedings of the National Academy of Sciences* 117, no. 35 (2020): 21194, https://doi.org/10.1073/pnas.1913405117.

73. Greenwood et al., "Physician–Patient Racial Concordance," 21195.

74. Alsan et al., "Does Diversity Matter for Health?," 4071; Frakes and Gruber, "Racial Concordance and the Quality of Medical Care," 30; Otte, "Improved Patient Experience," 471.

75. Megan Tenet, "Racial Inequality in Medicine: How Did We Get Here?," *Georgetown Medical Review* 5, no. 1 (2021): 1, https://doi.org/10.52504/001c.25142.

76. American Association of Colleges of Nursing, "Fact Sheet: Enhancing Diversity in the Nursing Workforce," last modified June 2024, https://www.aacnnursing.org/Portals/0/PDFs/Fact-Sheets/Enhancing-Diversity-Factsheet.pdf.

77. Meanwhile, 82 percent of white people have a white physician. Kristen Wilbur et al., "Developing Workforce Diversity in the Health Professions: A Social Justice Perspective," *Journal of Health Professions Education* 6, no. 2 (2020): 222, https://doi.org/10.1016/j.hpe.2020.01.002.

78. Ashton-James et al., "Understanding the Contribution," 223.

79. While black people are underrepresented in medicine and among registered nurses, they are not underrepresented in the healthcare field in general. Black people can be found in low-status jobs that do not involve providing care to patients. According to one set of researchers, "[C]lose evaluation of occupational data reveals that the majority of people of color in

healthcare jobs remain in entry-level and often lower-paying jobs with little opportunity for advancement, such as aides, assistants, and technicians." Wilbur et al., "Developing Workforce Diversity," 224.

80. Association of American Medical Colleges, "Action Plan 4: Increase the Diversity of Medical School Applicants and Matriculants," accessed August 2, 2024, https://www.aamc.org/about-us/strategic-plan/action-plan-4-increase-diversity-medical-school-applicants-and-matriculants.

81. Lauren A. Taylor et al., "Should a Healthcare System Facilitate Racially Concordant Care for Black Patients?," *Pediatrics* 148, no. 4 (2021): 6, https://doi.org/10.1542/peds.2021-051113.

82. Taylor et al., "Should a Healthcare System," 6.

83. Candice Tara Karber, "The Importance of Racial Concordance and the Childhood Experiences of Black Students and Practicing Clinicians in the Field of Social Work" (Master's thesis, Smith College, 2008): 15, https://scholarworks.smith.edu/theses/1242.

84. Taylor et al., "Should a Healthcare System," 6.

85. Taylor et al., "Should a Healthcare System," 6.

86. Greenwood et al., "Physician–Patient Racial Concordance," 21198.

87. Dána-Ain Davis, "Obstetric Racism: The Racial Politics of Pregnancy, Labor, and Birthing," *Medical Anthropology* 38, no. 7 (2019): 562, https://doi.org/10.1080/01459740.2018.1549389.

88. Amy Alspaugh et al., "'Patients Want to See People That Look Like Them': Aspiring Midwives of Color as Resistance to Racism through Concordant Care in the United States," *SSM—Qualitative Research in Health* 3, no. 100228 (2023): 3, https://doi.org/10.1016/j.ssmqr.2023.100226.

89. Taylor et al., "Should a Healthcare System," 4.

90. Cossette A. Kathawa et al., "Perspectives of Doulas of Color on Their Role in Alleviating Racial Disparities in Birth Outcomes: A Qualitative Study," *Journal of Midwifery and Women's Health* 67, no. 1 (2021): 31, https://doi.org/10.1111/jmwh.13305.

91. Kathawa et al., "Perspectives of Doulas of Color," 31.

92. Jennifer Nash, *Birthing Black Mothers* (Duke University Press, 2021), 90–91.

93. The Civil Rights Project, "Constitutional Requirements for Affirmative Action in Higher Education Admissions and Financial Aid," Harvard University, last modified September 23, 2002, https://civilrightsproject.ucla.edu/legal-developments/legal-memos/constitutional-requirements-for-affirmative-action-in-higher-education-admissions-and-financial-aid/constitutional-affirmative-action-financial-aid.pdf.

94. National Archives, "Affirmative Action: History and Rationale," accessed August 3, 2024, https://clintonwhitehouse3.archives.gov/WH/EOP/OP/html/aa/aa02.html.

95. *Regents of the University of California v. Bakke*, 438 U.S. 265, 320 (1978).

96. *Bakke*, 438 U.S. at 307.

97. Ian F. Haney López, "'A Nation of Minorities': Race, Ethnicity, and Reactionary Colorblindness," *Stanford Law Review* 59, no. 4 (2007): 985–1064; Kimberly Reyes, "Affirmative Action Shouldn't Be About Diversity," *The Atlantic*, December 27, 2018, https://www.theatlantic.com/ideas/archive/2018/12/affirmative-action-about-reparations-not-diversity/578005/.

98. Reyes, "Affirmative Action Shouldn't Be About Diversity."

99. *Grutter v. Bollinger*, 539 U.S. 306, 330 (2003).

100. *Students for Fair Admissions, Inc. v. President and Fellows of Harvard College*, 600 U.S. 181 (2023) (Thomas, J., concurring).

101. Noam Scheiber, "Affirmative Action Ruling May Upend Hiring Policies, Too," *New York Times*, June 30, 2023, https://www.nytimes.com/2023/06/30/business/economy/hiring-affirmative-action.html.

102. Jonathan Pidluzny, "Expert Insight: DEI Spells CRT: Legislation Restricting Diversity, Equity, and Inclusion Programs Will Improve the Intellectual Environment at Missouri Universities," America First Policy Institute, May 10, 2023, https://americafirstpolicy.com/issues/expert-insight-dei-spells-crt-legislation-restricting-diversity-equity-and-inclusion-programs-will-improve-the-intellectual-environment-at-missouri-universities.

103. Nicholas Confessore, "'America Is under Attack': Inside the Anti-DEI Crusade," *New York Times*, January 24, 2024, https://www.nytimes.com/interactive/2024/01/20/us/dei-woke-claremont-institute.html; Nicquel T. Ellis and Catherine Thorbecke, "DEI Efforts Are under Siege. Here's What Experts Say Is at Stake," CNN, January 11, 2024, https://www.cnn.com/2024/01/07/us/dei-attacks-experts-warn-of-consequences-reaj/index.html; Leah Watson, "Anti-DEI Efforts Are the Latest Attack on Racial Equity and Free Speech," ACLU, February 14, 2024, https://www.aclu.org/news/free-speech/anti-dei-efforts-are-the-latest-attack-on-racial-equity-and-free-speech.

104. Oni J. Blackstock et al., "Health Care Is the New Battlefront for Anti-DEI Attacks," *PLOS Global Public Health* 4, no. 4 (2024): e0003131, https://doi.org10.1371/journal.pgph.0003131.

105. Blackstock et al., "Health Care Is the New Battlefront," e0003131.

106. Antoinette Schoenthaler and Joseph Ravenell, "Understanding the Patient Experience through the Lenses of Racial/Ethnic and Gender Patient-Physician Concordance," *JAMA Network Open* 3, no. 11 (2020): 1–2, https://doi.org/10.1001/jamanetworkopen.2020.25349.

CONCLUSION

1. Jessica P. Cerdeña et al., "From Race-Based to Race-Conscious Medicine: How Anti-Racist Uprisings Call Us to Act," *Lancet* 396, no. 10257 (2020): 1125–1126, https://doi.org/10.1016/S0140-6736(20)32076-6; Joseph Friedman et al., "Assessment of Racial/Ethnic and Income Disparities in the Prescription of Opioids and Other Controlled Medications

in California," *JAMA Internal Medicine* 179, no. 4 (2019): 473; Adam W. Gaffney et al., "Are Lung Function Algorithms Perpetuating Health Disparities Experienced by Black People?," *Stat News*, September 15, 2020, https://www.statnews.com/2020/09/15/lung-function-algorithms-health-disparities-black-people/; Lucia Trimbur and Lundy Braun, "The NFL's Reversal on 'Race Norming' Reveals How Pervasive Medical Racism Remains," *NBC News*, June 8, 2021, https://www.nbcnews.com/think/opinion/nfl-s-reversal-race-norming-reveals-how-pervasive-medical-racismncna1269992; Darshali A. Vyas et al., "Hidden in Plain Sight: Reconsidering the Use of Race Correction in Clinical Algorithms," *New England Journal of Medicine* 383, no. 9 (2020): 875, https://doi.org/10.1056/NEJMms2004740.

Bibliography

Acevedo-Garcia, Dolores, Mah-J Soobader, and Lisa F. Berkman. "The Differential Effect of Foreign-Born Status on Low Birth Weight by Race/Ethnicity and Education." *Pediatrics* 115, no. 1 (2005): e20–e30. https://doi.org/10.1542/peds.2004-1306.

Agency for Healthcare Research and Quality. "Improving Cultural Competence to Reduce Health Disparities for Priority Populations." Effective Health Care Program. Archived July 8, 2014. https://effectivehealthcare.ahrq.gov/products/cultural-competence/research-protocol.

Agner, Joy. "Moving from Cultural Competence to Cultural Humility in Occupational Therapy: A Paradigm Shift." *American Journal of Occupational Therapy* 74, no. 4 (2020): 1–7. https://doi.org/10.5014/ajot.2020.038067.

Alameda Health System. "Black Centering Is a New Kind of Care Made for You and Your Baby." Accessed July 31, 2024. https://www.alamedahealthsystem.org/family-birthing-center/black-centering/.

Alang, Sirry, Donna D. McAlpine, and Rachel Hardeman. "Police Brutality and Mistrust in Medical Institutions." *Journal of Racial and Ethnic Health Disparities* 7, no. 4 (2020): 760–768. https://doi.org/10.1007/s40615-020-00706-w.

Alcindor, Yamiche. "Ben Carson Is Confirmed as HUD Secretary." *New York Times*, March 2, 2017. https://www.nytimes.com/2017/03/02/us/politics/ben-carson-housing-urban-development.html.

Alexander, Mariana, Charles Brecher, Patrick Orecki, and Kevin Medina. *A New Approach to Funding New York City Health + Hospitals*. Citizens Budget Commission, December 2019. https://cbcny.org/sites/default/files/media/files/CBCREPORT_Health%2BHospitals_12162019_1.pdf.

Alsan, Marcella, Owen Garrick, and Grant Graziani. "Does Diversity Matter for Health? Experimental Evidence from Oakland." *American Economic Review* 109, no. 12 (2019): 4071–4111. https://doi.org/10.1257/aer.20181446.

Alspaugh, Amy, Daniel F. M. Suárez-Baquero, Renee Mehra, et al. "'Patients Want to See People That Look Like Them': Aspiring Midwives of Color as Resistance to Racism through Concordant Care in the United States." *Qualitative Research in Health* 3, no. 5 (2023): 1–10. https://doi.org/10.1016/j.ssmqr.2023.100226.

American Anthropological Association. "AAA Statement on Race." https://americananthro.org/about/policies/statement-on-race/.

American Association of Colleges of Nursing. "Fact Sheet: Enhancing Diversity in the Nursing Workforce." Last modified June 2024. https://www.aacnnursing.org/Portals/0/PDFs/Fact-Sheets/Enhancing-Diversity-Factsheet.pdf.

American Hospital Association. "Metropolitan Anchor Hospital (MAH) Case Study." June 2022. https://aha.org/case-studies/2022-11-22-nyc-health-hospitals-new-york.

American Midwifery Certification Board. *2023 Demographic*. 2024. https://www.amcbmidwife.org/docs/default-source/default-document-library/demographic-report-2023.pdf?sfvrsn=432df54b_0.

Ammon, Francesca Russello. "Commemoration Amid Criticism: The Mixed Legacy of Urban Renewal in Southwest Washington, D.C." *Journal of Planning and History* 8, no. 3 (2009): 175–220. https://doi.org/10.1177/1538513209340630.

Anderson, Brittney T. "Access to Quality, Culturally Appropriate Health Care." In *Black Health in the South*, edited by Steven S. Coughlin, Lovoria Williams, and Tabia Henry Akintobi. Johns Hopkins University Press, 2023.

Andrews-Dyer, Helena. "This Isn't Another Horror Story About Black Motherhood." *Washington Post*, September 4, 2019. https://www.washingtonpost.com/graphics/2019/lifestyle/black-motherhood/.

Ashton-James, Claire E., Steven R. Anderson, and Adam T. Hirsch. "Understanding the Contribution of Racially and Ethnically Discordant Interactions to Pain Disparities: Proximal Mechanisms and Potential Solutions." *Pain* 164, no. 2 (2023): 223–229. https://doi.org/10.1097/j.pain.0000000000002698.

Association of American Medical Colleges. "Action Plan 4: Increase the Diversity of Medical School Applicants and Matriculants." Accessed August 2, 2024. https://www.aamc.org/about-us/strategic-plan/action-plan-4-increase-diversity-medical-school-applicants-and-matriculants.

Bajaj, Simar S., Ahmed M. Ahmed, and Valerie E. Stone. "Medicine's DEI Backlash Offers an Opportunity to Refocus on Evidence-Based Approaches." *Nature Medicine* 30 (2024): 3040–3041. https://doi.org/10.1038/s41591-024-03236-8.

Bajaj, Simar Singh, and Fatima Cody Stanford. "Beyond Tuskegee: Vaccine Distrust and Everyday Racism." *New England Journal of Medicine* 384, no. 5 (2021): e12(1)–e12(2). https://doi.org/10.1056/NEJMpv2035827.

Barker, Kristin K. "A Ship upon a Stormy Sea: The Medicalization of Pregnancy." *Social Science and Medicine* 47, no. 8 (1998): 1067–1076. https://doi.org/10.1016/S0277-9536(98)00155-5.

Barrientos, Carlos. "25 Popular San Francisco Neighborhoods: Where to Live in San Francisco in 2025." Redfin, April 22, 2024. https://www.redfin.com/blog/san-francisco-ca-neighborhoods/.

Beaulac, Julie, Elizabeth Kristjansson, and Steven Cummins. "A Systematic Review of Food Deserts, 1966–2007." *Preventing Chronic Disease* 6, no. 3 (2009): 1–10. http://www.cdc.gov/pcd/issues/2009/jul/08_0163.htm.

Benjamin, Ruha. "Cultura Obscura: Race, Power, and 'Culture Talk' in the Health Sciences." *American Journal of Law and Medicine* 43, no. 2–3 (2017): 225–238. https://doi.org/10.1177/0098858817723661.

Berger, Jeffrey T., and Dana Ribeiro Miller. "Health Disparities, Systemic Racism, and Failures of Cultural Competence." *American Journal of Bioethics* 21, no. 4 (2021): 4–10. https://doi.org/10.1080/15265161.2021.1915411.

Bersted, Kyle A., Kerri M. Lockhart, Janet Yarboi, et al. "A Path toward Equity and Inclusion: Establishing a DEI Committee in a Department of Pediatrics." *Journal of Clinical Psychology in Medical Settings* 30 (2023): 342–345. https://doi.org/10.1007/s10880-022-09929-x.

Betancourt, Joseph R. "Cultural Competence and Medical Education: Many Names, Many Perspectives, One Goal." *Academic Medicine* 81, no. 6 (2006): 499–501. https://doi.org/10.1097/01.ACM.0000225211.77088.cb.

Blackstock, Oni J., Jessica E. Isom, and Rupinder K. Legha. "Health Care Is the New Battlefront for Anti-DEI Attacks." *PLOS Global Public Health* 4, no. 4 (2024): e0003131. https://doi.org/10.1371/journal.pgph.0003131.

Blackstock, Uché. "'At the Private Hospital, the Disrespect Was Just More Subtle': A Tale of America's Two Healthcare Systems." *The Guardian*, January 23, 2024. https://www.theguardian.com/wellness/2024/jan/23/us-hospital-segregation-racism-public-private.

Brancaccio-Taras, Loretta, Judy Awong-Taylor, Monica Linden, Kate Marley, Gary C. Reiness, and J. Akif Uzman. "The PULSE Diversity Equity and Inclusion (DEI) Rubric: A Tool to Help Assess Departmental DEI Efforts." *Journal of Microbiology and Biology Education* 23, no. 3 (2022): 1–8. https://doi.org/10.1128/jmbe.00057-22.

Brandt, Allan M. "Racism and Research: The Case of the Tuskegee Syphilis Study." *Hastings Center Report* 8, no. 6 (1978): 21–29. https://doi.org/10.2307/3561468.

Braveman, Paula, Susan Egerter, and David R. Williams. "The Social Determinants of Health: Coming of Age." *Annual Review of Public Health* 32, no. 1 (2011): 381–398. https://doi.org/10.1146/annurev-publhealth-031210-101218.

Bridges, Khiara M. *Critical Race Theory: A Primer*. West Academic Publishing, 2018.

Bridges, Khiara M. "Racial Disparities in Maternal Mortality." *New York University Law Review* 95, no. 5 (2020): 1229–1318.

Bridges, Khiara M. *Reproducing Race: An Ethnography of Pregnancy as a Site of Racialization*. University of California Press, 2011.

Bridges, Khiara, and Douglas White. "COVID-19 Is Not an Equalizer: Early Data Shows African Americans Are Dying at Higher Rates." Interview by Lizzie O'Leary, *The Takeaway*, April 6, 2020. WNYC Studios and WGBH. https://www.wnycstudios.org/podcasts/takeaway/segments/covid19-black-people-dying-at-higher-rates.

Brinklow, Adam. "San Francisco Has Done Everything to the Bayview Except Fix Problems." *Curbed SF*, February 18, 2020. https://sf.curbed.com/2020/2/18/21142590/bayview-black-population-sfmta-transit-report.

Brubaker, Sarah Jane. "Denied, Embracing, and Resisting Medicalization: African American Teen Mothers' Perceptions of Formal Pregnancy and Childbirth Care." *Gender & Society* 21, no. 4 (2007): 528–552. https://doi.org/10.1177/0891243207304972.

Bruch, Joseph D., and David Bellamy. "Charity Care: Do Nonprofit Hospitals Give More than For-Profit Hospitals?" *Journal of General Internal Medicine* 36, no. 10 (2020). https://doi.org/10.1007/s11606-020-06147-9.

Bryant, Allison S., Ayaba Worjoloh, Aaron B. Caughey, and A. Eugene Washington. "Racial/Ethnic Disparities in Obstetric Outcomes and Care: Prevalence and Determinants." *American Journal of Obstetrics and Gynecology* 202, no. 4 (2010): 335–343. https://doi.org/10.1016/j.ajog.2009.10.864.

Bryant, Cierra, and Brooke Muya. "We Must Treat the Black Maternal Health Crisis with the Urgency It Deserves." *Newsweek*, July 7, 2023. https://www.newsweek.com/we-must-treat-black-maternal-health-crisis-urgency-it-deserves-opinion-1811127.

Burfoot, Annette, and Derya Güngör. "The Medicalization of Pregnancy and Birth." In *Women and Reproductive Technologies: The Socio-Economic Development of Technologies Changing the World*. Routledge, 2022.

Burke, Minvonne. "She Was a Black Pediatrician But Still Died after Giving Birth to Her 1st Child." *Today*, November 6, 2022. https://www.today.com/health/she-was-black-pediatrician-still-died-after-giving-birth-her-t198011.

Cabral, Howard, Lise E. Fried, Suzette Levenson, Hortensia Amaro, and Barry Zuckerman. "Foreign-Born and US-Born Black Women: Differences in Health Behaviors and Birth Outcomes." *American Journal of Public Health* 80, no. 1 (1990): 70–72. https://doi.org/10.2105/AJPH.80.1.70.

Cahill, Heather A. "Male Appropriation and Medicalization of Childbirth: An Historical Analysis." *Journal of Advanced Nursing* 33, no. 3 (2001): 334–342.

California Department of Health Care Access and Information. "Hospital Profile." Accessed August 17, 2024. [url redacted].

California Department of Health Care Access and Information. "Hospital Profile: [name redacted]." Accessed August 17, 2024. [url redacted].

California Department of Health Care Access and Information. "Hospital Profile: [name redacted]." Accessed August 17, 2024. [url redacted].

California Department of Health Care Access and Information. "[redacted] Hospital—San Francisco." Accessed August 17, 2024. [url redacted].

California Department of Health Care Services. "Federally Qualified Health Centers and Rural Health Clinics." https://www.dhcs.ca.gov/services/medi-cal/Pages/FQHC_RHC.aspx.

California Department of Health Care Services. "Information on the Presumptive Eligibility for Pregnant Women." Accessed February 11, 2025. https://www.dhcs.ca.gov/services/medi-cal/eligibility/Pages/PE_Info_women.aspx.

California Department of Health Care Services. "Medi-Cal Resources." Accessed August 15, 2024. https://www.dhcs.ca.gov/services/medi-cal/Pages/default.aspx.

California Maternal Quality Care Collaborative. "California Hospital Membership." Accessed January 24, 2025. https://www.cmqcc.org/about-cmqcc/member-hospitals/california-hospital-membership.

California Maternal Quality Care Collaborative. "Toolkits." Accessed August 1, 2024. https://www.cmqcc.org/resources-tool-kits/toolkits.

California Maternal Quality Care Collaborative. "Who We Are." Accessed August 1, 2024. https://www.cmqcc.org/who-we-are.

Campbell, Colleen. "Medical Violence, Obstetric Racism, and the Limits of Informed Consent for Black Women," *Michigan Journal of Race and Law* 26, special issue (2021): 47–75. https://doi.org/10.36643/mjrl.26.sp.medical.

Canopy Health. "Canopy Health, San Francisco Health Network Announce Collaboration That Will Expand Hospital-Based Midwifery Access in San Francisco." Last modified August 5, 2019. https://www.canopyhealth.com/canopy-health-san-francisco-health-network-announce-collaboration-that-will-expand-hospital-based-midwifery-access-in-san-francisco/.

"CDC on Infant and Maternal Mortality in the United States: 1900–99." *Population and Development Review* 25, no. 4 (1999): 821–826. https://www.jstor.org/stable/172510.

Cerdeña, Jessica P., Marie V. Plaisime, and Jennifer Tsai. "From Race-Based to Race-Conscious Medicine: How Anti-Racist Uprisings Call Us to Act." *Lancet* 396, no. 10257 (2020): 1125–1128. https://doi.org/10.1016/S0140-6736(20)32076-6.

Chang, Ailsa, Rachel Martin, and Eric Marrapodi, hosts. *Summer of Racial Reckoning*. Podcast, season 1, episode 1, "The Match Lit." NPR, August 16, 2020. https://www.npr.org/2020/08/16/902179773/summer-of-racial-reckoning-the-match-lit.

Chang, Alisa, Jonaki Mehta, and Christopher Intagliata. "Beneath the Santa Monica Freeway Lies the Erasure of Sugar Hill." NPR, May 4, 2021. https://www.npr.org/2021/05/04/993605428/beneath-the-santa-monica-freeway-lies-the-erasure-of-sugar-hill.

Chang, Hetty. "Combating Vaccine Hesitancy among Black Americans after Mistrust Caused by Unethical Study." NBC Los Angeles, September 11, 2021. https://www.nbclosangeles.com/news/local/combating-vaccine-hesitancy-among-black-americans-after-mistrust-caused-by-unethical-study/2690303/.

Chen, Shawna, Alex Fitzpatrick, and Kavya Beheraj. "How San Francisco's Racial Demographics Have Changed since 2000." *Axios San Francisco*, July 6, 2023. https://www.axios.com/local/san-francisco/2023/07/06/san-francisco-demographic-trends.

Chetty, Raj, Nathaniel Hendren, Maggie R. Jones, and Sonya R. Porter. "Race and Economic Opportunity in the United States: An Intergenerational Perspective." Working Paper No. 24441. National Bureau of Economic Research, December 2019. https://doi.org/10.3386/w24441.

Chou, Christopher. "Land Use and the Chinatown Problem." *UCLA Asian Pacific American Law Journal* 19 (2014): 29–75. https://doi.org/10.5070/P3191024222.

Civil Rights Project. "Constitutional Requirements for Affirmative Action in Higher Education Admissions and Financial Aid." Harvard University. Last updated September 23, 2002. https://civilrightsproject.ucla.edu/legal-developments/legal-memos/constitutional-requirements-for-affirmative-action-in-higher-education-admissions-and-financial-aid/constitutional-affirmative-action-financial-aid.pdf.

Clay-Murray, Denise. "The HBCU Endowment Gap: Why Black Colleges Lag So Far behind PWIs." *BET*, October 7, 2022. https://www.bet.com/article/3d5ktm/black-colleges-endowment-gap.

Cohen, Michael, Jared Maeda, and Daria Pelech. *The Prices That Commercial Health Insurers and Medicare Pay for Hospitals' and Physicians' Services*. Congressional Budget Office, January 2022. https://www.cbo.gov/system/files/2022-01/57422-medical-prices.pdf.

Cole, Haile Eshe. "Reproduction on Display: Black Maternal Mortality and the Newest Case for National Action." *Journal of the Motherhood Initiative for Research and Community Involvement* 9, no. 2 (2018): 89–101. https://jarm.journals.yorku.ca/index.php/jarm/article/view/40511.

Collins, James W., Jr., Shou-Yien Wu, and Richard J. David. "Differing Intergenerational Birth Weights among the Descendants of US-Born and Foreign-Born Whites and African Americans in Illinois." *American Journal of Epidemiology* 155, no. 3 (2002): 210–216. https://doi.org/10.1093/aje/155.3.210.

Colliver, Victoria. "For-Profit Hospitals Give Back as Much as Nonprofits, Study Finds." *SFGate*, August 4, 2015. https://www.sfgate.com/health/article/For-profit-hospitals-give-back-as-much-as-6422790.php.

Committee on African American Parity of the Human Rights Commission of San Francisco. *The Unfinished Agenda: The Economic Status of African Americans in San Francisco 1964–1990*. Polaris Research and Development, 1993.

Confessore, Nicholas. "'America Is under Attack': Inside the Anti-DEI Crusade." *New York Times*, January 24, 2024. https://www.nytimes.com/interactive/2024/01/20/us/dei-woke-claremont-institute.html.

Connolly, N. D. B. "Colored, Caribbean, and Condemned: Miami's Overtown District and the Cultural Expense of Progress, 1940–1970." *Caribbean Studies* 34, no. 1 (2006): 3–60. https://www.redalyc.org/pdf/392/39211247001.pdf.

Cooper, Lisa A., and Neil R. Powe. "Disparities in Patient Experiences, Health Care Processes, and Outcomes: The Role of Patient-Provider Racial, Ethnic, and Language Concordance." The Commonwealth Fund, July 1, 2004. https://www.commonwealthfund.org/publications/fund-reports/2004/jul/disparities-patient-experiences-health-care-processes-and.

Coughlin, Steven S., Lovoria B. Williams, and Tabia Henry Akintobi, eds. *Black Health in the South*. Johns Hopkins University Press, 2023.

Cox, Joy Arlene Renee. *Fat Girls in Black Bodies: Creating Communities of Our Own*. North Atlantic Books, 2020.

Cox, Rachel, Samantha Bernstein, and Kaveri Roy. "A Guide to Application of Diversity, Equity, and Inclusion (DEI) Principles for Prelicensure Nursing Education." *Journal of Professional Nursing* 46 (2023): 146–154. https://doi.org/10.1016/j.profnurs.2023.03.002.

Craven, Julia. "How Do Black Patients and White Patients Get Different Doctors in the Same Hospitals?" *Slate*, May 26, 2021. https://slate.com/technology/2021/05/hospital-segregation-study.html.

Cuevas, Adolfo G., and Kerth O'Brien. "Racial Centrality May Be Linked to Mistrust in Healthcare Institutions for African Americans." *Journal of Health Psychology* 24, no. 14 (2019): 2022–2030. https://doi.org/10.1177/1359105317715092.

Custodio, Jonathan. "This Bronxite Died Weeks after an Emergency C-Section. Her Family Wants Answers, and Changes." *The City*, September 24, 2023. https://www.thecity.nyc/2023/09/24/bronxcare-maternal-mortality-elaina-boone-death/.

Davis, Dána-Ain. "Obstetric Racism: The Racial Politics of Pregnancy, Labor, and Birthing." *Medical Anthropology* 38, no. 7 (2019): 560–573. https://doi.org/10.1080/01459740.2018.1549389.

Davis, Dána-Ain. *Reproductive Injustice: Racism, Pregnancy, and Premature Birth*. New York University Press, 2019.

Davis-Floyd, Robbie E. "The Technocratic Body: American Childbirth as Cultural Expression." *Social Science and Medicine* 38, no. 8 (1994): 1125–1140. https://doi.org/10.1016/0277-9536(94)90228-3.

Demby, Gene. "The Truth behind the Lies of the Original 'Welfare Queen.'" NPR, December 20, 2013. https://www.npr.org/sections/codeswitch/2013/12/20/255819681/the-truth-behind-the-lies-of-the-original-welfare-queen.

De Rooij, Susanne R., Laura S. Bleker, Rebecca C. Painter, Anita C. Ravelli, and Tessa J. Roseboom. "Lessons Learned from 25 Years of Research into Long-Term Consequences of Prenatal Exposure to the Dutch Famine 1944–45: The Dutch Famine Birth Cohort." *International Journal of Environmental Health Research* 32, no. 7 (2022): 1432–1446. https://doi.org/10.1080/09603123.2021.1888894.

Detrow, Scott. "Trump Says African-American Communities in 'Worst Shape' Ever; Data Disagree." NPR, September 21, 2016. https://www.npr.org/2016/09/21/494883725/trump-says-african-americans-are-in-their-worst-shape-ever-the-data-disagrees.

Devienne, Elsa. "The Right to the Beach? Urban Renewal, Public Space Policing and the Definition of a Beach Public in Postwar Los Angeles, 1940s–1960s." *Revue française d'études américaines* 148, no. 3 (2016): 31–51. https://doi.org/10.3917/rfea.148.0031.

Devine, Patricia G., and Tory L. Ash. "Diversity Training Goals, Limitations, and Promise: A Review of the Multidisciplinary Literature." *Annual Review of Psychology* 73, no. 1 (2022): 403–429. https://doi.org/10.1146/annurev-psych-060221-122215.

Dluhy, Milan, Keith Revell, and Sidney Wong. "Creating a Positive Future for a Minority Community: Transportation and Urban Renewal Politics in Miami." *Journal of Urban Affairs* 24, no. 1 (2002): 75–95. https://doi.org/10.1111/1467-9906.00115.

Drame, Imbi, Caitlin M. Gibson, Nkem P. Nonyel, et al. "Strategies for Incorporating Health Disparities and Cultural Competency Training into the Pharmacy Curriculum and Co-Curriculum." *American Journal of Pharmaceutical Education* 86, no. 3 (2022): 199–206. https://doi.org/10.5688/ajpe8631.

Dressler, William, Kathryn S. Oths, and Clarence C. Gravlee. "Race and Ethnicity in Public Health Research: Models to Explain Health Disparities." *Annual Review of Anthropology* 34, no. 1 (October 2005): 231–252. https://doi.org/10.1146/annurev.anthro.34.081804.120505.

Ebrahimji, Alisha. "Some Say Sharing Videos of Police Brutality against Black People Is Just 'Trauma Porn.'" CNN, August 25, 2020. https://www.cnn.com/2020/08/25/us/police-brutality-videos-trauma-porn-trnd/index.html.

Edgoose, Jennifer, Joedrecka Brown Speights, Tanya White-Davis, et al. "Teaching About Racism in Medical Education: A Mixed-Method Analysis of a Train-the-Trainer Faculty Development Workshop." *Family Medicine* 53, no. 1 (2021): 23–31. https://doi.org/10.22454/FamMed.2021.408300.

Eiser, Arnold R., and Glenn Ellis. "Cultural Competence and the African American Experience with Health Care: The Case for Specific Content in Cross-Cultural Education." *Academic Medicine* 82, no. 2 (2007): 176–183. https://doi.org/10.1097/ACM.0b013e31802d92ea.

Ellis, Nicquel T., and Catherine Thorbecke. "DEI Efforts Are under Siege. Here's What Experts Say Is at Stake." CNN, January 11, 2024. https://www.cnn.com/2024/01/07/us/dei-attacks-experts-warn-of-consequences-reaj/index.html.

Eltoukhi, Heba M., Monica N. Modi, Meredith Weston, Alicia Y. Armstrong, and Elizabeth A. Stewart. "The Health Disparities of Uterine Fibroid Tumors for African American Women: A Public Health Issue." *American Journal of Obstetrics and Gynecology* 210, no. 3 (2014): 194–199. https://doi.org/10.1016/j.ajog.2013.08.008.

Eneanya, Nwamaka D., Wei Yang, and Phillip P. Reese. "Reconsidering the Consequence of Using Race to Estimate Kidney Function." *JAMA* 322, no. 2 (2019): 113–114. https://doi.org/10.1001/jama.2019.5774.

Energy and Commerce Committee Democrats. Hearing on "Better Data and Better Outcomes: Reducing Maternal Mortality in the U.S." Subcommittee on Health, September 27, 2018. https://democrats-energycommerce.house.gov/committee-activity/hearings/hearing-on-better-data-and-better-outcomes-reducing-maternal-mortality.

Equal Justice Initiative. "Bloody Sunday: Civil Rights Activists Brutally Attacked in Selma." Accessed February 11, 2025. https://calendar.eji.org/racial-injustice/mar/7#:~:text=On%20March%207%2C%201965%2C%20state,the%20state%20capitol%20in%20Montgomery.

Fernández, Lilia. *Brown in the Windy City: Mexicans and Puerto Ricans in Postwar Chicago.* University of Chicago Press, 2012.

Flagg, Barbara J. "'Was Blind, But Now I See': White Race Consciousness and the Requirement of Discriminatory Intent." *Michigan Law Review* 91, no. 5 (1993): 953–1017. https://doi.org/10.2307/1289678.

Forna, Fatu, Denise J. Jamieson, D. Sanders, and Michael K. Lindsay. "Pregnancy Outcomes in Foreign-Born and US-Born Women." *International Journal of Gynecology and Obstetrics* 83, no. 3 (2003): 257–265. https://doi.org/10.1016/S0020-7292(03)00307-2.

Frakes, Michael D., and Jonathan Gruber. "Racial Concordance and the Quality of Medical Care: Evidence from the Military." Working Paper No. 30767. National Bureau of Economic Research, December 2022. http://www.nber.org/papers/w30767.

Francisco, Crilhien R. *Report on the Fiscal 2024 Preliminary Plan and the Fiscal 2023 Mayor's Management Report for the New York City Health + Hospitals*. New York City Council Finance Division, 2023. https://council.nyc.gov/budget/wp-content/uploads/sites/54/2023/03/HH.pdf.

Fraser, Gertrude Jacinta. *African American Midwifery in the South: Dialogues of Birth, Race, and Memory*. Harvard University Press, 1998.

Frazin, Rachel. "Warren Unveils Plan to Reward Hospitals That Make Childbirth Safer for Black Women." *The Hill*, April 25, 2019. https://thehill.com/homenews/campaign/440629-warren-unveils-plan-to-reward-hospitals-that-make-childbirth-safer-for/.

Friedman, Jospeh, David Kim, and Todd Schneberk. "Assessment of Racial/Ethnic and Income Disparities in the Prescription of Opioids and Other Controlled Medications in California." *JAMA Internal Medicine* 179, no: 4 (2019): 469–476.

Fry, Richard. "Are You in the American Middle Class? Find Out with Our Income Calculator." Pew Research Center, September 16, 2024. https://www.pewresearch.org/short-reads/2020/07/23/are-you-in-the-american-middle-class/.

Fuller, Thomas. "The Loneliness of Being Black in San Francisco." *New York Times*, July 20, 2016. https://www.nytimes.com/2016/07/21/us/black-exodus-from-san-francisco.html.

Gaffney, Adam W., Steffie Woolhandler, and David U. Himmelstein. "Are Lung Function Algorithms Perpetuating Health Disparities Experienced by Black People?" *Stat News*, September 15, 2020. https://www.statnews.com/2020/09/15/lung-function-algorithms-health-disparities-black-people/.

Ganju, Kartik K., Hilal Atasoy, Jeffrey McCullough, and Brad N. Greenwood. "The Role of Decision Support Systems in Attenuating Biases in Healthcare Delivery." *Fox School of Business Research Paper* (2019): 1–36. https://doi.org/10.2139/ssrn.3465839.

Geronimus, Arline T. "The Effects of Race, Residence, and Prenatal Care on the Relationship of Maternal Age to Neonatal Mortality." *American Journal of Public Health* 76, no. 12 (1986): 1416–1421. https://doi.org/10.2105/ajph.76.12.1416.

Geronimus, Arline T. "Making the Case That Discrimination Is Bad for Your Health." Interview by Gene Demby. *Code Switch*, NPR, January 14, 2018. https://www.npr.org/sections/codeswitch/2018/01/14/577664626/making-the-case-that-discrimination-is-bad-for-your-health.

Geronimus, Arline T. *Weathering: The Extraordinary Stress of Ordinary Life in an Unjust Society.* Little, Brown Spark, 2023.

Geronimus, Arline T., Margaret Hicken, Danya Keene, and John Bound. "'Weathering' and Age Patterns of Allostatic Load Scores among Blacks and Whites in the United States." *American Journal of Public Health* 96, no. 5 (2006): 826–833. https://doi.org/10.2105/AJPH.2004.060749.

Gibbens, Sarah. "A Brief History of How Plastic Straws Took Over the World." *National Geographic*, January 2, 2019. https://www.nationalgeographic.com/environment/article/news-plastic-drinking-straw-history-ban.

Gleicher, Sonya T., Morgen A. Chalmiers, Beverly Aiyanyor, Rohini Jain, Nikhil Kotha, Robert S. Song, Jennifer Tram, Caresse L. Vuong, and Jennifer Kesselheim. "Confronting Implicit Bias toward Patients: A Scoping Review of Post-graduate Physician Curricula." *BMC Medical Education* 22, no. 1 (2022): 1–12. https://doi.org/10.1186/s12909-022-03720-0.

Godwin, Jamie, Zachary Levinson, and Scott Hulver. "Understanding Mergers between Hospitals and Health Systems in Different Markets." KFF, August 23, 2023. https://www.kff.org/health-costs/issue-brief/understanding-mergers-between-hospitals-and-health-systems-in-different-markets/.

Gold, Jenny, and Sarah Kliff. "A Baby Was Treated with a Nap and a Bottle of Formula. His Parents Received an $18,000 Bill." *Vox*, July 20, 2018. https://www.vox.com/2018/6/28/17506232/emergency-room-bill-fees-health-insurance-baby.

Golsby, Jacqueline. *A Spectacular Secret: Lynching in American Life and Literature.* University of Chicago Press, 2006.

Gorn, David. "San Francisco Plastic Bag Ban Interests Other Cities." NPR, March 27, 2008. https://www.npr.org/2008/03/27/89135360/san-francisco-plastic-bag-ban-interests-other-cities.

Green, Erica L. "'I Don't Want to Die': Fighting Maternal Mortality among Black Women." *New York Times*, January 18, 2023. https://www.nytimes.com/2023/01/18/us/doula-black-women.html.

Greenwood, Brad N., Rachel R. Hardeman, Laura Huang, and Aaron Sojourner. "Physician-Patient Racial Concordance and Disparities in Birthing Mortality for Newborns." *Proceedings of the National Academy of Sciences* 117, no. 35 (2020): 21194–21200. https://doi.org/10.1073/pnas.1913405117.

Gregory, Kia. "How Videos of Police Brutality Traumatize African Americans and Undermine the Search for Justice." *New Republic*, February 13, 2019. https://newrepublic.com/article/153103/videos-police-brutality-traumatize-african-americans-undermine-search-justice.

Greve, Joan E. "Senate Passes $739 Bn Healthcare and Climate Bill after Months of Wrangling." *The Guardian*, August 7, 2022. https://www.theguardian.com/us-news/2022/aug/07/inflation-reduction-act-senate-democrats-pass.

Grose, Jessica. "Black Maternal Mortality Is Still a Crisis." *New York Times*, June 22, 2022. https://www.nytimes.com/2022/06/22/opinion/black-maternal-mortality.html.

Gruber, Jonathan, and Benjamin D. Sommers. "Fiscal Federalism and the Budget Impacts of the Affordable Care Act's Medicaid Expansion." Working Paper No. 26862. National Bureau of Economic Research, March 2020. https://doi.org/10.3386/w26862.

Grutter v. Bollinger, 539 U.S. 306 (2003).

Gunja, Munira Z., Evan D. Gumas, Relebohile Masitha, and Laurie C. Zephyrin. "Insights into the U.S. Maternal Mortality Crisis: An International Comparison." The Commonwealth Fund, June 4, 2024. https://www.commonwealthfund.org/publications/issue-briefs/2024/jun/insights-us-maternal-mortality-crisis-international-comparison.

Gunja, Munira Z., Evan D. Gumas, and Reginald D. Williams II. "U.S. Health Care from a Global Perspective, 2022: Accelerating Spending, Worsening Outcomes." The Commonwealth Fund, January 31, 2023. https://www.commonwealthfund.org/publications/issue-briefs/2023/jan/us-health-care-global-perspective-2022.

Hagen-Smith, Zachary. "Salience Bias: The 24-Hour News Cycle Is a Market Failure." *Berkeley Economic Review*, April 25, 2022. https://econreview.studentorg.berkeley.edu/salience-bias-the-24-hour-news-cycle-is-a-market-failure/.

Haney López, Ian F. "'A Nation of Minorities': Race, Ethnicity, and Reactionary Colorblindness." *Stanford Law Review* 59, no. 4 (2007): 985–1064.

Harrison, Da'Shaun L. *Belly of the Beast: The Politics of Anti-Fatness as Anti-Blackness*. North Atlantic Books, 2021.

Hartman, Saidiya. *Scenes of Subjection: Terror, Slavery, and Self-Making in Nineteenth-Century America*. W. W. Norton, 1997.

Harvey, David. *A Brief History of Neoliberalism*. Oxford University Press, 2005.

"Harvey Milk Becomes the First Openly Gay Person Elected to Public Office in California." *History*, August 28, 2019. https://www.history.com/this-day-in-history/harvey-milk-first-openly-gay-person-elected-in-california.

Haskell, Rob. "Serena Williams on Motherhood, Marriage, and Making Her Comeback." *Vogue*, January 10, 2018. https://www.vogue.com/article/serena-williams-vogue-cover-interview-february-2018.

Haviland, Lyndon. "Regardless of Income, Black Women Face Death to Give Birth in America." *The Hill*, March 1, 2023. https://thehill.com/opinion/healthcare/3879248-regardless-of-income-black-women-face-death-to-give-birth-in-america/.

Herring, Bradley, Darrell Gaskin, Hossein Zare, and Gerard Anderson. "Comparing the Value of Nonprofit Hospitals' Tax Exemption to Their Community Benefits." *Inquiry* 55 (2018).

Higuera, Valencia. "What to Expect from a Foley Bulb Induction." *Healthline*, December 10, 2018. https://www.healthline.com/health/pregnancy/foley-bulb-induction.

Hill, Latoya, Alisha Rao, Samantha Artiga, and Usha Ranji. "Racial Disparities in Maternal and Infant Health: Current Status and Efforts to Address Them." KFF, October 25, 2024. https://www

.kff.org/racial-equity-and-health-policy/issue-brief/racial-disparities-in-maternal-and-infant-health-current-status-and-efforts-to-address-them/.

Holcomb, Jesse, Amy Mitchell, Jan Lauren Boyles, Emily Guskin, Mark Jurkowitz, and Katerina-Eva Matsa. "The Revenue Picture for American Journalism and How It Is Changing." Pew Research Center, March 26, 2014. https://www.pewresearch.org/wp-content/uploads/sites/8/2014/03/Revnue-Picture-for-American-Journalism.pdf.

Hoskin, Maia Niguel. "Black Women Are Dying during Childbirth and No One Seems to Care." *Forbes*, February 20, 2023. https://www.forbes.com/sites/maiahoskin/2023/02/20/black-mothers-report-feeling-ignored-or-dismissed-by-health-care-providers-as-maternal-health-disparities-persist/?sh=2737e681d857.

Hossain, Anushay. "We Should All Be Talking About America's Black Maternal Health Crisis." *Harper's Bazaar*, November 5, 2021. https://www.harpersbazaar.com/culture/features/a38094736/americas-black-maternal-health-crisis/.

Howell, Elizabeth A. "Reducing Disparities in Severe Maternal Morbidity and Mortality." *Clinical Obstetrics and Gynecology* 61, no. 2 (2018): 387–399. https://doi.org/10.1097/GRF.0000000000000349.

Howell, Elizabeth A., Natalia Egorova, Amy Balbierz, Jennifer Zeitlin, and Paul L. Hebert. "Black-White Differences in Severe Maternal Morbidity and Site of Care." *American Journal of Obstetrics and Gynecology* 214, no. 1 (2016): 122.e1–122.e7. https://doi.org/10.1016/j.ajog.2015.08.019.

Howell, Elizabeth A., Natalia N. Egorova, Amy Balbierz, Jennifer Zeitlin, and Paul L. Hebert. "Site of Delivery Contribution to Black–White Severe Maternal Morbidity Disparity." *American Journal of Obstetrics and Gynecology* 215, no. 2 (2016): 143–152. https://doi.org/10.1016/j.ajog.2016.05.007.

Irth (@irthapp). "Rest in Peace Elaina Boone." TikTok, September 15, 2023. https://www.tiktok.com/@irthapp/video/7279295156648414510.

Jackson, Christina, and Nikki Jones, "Remember the Fillmore: The Lingering History of Urban Renewal in Black San Francisco." In *Black California Dreamin': The Crises of California's African American Communities*, edited by C. Woods. UCSB Center for Black Studies Research, 2012. https://escholarship.org/uc/item/63g6128j.

James, Osamudia. "The 'Innocence' of Bias." *Michigan Law Review* 119, no. 6 (2021): 1345–1364. https://doi.org/10.36644/mlr.119.6.innocence.

Jellins, Tennyson S., Tyler L. Borko, Raylee Otero-Bell, et al. "Diversity, Equity, and Inclusion (DEI) in Medical Education: DEI at the Bedside." *Journal of the Neurological Sciences* 459 (2024): 1–7. https://doi.org/10.1016/j.jns.2024.122946.

Jelsing, Nadine. "How a 1934 Waterfront Strike Was a Major Turning Point for West Coast Labor." *Oregon Public Broadcasting*, July 11, 2022. https://www.opb.org/article/2022/07/11/1934-west-coast-ilwu-longshore-big-strike-labor-victory/.

Johnson, Marilynn S. *The Second Gold Rush: Oakland and the East Bay in World War II*. University of California Press, 1993.

Johnson, Nia. "From a Reckoning to Racial Concordance: A Strategy to Protect Black Mothers, Children, and Infants." *Hastings Center Report* 52, no. 2 (2022): S32–S34. https://doi.org/10.1002/hast.1366.

Jones, Rachel. "Maternal Mortality is Shockingly High in the U.S.—Especially If You're Black." *National Geographic*, June 22, 2023. https://www.nationalgeographic.com/premium/article/maternal-mortality-usa-health-motherhood.

Jongen, Crystal, Janya McCalman, Roxanne Bainbridge, and Anton Clifford. *Cultural Competence in Health: A Review of the Evidence*. Springer, 2018.

Joshi, Shriya, Chakravarthy Garlapati, and Ritu Aneja. "Epigenetic Determinants of Racial Disparity in Breast Cancer: Looking beyond Genetic Alterations." *Cancers* 14, no. 8 (2022). https://doi.org/10.3390/cancers14081903.

Kamin, Debra Kamin. "Cole Valley, San Francisco: Where High Prices Meet Low Inventory." *New York Times*, December 31, 2019. https://www.nytimes.com/2019/12/31/realestate/cole-valley-san-francisco-where-high-prices-meet-low-inventory.html.

Kanherkar, Riya R., Naina Bhatia-Dey, and Antonei B. Csoka. "Epigenetics across the Human Lifespan." *Frontiers in Cell and Developmental Biology* 2, no. 49 (2014): 1–19. https://doi.org/10.3389/fcell.2014.00049.

Karber, Candice Tara. "The Importance of Racial Concordance and the Childhood Experiences of Black Students and Practicing Clinicians in the Field of Social Work." Master's thesis, Smith College, 2008. https://scholarworks.smith.edu/theses/1242.

Kathawa, Cossette A., Kavita Shah Arora, Ruth Zielinski, and Lisa Kane Low. "Perspectives of Doulas of Color on Their Role in Alleviating Racial Disparities in Birth Outcomes: A Qualitative Study." *Journal of Midwifery and Women's Health* 67, no. 1 (2021): 31–38. https://doi.org/10.1111/jmwh.13305.

Kennedy-Moulton, Kate, Sarah Miller, Petra Persson, Maya Rossin-Slater, Laura Wherry, and Gloria Aldana. "Maternal and Infant Health Inequality: New Evidence from Linked Administrative Data." Working Paper No. 30693. National Bureau of Economic Research, September 2023. https://doi.org/10.3386/w30693.

KFF. "Medicaid Postpartum Coverage Extension Tracker." Last modified January 17, 2025. https://www.kff.org/medicaid/issue-brief/medicaid-postpartum-coverage-extension-tracker/.

KFF. "Poverty Rate by Race/Ethnicity." Accessed August 14, 2024. https://www.kff.org/other/state-indicator/poverty-rate-by-raceethnicity/.

Kindelan, Katie, Jade Cobern, and Shiela Beroukhim Afrahimi. "US Olympian Dies from Pregnancy Complication That Disproportionately Impacts Black Women." ABC News, June 13, 2023. https://abcnews.go.com/GMA/Wellness/us-olympian-dies-pregnancy-complication-disproportionately-impacts-black/story?id=100045363.

King, Debra Walker. *African Americans and the Culture of Pain*. University of Virginia Press, 2008.

Kliff, Sarah. "Hit by a City Bus—and Hit with a $27,660 City Hospital Bill." *Vox*, February 19, 2019. https://www.vox.com/2019/2/19/18213948/zuckerberg-hospital-emergency-room-bill-bus-accident.

Kliff, Sarah. "Prices at Zuckerberg Hospital's Emergency Room Are Higher than Anywhere Else in San Francisco." *Vox*, January 22, 2019. https://www.vox.com/2019/1/22/18183534/zuckerberg-san-francisco-general-hospital-er-prices.

Kliff, Sarah. "A $20,243 Bike Crash: Zuckerberg Hospital's Aggressive Tactics Leave Patients with Big Bills." *Vox*, January 24, 2019. https://www.vox.com/policy-and-politics/2019/1/7/18137967/er-bills-zuckerberg-san-francisco-general-hospital.

Kliff, Sarah, and Jessica Silver-Greenberg. "'Major Trustee, Please Prioritize': How [redacted]'s E.R. Favors the Rich." *New York Times*, December 22, 2022. [url redacted].

Knowles-Carter, Beyoncé, dir. *Homecoming: A Film by Beyoncé*. Parkwood Entertainment, 2019. 2 hr., 17 min. https://www.netflix.com/title/81013526.

Kogan, Michael D., Milton Kotelchuck, Greg R. Alexander, and Wayne E. Johnson. "Racial Disparities in Reported Prenatal Care Advice from Health Care Providers." *American Journal of Public Health* 84, no. 1 (1994): 82–88. https://doi.org/10.2105/AJPH.84.1.82.

Krauthammer, Charles. "Children of Cocaine." *Washington Post*, July 30, 1989.

Kripalani, Sunil, Jada Bussey-Jones, Marra G. Katz, and Inginia Genao. "A Prescription for Cultural Competence in Medical Education." *Journal of General Internal Medicine* 21, no. 10 (2006): 1116. https://doi.org/10.1111/j.1525-1497.2006.00557.x.

Kuzawa, Christopher W., and Elizabeth Sweet. "Epigenetics and the Embodiment of Race: Developmental Origins of US Racial Disparities in Cardiovascular Health." *American Journal of Human Biology* 21, no. 1 (2009): 2–15. https://doi.org/10.1002/ajhb.20822.

Lacy, Karyn. *Blue-Chip Black: Race, Class, and Status in the New Black Middle Class*. University of California Press, 2007.

Lazarus, Ellen S. "What Do Women Want? Issues of Choice, Control, and Class in Pregnancy and Childbirth." *Medical Anthropology Quarterly* 8, no.1 (1994): 25–46. https://doi.org/10.1525/maq.1994.8.1.02a00030.

Levins, Hoag Levins. "Hospital Consolidation Continues to Boost Costs, Narrow Access, and Impact Care Quality." University of Pennsylvania Leonard Davis Institute of Health Economics, January 19, 2023. https://ldi.upenn.edu/our-work/research-updates/hospital-consolidation-continues-to-boost-costs-narrow-access-and-impact-care-quality/.

Liaison Committee on Medical Education. "Functions and Structure of a Medical School: Standards for Accreditation of Medical Education Programs Leading to the MD Degree." November 2023.

Library of Congress. "Today in History—March 7: First March from Selma." Accessed August 1, 2024. https://www.loc.gov/item/today-in-history/march-07/.

Lim, Dion, and Ken Miguel. "San Francisco Bans Some Commonly Used Plastic Items." *ABC7 News*, July 1, 2019. https://abc7news.com/san-francisco-plastic-ban-plastics-straw/5368614/.

Lin, Jessica. "Lincoln Square Renewal Project (New York, 1955–1969)." *ArcGIS StoryMaps*, December 16, 2020. https://storymaps.arcgis.com/stories/d6c942630bee454bae0c7b459a081f07.

Lomax, Michael L. "Why HBCUs Still Matter." United Negro College Fund. https://uncf.org/the-latest/why-hbcus-still-matter#:~:text=While%20Black%20and%20White%20students,STEM%20degrees%20come%20from%20HBCUs.

Lowery, Wesley. "A Test of the News, Objectivity, Democracy, and the American Mosaic." *Columbia Journalism Review*, April 25, 2023. https://www.cjr.org/analysis/a-test-of-the-news-wesley-lowery-objectivity.php.

Madison, Tianna. "I Survived the Black Maternal Health Crisis. My Friend Didn't." *Newsweek*, June 26, 2023. https://www.newsweek.com/black-maternity-crisis-tori-bowie-1808651.

Maina, Ivy W., Tanisha D. Belton, Sara Ginzberg, Ajit Singh, and Tiffani J. Johnson. "A Decade of Studying Implicit Racial/Ethnic Bias in Healthcare Providers Using the Implicit Association Test." *Social Science and Medicine* 199 (2018): 219–229. https://doi.org/10.1016/j.socscimed.2017.05.009.

Mann, Cindy, and Adam Striar. "How Differences in Medicaid, Medicare, and Commercial Health Insurance Payment Rates Impact Access, Health Equity, and Cost." The Commonwealth Fund, August 17, 2022. https://www.commonwealthfund.org/blog/2022/how-differences-medicaid-medicare-and-commercial-health-insurance-payment-rates-impact.

Marmot, Michael, and Richard Wilkinson, eds. *Social Determinants of Health*. 2nd ed. Oxford University Press, 2005.

Martin, Chantel L., Lea Ghastine, Evans K. Lodge, Radhika Dhingra, and Cavin K. Ward-Caviness. "Understanding Health Inequalities through the Lens of Social Epigenetics." *Annual Review of Public Health* 43 (2022): 235–254. https://doi.org/10.1146/annurev-publhealth-052020-105613.

Martin, Nina, and Renee Montagne. "Black Mothers Keep Dying after Giving Birth. Shalon Irving's Story Explains Why." NPR, December 7, 2017. https://www.npr.org/2017/12/07/568948782/black-mothers-keep-dying-after-giving-birth-shalon-irvings-story-explains-why.

Martin, Nina, and Renee Montagne. "Lost Mothers: Maternal Mortality in the U.S." NPR, 2017. https://www.npr.org/series/543928389/lost-mothers.

Martin, Nina, and Renee Montagne. "Nothing Protects Black Women from Dying in Pregnancy and Childbirth." *ProPublica*, December 7, 2017. https://www.propublica.org/article/nothing-protects-black-women-from-dying-in-pregnancy-and-childbirth.

Massey, Douglas S., and Nancy A. Denton. *American Apartheid: Segregation and the Making of the Underclass*. Harvard University Press, 1998.

Mayo Clinic. "Vaginal Tears in Childbirth." Accessed August 31, 2024. https://www.mayoclinic.org/healthy-lifestyle/labor-and-delivery/in-depth/vaginal-tears/art-20546855.

McCarthy, Douglas, and Kimberly Mueller. "The New York City Health and Hospitals Corporation: Transforming a Public Safety Net Delivery System to Achieve Higher Performance." The Commonwealth Fund, October 2008. https://www.commonwealthfund.org/sites/default/files/documents/___media_files_publications_fund_report_2008_oct_the_new_york_city_health_and_hospitals_corporation__transforming_a_public_safety_net_delivery_system_mccarthy_nychlthospitalscorpcasestudy_1154_pdf.pdf.

McClellan, Frank M., James E. Wood Jr., and Sherin Fahmy. "It Takes a Village: Reforming Law to Promote Health Literacy and Reduce Orthopedic Health Disparities." *Journal of Health and Biomedical Law* 8, no. 3 (2013): 333–375. https://doi.org/10.2139/ssrn.2275424.

McElwee, Sean. "One Big Reason Congress Ignores the Poor: They Don't Vote." *Vox*, September 24, 2015. https://www.vox.com/2015/9/24/9388045/2014-voter-turnout-redistribution.

McEwen, Bruce S., and Elliot Stellar. "Stress and the Individual: Mechanisms Leading to Disease." *Archives of Internal Medicine* 157, no. 22 (1993): 2093–2101. https://doi.org/10.1001/archinte.1993.00410180039004.

McMorrow, Stacey, Robert A. Berenson, and John Holahan. "Commercial Health Insurance Markups over Medicare Prices for Physician Services Vary Widely by Specialty." Urban Institute, 2021. https://www.urban.org/sites/default/files/publication/104945/commercial-health-insurance-markups-over-medicare-prices-for-physician-services-vary-widely-by-specialty_0.pdf.

Medicaid. "Medicaid." Accessed August 15, 2024. https://www.medicaid.gov/medicaid/index.html.

Medicaid and CHIP Payment and Access Commission. "Medicaid Hospital Payment: A Comparison across States and to Medicare." Updated April 2017. https://www.macpac.gov/publication/medicaid-hospital-payment-a-comparison-across-states-and-to-medicare/.

Menendian, Stephen, and Samir Gambhir. "Racial Segregation in the San Francisco Bay Area, Part 2." Othering & Belonging Institute, February 7, 2019. https://belonging.berkeley.edu/racial-segregation-san-francisco-bay-area-part-2.

Metzl, Jonathan M. "Structural Competency." *American Quarterly* 64, no. 2 (2012): 213–218. http://www.jstor.org/stable/23273514.

Metzl, Jonathan M., and Helena Hansen. "Structural Competency and Psychiatry." *JAMA Psychiatry* 75, no. 2 (2018): 115–117. https://doi.org/10.1001/jamapsychiatry.2017.3891.

Metzl, Jonathan M., and Helena Hansen. "Structural Competency: Theorizing a New Medical Engagement with Stigma and Inequality." *Social Science and Medicine* 103, no. 126 (2014): 126–133. https://doi.org/10.1016/j.socscimed.2013.06.032.

Metzl, Jonathan M., Aletha Maybank, and Fernando De Maio. "Responding to the COVID-19 Pandemic: The Need for a Structurally Competent Health Care System." *JAMA* 324, no. 3 (2020): 231–232. https://doi.org/10.1001/jama.2020.9289.

Metzl, Jonathan M., JuLeigh Petty, and Oluwatunmise V. Olowojoba. "Using a Structural Competency Framework to Teach Structural Racism in Pre-health Education." *Social Science and Medicine* 199 (2018): 189–201. https://doi.org/10.1016/j.socscimed.2017.06.029.

Miller, Ann Neville, Andrew Todd, Robert Toledo, et al. "The Relationship of Ethnic, Racial, and Cultural Concordance to Physician-Patient Communication: A Mixed-Methods Systematic Review Protocol, Health Communication." *Health Communication* 38, no. 11 (2022): 2370–2376. https://doi.org/10.1080/10410236.2022.2070449.

Miller, Claire Cain, Sarah Kliff, and Larry Buchanan. "Childbirth Is Deadlier for Black Families Even When They're Rich, Expansive Study Finds." *New York Times*, February 12, 2023. https://www.nytimes.com/interactive/2023/02/12/upshot/child-maternal-mortality-rich-poor.html.

Minow, Martha. *Saving the News: Why the Constitution Calls for Government Action to Preserve Freedom of Speech*. Oxford University Press, 2021.

Mondestin, Tanesha. "State Momentum on Medicaid Doula Coverage, Rate Increases." Center for Children & Families at the Georgetown University McCourt School of Public Policy, April 11, 2024. https://ccf.georgetown.edu/2024/04/11/state-momentum-on-medicaid-doula-coverage-rate-increases/.

Montagu, Ashley. *Statement on Race: An Extended Discussion in Plain Language of the UNESCO Statement by Experts on Race Problems*. Schuman, 1951.

Moore, Eli, Nicole Montojo, and Nicole Mauri. *Roots, Race, and Place: A History of Racially Exclusionary Housing in the San Francisco Bay Area*. Haas Institute for a Fair and Inclusive Society Public Education Report, 2019.

Mowatt, Rasul A. "Black Lives as Snuff: The Silent Complicity in Viewing Black Death." *Biography* 41, no. 4 (September 2018): 777–806, https://doi.org/10.1353/bio.2018.0079.

Moynihan, Daniel Patrick. *The Negro Family: The Case for National Action*. United States Department of Labor, 1965. https://web.stanford.edu/~mrosenfe/Moynihan's%20The%20Negro%20Family.pdf.

Mszar, Reed, Dipika J. Gopal, Rupa Chowdary, et al. "Racial/Ethnic Disparities in Screening for and Awareness of High Cholesterol among Pregnant Women Receiving Prenatal Care." *Journal of the American Heart Association* 10, no. 1 (2021): 1–11. https://doi.org/10.1161/JAHA.120.017415.

Mullings, Leith, and Alaka Wali. *Stress and Resilience: The Social Context of Reproduction in Central Harlem*. Springer Nature, 2001.

MyChart. "Home." Accessed August 19, 2024. https://www.mychart.org/.

Mystal, Elie. "Let's Talk About the Taking of Black Land." *The Nation*, March 7/14, 2022. https://www.thenation.com/article/society/black-land-seneca-village/.

Nash, Jennifer C. *Birthing Black Mothers*. Duke University Press, 2021.

National Archives. "Affirmative Action: History and Rationale." Accessed August 3, 2024. https://clintonwhitehouse3.archives.gov/WH/EOP/OP/html/aa/aa02.html.

Neely, Megan Tobias, Patrick Sheehan, and Christine L. Williams. "Social Inequality in High Tech: How Gender, Race, and Ethnicity Structure the World's Most Powerful Industry." *Annual Review of Sociology* 49 (2023): 319–338. https://doi.org/10.1146/annurev-soc-031021-034202.

New York City Health + Hospitals. *Community Health Needs Assessment 2022*. 2022. https://hhinternet.blob.core.windows.net/uploads/2022/07/community-health-needs-asssessment-2022.pdf.

New York State Department of Health. "Safety Net Definition." Revised February 2016. https://www.health.ny.gov/health_care/medicaid/redesign/dsrip/safety_net_definition.htm.

Noble, Safiya Umoja. "Critical Surveillance Literacy in Social Media: Interrogating Black Death and Dying Online." *Black Camera* 9, no. 2 (2018): 147–160. https://doi.org/10.2979/blackcamera.9.2.10.

Noble, Safiya Umoja. "Media Coverage and the Political Economy of Black Death," Interview by Jared Ball. *¡MWiL!*, July 14, 2016. Video, 19:43. https://imixwhatilike.org/2016/07/14/media-coverage-and-the-political-economy-of-black-death/.

Noble, Safiya Umoja. "Teaching Trayvon: Race, Media, and the Politics of Spectacle." *Black Scholar* 44. no. 1 (2014): 12–29. https://www.jstor.org/stable/10.5816/blackscholar.44.1.0012.

Olsen, Niklas. *The Sovereign Consumer: A New Intellectual History of Neoliberalism*. Palgrave MacMillan, 2019.

Oparah, Julia Chinyere, Helen Arega, Dantia Hudson, Linda Jones, and Talita Oseguera. *Battling over Birth: Black Women and Maternal Health Care Crisis*. Praeclarus Press, 2017.

Otte, Sonia V. "Improved Patient Experience and Outcomes: Is Patient–Provider Concordance Key?" *Journal of Patient Experience* 9 (2022): 1–7. https://doi.org/10.1177/23743735221103033.

Ozimek, John A., and Sarah J. Kilpatrick. "Maternal Mortality in the Twenty-First Century." *Obstetrics and Gynecology Clinics of North America* 45, no. 2 (2018). https://doi.org/10.1016/j.ogc.2018.01.004.

Patterson, Thomas E. "Time and News: The Media's Limitations as an Instrument of Democracy." *International Political Science Review* 19, no. 1 (1998): 55–67.

Paul, David A., Robert Locke, Kelly Zook, Kathleen H. Leef, John L. Stefano, and Garrett Colmorgen. "Racial Differences in Prenatal Care of Mothers Delivering Very Low Birth Weight Infants." *Journal of Perinatology* 26 (January 2006): 74–78. https://doi.org/10.1038/sj.jp.7211428.

Pearce, Robin. *The Sick Side of Town: How Place Shapes Disparities in Health*. Haas Institute for a Fair and Inclusive Society, 2018. https://belonging.berkeley.edu/sites/default/files/haasinstitute_thesicksideoftown_healthdisparitiesweb.pdf?file=1&force=1.

Petersen, Emily E., Nicole L. Davis, David Goodman, et al. "Racial/Ethnic Disparities in Pregnancy-Related Deaths—United States, 2007–2016." *Morbidity and Mortality Weekly Report* 68, no. 35 (2019): 762–765. http://dx.doi.org/10.15585/mmwr.mm6835a3.

Pfau, Ann, Kathleen Lawlor, David Hochfelder, and Stacy Kinlock Sewell. "Using Urban Renewal Records to Advance Reparative Justice." *Russell Sage Foundation Journal of the Social Sciences* 10, no. 2 (2024): 113–131. https://doi.org/10.7758/RSF.2024.10.2.05.

Phelps, Michelle S., and Amber M. Hamilton. "Visualizing Injustice or Reifying Racism? Images in the Digital Media Coverage of the Killing of Michael Brown." *Sociology of Race and Ethnicity* 8, no. 1 (2021): 160–175. https://doi.org/10.1177/23326492211015696.

Pidluzny, Jonathan. "Expert Insight: DEI Spells CRT: Legislation Restricting Diversity, Equity, and Inclusion Programs Will Improve the Intellectual Environment at Missouri Universities." America First Policy Institute, May 10, 2023. https://americafirstpolicy.com/issues/expert-insight-dei-spells-crt-legislation-restricting-diversity-equity-and-inclusion-programs-will-improve-the-intellectual-environment-at-missouri-universities.

Pilgrim, David. "The Mammy Caricature." Jim Crow Museum, October 2000. Last modified 2024. https://jimcrowmuseum.ferris.edu/mammies/homepage.htm.

Purnell, Derecka. "If Even Beyoncé Had a Rough Pregnancy, What Hope Do Other Black Women Have?" *The Guardian*, April 23, 2019. https://www.theguardian.com/commentisfree/2019/apr/23/beyonce-pregnancy-black-women.

Racehorse, Vanessa, and Anna Hohag. "Achieving Climate Justice through Land Back: An Overview of Tribal Dispossession, Land Return Efforts, and Practical Mechanisms for #LandBack." *Colorado Environmental Law Journal* 34, no. 2 (2023): 175–212.

Redfin. "Cole Valley, CA Housing Market." Accessed August 30, 2024. https://www.redfin.com/neighborhood/548/CA/San-Francisco/Cole-Valley/housing-market.

Regents of the University of California v. Bakke, 438 U.S. 265 (1978).

Reyes, Kimberly. "Affirmative Action Shouldn't Be About Diversity." *The Atlantic*, December 27, 2018. https://www.theatlantic.com/ideas/archive/2018/12/affirmative-action-about-reparations-not-diversity/578005/.

Richardson, L. Song, and Phillip A. Goff. "Implicit Racial Bias in Public Defender Triage." *Yale Law Journal* 122, no. 8 (2013): 2626–2649. https://www.jstor.org/stable/23528687.

Rios, Edwin. "'Birthing While Black' Is a National Crisis for the US. Here's What Black Lawmakers Want to Do about It." *The Guardian*, April 19, 2022. https://www.theguardian.com/us-news/2022/apr/19/black-mothers-birth-maternal-mortality.

Roberts, Dorothy. *Fatal Invention: How Science, Politics, and Big Business Re-Create Race in the Twenty-First Century*. New Press, 2011.

Roberts, Dorothy. "What's Wrong with Race-Based Medicine? Genes, Drugs, and Health Disparities." *Minnesota Journal of Law, Science & Technology* 12, no. 1 (2011): 1–21. https://scholarship.law.umn.edu/mjlst/vol12/iss1/3.

Robles, Frances. "The Citizen's Arrest Law Cited in Arbery's Killing Dates Back to the Civil War." *New York Times*, May 13, 2020. https://www.nytimes.com/article/ahmaud-arbery-citizen-arrest-law-georgia.html.

Rose, Patti Renee. *Health Equity Diversity, and Inclusion: Context, Controversies, and Solutions*. Jones & Bartlett Learning, 2021.

Rosenberg, Howard, and Charles S. Feldman. *No Time to Think: The Menace of Media Speed and the 24-Hour News Cycle.* Bloomsbury Publishing, 2009.

Rothstein, Richard. *The Color of Law: A Forgotten History of How Our Government Segregated America.* Liveright, 2017.

Royce, Celeste S., Helen Kang Morgan, Laura Baecher-Lind, et al. "The Time Is Now: Addressing Implicit Bias in Obstetrics and Gynecology Education." *American Journal of Obstetrics and Gynecology* 228, no. 4 (2023): 369–381. https://doi.org/10.1016/j.ajog.2022.12.016.

Saito, Leland T. *Building Downtown Los Angeles: The Politics of Race and Place in Urban America.* Stanford University Press, 2022.

Sapkota, Yadav, Na Qin, Matthew J. Ehrhardt, et al. "Genetic Variants Associated with Therapy-Related Cardiomyopathy among Childhood Cancer Survivors of African Ancestry." *Cancer Research* 81, no. 9 (2021): 2556–2565. https://doi.org/10.1158/0008-5472.CAN-20-2675.

Scheiber, Noam. "Affirmative Action Ruling May Upend Hiring Policies, Too." *New York Times,* June 30, 2023. https://www.nytimes.com/2023/06/30/business/economy/hiring-affirmative-action.html.

Schoenthaler, Antoniette, and Joseph Ravenell. "Understanding the Patient Experience through the Lenses of Racial/Ethnic and Gender Patient-Physician Concordance." *JAMA Network Open* 3, no. 11 (2020): 1–2. https://doi.org/10.1001/jamanetworkopen.2020.25349.

Scott, Brianna, Jeanette Woods, and Scott Detrow. "The Rates of Death for Pregnant Black Women Have Doubled the Last 20 Years." NPR, July 7, 2023. https://www.npr.org/2023/07/07/1186531829/the-rates-of-death-for-pregnant-black-women-have-doubled-the-last-20-years.

Semuels, Alana. "No, Most Black People Don't Live in Poverty—or Inner Cities." *The Atlantic,* October 12, 2016. https://www.theatlantic.com/business/archive/2016/10/trump-african-american-inner-city/503744/.

Shange, Savannah. *Progressive Dystopia: Abolition, Antiblackness, and Schooling in San Francisco.* Duke University Press, 2019.

Shen, Megan Johnson, Emily B. Peterson, Rosario Costas-Muñiz, et al. "The Effects of Race and Racial Concordance on Patient–Physician Communication: A Systematic Review of the Literature." *Journal of Racial and Ethnic Health Disparities* 5, no. 1 (2018): 117–140. https://doi.org/10.1007/s40615-017-0350-4.

Shepherd, Stephane. "Cultural Awareness Workshops: Limitations and Practical Consequences." *BMC Medical Education* 19, no. 1 (2019): 1–10. https://doi.org/10.1186/s12909-018-1450-5.

Shmerling, Robert H. "Is Our Healthcare System Broken?" *Harvard Health Publishing,* July 13, 2021. https://www.health.harvard.edu/blog/is-our-healthcare-system-broken-202107132542#:~:text=Despite%20spending%20far%20more%20on,relatively%20low%20in%20the%20US.

Silver-Greenberg, Jessica, and Katie Thomas. "They Were Entitled to Free Care. Hospitals Hounded Them to Pay." *New York Times,* last updated December 15, 2022. https://www.nytimes.com/2022/09/24/business/nonprofit-hospitals-poor-patients.html.

Simmons, Ann M. "The Quiet Crisis among African Americans: Pregnancy and Childbirth Are Killing Women at Inexplicable Rates." *Los Angeles Times*, October 26, 2017. https://www.latimes.com/world/global-development/la-na-texas-black-maternal-mortality-2017-htmlstory.html.

Simon, Melora. "Medi-Cal Explained: Paying for Maternity Services." California Health Care Foundation, September 2020. https://www.chcf.org/wp-content/uploads/2020/09/MediCal ExplainedPayingMaternityServices.pdf.

Singh, Gopal K., and Stella M. Yu. "Adverse Pregnancy Outcomes: Differences between US- and Foreign-Born Women in Major US Racial and Ethnic Groups." *American Journal of Public Health* 86, no. 6 (1996): 837–843. https://doi.org/10.2105/AJPH.86.6.837.

Smith, William A., Tara J. Yosso, and Daniel G. Solórzano. "Challenging Racial Battle Fatigue on Historically White Campuses: A Critical Race Examination of Race-Related Stress." In *Faculty of Color: Teaching in Predominately White Colleges and Universities*, edited by Christine A. Stanley. Anker Publishing, 2007.

Social Explorer. "ACS 2021 (5-Year Estimates), San Francisco City, California: Household Income in the Past 12 Months (in 2021 Inflation-Adjusted Dollars)." Accessed February 16, 2023. https://www.socialexplorer.com/tables/ACS2021_5yr/R13302533.

Solomon, Sonja R., Alev J. Atalay, and Nora Y. Osman. "Diversity Is Not Enough: Advancing a Framework for Antiracism in Medical Education." *Academic Medicine* 96, no. 11 (2021): 1513–1517. https://doi.org/10.1097/acm.0000000000004251.

Spellmeyer, Quinlyn R. "Southwest DC: A Cycle of Urban Renewal and 'Revitalization.'" *ArcGIS StoryMaps*, December 16, 2020. https://storymaps.arcgis.com/stories/f43a96703b3e4d098b7c242d680e3498.

Starbucks. "Starbucks to Close All Stores Nationwide for Racial-Bias Education on May 29." Accessed December 11, 2024. https://stories.starbucks.com/press/2018/starbucks-to-close-stores-nationwide-for-racial-bias-education-may-29/.

Stone, Jeff, and Gordon B. Moskowitz. "Non-Conscious Bias in Medical Decision Making: What Can Be Done to Reduce It?" *Medical Education* 45, no. 8 (2011): 768–776. https://doi.org/10.1111/j.1365-2923.2011.04026.x.

Stonington, Scott D., Seth M. Holmes, Helena Hansen, et al. "Case Studies in Social Medicine: Attending to Structural Forces in Clinical Practice." *New England Journal of Medicine* 379, no. 20 (2018): 1958–1961. https://doi.org/10.1056/NEJMms1814262.

Strings, Sabrina. *Fearing the Black Body: The Racial Origins of Fat Phobia*. New York University Press, 2018.

Students for Fair Admissions, Inc. v. President and Fellows of Harvard College, 600 U.S. 181 (2023) (Thomas, J., concurring).

Sumchai, Ahimsa Porter. "Reflections . . . On the Unspeakable History of Animal Cruelty at the Hunters Point Naval Shipyard." *Medium*, August 25, 2021. https://ahimsaportersumchaimd.medium.com/reflections-efc3cc6156ac.

Sutherland, Tonia. "Making a Killing: On Race, Ritual, and (Re)Membering in Digital Culture." *Preservation, Digital Technology & Culture* 46, no. 1 (2017): 32–40. https://doi.org/10.1515/pdtc-2017-0025.

Tam, Katherine. "Expanded Partnership at [redacted] to Advance Care for Publicly Insured Pregnant Patients." *Science of Caring*, January 25, 2023. [url redacted].

Taylor, Bianca. "Why San Francisco's Fillmore District Is No Longer the 'Harlem of the West.'" KQED, June 25, 2010. https://www.kqed.org/news/11825401/how-urban-renewal-decimated-the-fillmore-district-and-took-jazz-with-it.

Taylor, Lauren A., Osaze Udeagbala, Adam Biggs, Helen-Maria Lekas, and Keisha Ray. "Should a Healthcare System Facilitate Racially Concordant Care for Black Patients?" *Pediatrics* 148, no. 4 (2021): 1–7. https://doi.org/10.1542/peds.2021-051113.

Tenet, Megan. "Racial Inequality in Medicine: How Did We Get Here?" *Georgetown Medical Review* 5, no. 1 (2021): 1–6. https://doi.org/10.52504/001c.25142.

Thompson, Walter. "How Urban Renewal Destroyed the Fillmore in Order to Save It." *Hoodline*, January 3, 2016. https://hoodline.com/2016/01/how-urban-renewal-destroyed-the-fillmore-in-order-to-save-it/.

Tobbell, Dominique, and Patricia D'Antonio. "The History of Racism in Nursing: A Review of Existing Scholarship." National Commission to Address Racism in Nursing, 2022. https://www.nursingworld.org/globalassets/practiceandpolicy/workforce/commission-to-address-racism/1thehistoryofracisminnursing.pdf.

Tobi, Elmar W., Jelle J. Goeman, Ramin Monajemi, et al. "DNA Methylation Signatures Link Prenatal Famine Exposure to Growth and Metabolism." *Nature Communications* 5 (2014):1–13. https://doi.org/10.1038/ncomms6592.

Trimbur, Lucia, and Lundy Braun. "The NFL's Reversal on 'Race Norming' Reveals How Pervasive Medical Racism Remains." NBC News, June 8, 2021. https://www.nbcnews.com/think/opinion/nfl-s-reversal-race-norming-reveals-how-pervasive-medical-racismncna1269992.

Truven Health Analytics. *The Cost of Having a Baby in the United States*. January 2013. https://nationalpartnership.org/wp-content/uploads/2023/02/the-cost-of-having-a-baby-in-the-us.pdf.

Tsai, Jinyun. "One in Three Homes in This San Francisco Neighborhood Lives below the Poverty Line." *San Francisco Standard*, December 8, 2022. https://sfstandard.com/2022/12/08/san-francisco-neighborhood-new-census-data-maps/.

Tubbs, Anna Malaika. "'I Knew How Dangerous Things Could Become': The Perils of Childbirth as a Black Woman." *The Guardian*, June 26, 2021. https://www.theguardian.com/lifeandstyle/2021/jun/26/i-knew-how-dangerous-things-could-become-perils-of-childbirth-as-a-black-woman.

Tummala, Lakshmi S., Akanksha Agrawal, and Gina Lundberg. "Management Considerations for Lipid Disorders during Pregnancy." *Current Treatment Options in Cardiovascular Medicine* 23, no. 50 (2021): 1–12. https://doi.org/10.1007/s11936-021-00926-1.

United States Census Bureau. "Black Individuals Had Record Low Official Poverty Rate in 2022." September 12, 2023. https://www.census.gov/library/stories/2023/09/black-poverty-rate.html.

United States Census Bureau. "Quick Facts: San Francisco City, California—Race and Hispanic Origin." https://www.census.gov/quickfacts/fact/table/sanfranciscocitycalifornia/PST045222.

United States Centers for Disease Control and Prevention. "Pregnancy Mortality Surveillance System." Accessed August 31, 2024. https://www.cdc.gov/maternal-mortality/php/pregnancy-mortality-surveillance/index.html.

United States Department of Health and Human Services. "Who's Eligible for Medicare?" Last modified December 8, 2022. https://www.hhs.gov/answers/medicare-and-medicaid/who-is-eligible-for-medicare/index.html.

United States Department of the Interior. "National Register of Historic Places Multiple Property Documentation Form for African Americans in California, 1850–1974." https://ohp.parks.ca.gov/pages/1067/files/CA_Multiple percent20Counties_African percent20Americans percent20in percent20CA percent20MPDF_DRAFT.pdf.

UC Berkeley's Urban Displacement Project and the California Housing Partnership. "Rising Costs and Re-Segregation in the San Francisco Bay Area." Accessed August 2021. https://www.urbandisplacement.org/wp-content/uploads/2021/08/bay_area_re-segregation_rising_housing_costs_report_2019.pdf.

University of California Health. "Our Commitment to Medi-Cal." Accessed August 19, 2024. https://health.universityofcalifornia.edu/about-us/our-commitment-medi-cal.

Valdes, Elise G. "Examining Cesarean Delivery Rates by Race: A Population-Based Analysis Using the Robson Ten-Group Classification System." *Journal of Racial and Ethnic Health Disparities* 8, no. 4 (2021): 844–851. https://doi.org/10.1007/s40615-020-00842-3.

Veenendaal, M. V. E., Rebecca C. Painter, Susanne R. de Rooij, et al. "Transgenerational Effects of Prenatal Exposure to the 1944–45 Dutch Famine." *BJOG: An International Journal of Obstetrics & Gynaecology* 120, no. 5 (2013): 548–554. https://doi.org/10.1111/1471-0528.12136.

Vela, Monica B., Amarachi I. Erondu, Nichole A. Smith, Monica E. Peek, James N. Woodruff, and Marshall H. Chin. "Eliminating Explicit and Implicit Biases in Health Care: Evidence and Research Needs." *Annual Review of Public Health* 43 (2022): 477–501. https://doi.org/10.1146/annurev-publhealth-052620-103528.

Vella, Elizabeth, Victoria M. White, and Patricia Livingston. "Does Cultural Competence Training for Health Professionals Impact Culturally and Linguistically Diverse Patient Outcomes? A Systematic Review of the Literature." *Nurse Education Today* 118, no. 1 (2022). https://doi.org/10.1016/j.nedt.2022.105500.

Vernon, Marlo, Colleen Walters, Samantha Sojourner, and Candace Best. "Maternal Mortality." In *Black Health in the South*, edited by Steven S. Coughlin, Lovoria B. Williams, and Tabia Henry Akintobi. Johns Hopkins University Press, 2023.

Villarosa, Linda. *Under the Skin: The Hidden Toll of Racism on American Lives and on the Health of Our Nation*. Vintage, 2023.

Villarosa, Linda. "Why America's Black Mothers and Babies Are in a Life-or-Death Crisis." *New York Times*, April 11, 2018. https://www.nytimes.com/2018/04/11/magazine/black-mothers-babies-death-maternal-mortality.html.

Vincenty, Samantha. "Kamala Harris Is Fighting to Protect Black Mothers from Medical Bias." *Oprah Daily*, August 13, 2020. https://www.oprahdaily.com/entertainment/a33577853/kamala-harris-black-maternal-health-care-crisis/.

Vora, Samreen, Brittany Dahlen, Mark Adler, et al. "Recommendations and Guidelines for the Use of Simulation to Address Structural Racism and Implicit Bias." *Simulation in Healthcare: The Journal of the Society for Simulation in Healthcare* 16, no. 4 (2021): 275–284. https://doi.org/10.1097/SIH.0000000000000591.

Vyas, Darshali A., Leo G. Eisenstein, and David S. Jones. "Hidden in Plain Sight: Reconsidering the Use of Race Correction in Clinical Algorithms." *New England Journal of Medicine* 383, no. 9 (2020): 874–882. https://doi.org/10.1056/NEJMms2004740.

Walker, Denetra, and Kelli Boling. "Black Maternal Mortality in the Media: How Journalists Cover a Deadly Racial Disparity." *Journalism* 24, no. 7 (2023): 1536–1553. https://doi.org/10.1177/14648849211063361.

Watson, Leah. "Anti-DEI Efforts Are the Latest Attack on Racial Equity and Free Speech." ACLU, February 14, 2024. https://www.aclu.org/news/free-speech/anti-dei-efforts-are-the-latest-attack-on-racial-equity-and-free-speech.

Weingroff, Richard F. "Federal-Aid Highway Act of 1956: Creating the Interstate System." *Public Roads* 60, no. 1 (1996). https://highways.dot.gov/public-roads/summer-1996/federal-aid-highway-act-1956-creating-interstate-system-sidebars.

Whalen, Andrew. "Zuckerberg Hospital ER Doesn't Take Private Insurance, Sticking San Francisco Patients with Huge Bills." *Newsweek*, January 7, 2019. https://www.newsweek.com/zuckerberg-hospital-er-private-insurance-medicare-medicaid-mark-facebook-san-1282274.

White House, The. "Fact Sheet: Vice President Kamala Harris Announces Call to Action to Reduce Maternal Mortality and Morbidity." December 7, 2021. https://web.archive.org/web/20250116071958/https://www.whitehouse.gov/briefing-room/statements-releases/2021/12/07/fact-sheet-vice-president-kamala-harris-announces-call-to-action-to-reduce-maternal-mortality-and-morbidity/.

Wilbur, Kristen, Cyndy Snyder, Alison C. Essary, Swapna Reddy, Kristen K. Will, and Mary Saxon. "Developing Workforce Diversity in the Health Professions: A Social Justice Perspective." *Journal of Health Professions Education* 6, no. 2 (2020): 222–229. https://doi.org/10.1016/j.hpe.2020.01.002.

Wilkinson, Rachel, Zina Huxley-Reicher, G. W. Conner Fox, et al. "Leveraging Clerkship Experiences to Address Segregated Care: A Survey-Based Approach to Student-Led Advocacy." *Teaching and Learning in Medicine* 35, no. 4 (2022): 381–388. https://doi.org/10.1080/10401334.2022.2088538.

Williams, Michelle A. "The Cost of Bearing Witness: Watching and Sharing Videos of Police Brutality Online." *BMJ*, March 16, 2023. https://doi.org/10.1136/bmj.p616.

Williamson, Lillie D. "Beyond Personal Experiences: Examining Mediated Vicarious Experiences as an Antecedent of Medical Mistrust." *Health Communication* 37, no. 9 (2022): 1061–1074. https://doi.org/10.1080/10410236.2020.1868744.

Wood, Amy Louise. *Lynching and Spectacle: Witnessing Racial Violence in America, 1890–1940.* University of North Carolina Press, 2009.

World Health Organization. "Social Determinants of Health." Accessed August 2, 2024. https://www.who.int/health-topics/social-determinants-of-health#tab=tab_1.

Wright, Maya A., Kemi M. Doll, Evan Myers, William R. Carpenter, Danielle R. Gartner, and Whitney R. Robinson. "Changing Trends in Black–White Racial Differences in Surgical Menopause: A Population-Based Study." *American Journal of Obstetrics and Gynecology* 225, no. 5 (2021): 502.e1–502.e13. https://doi.org/10.1016/j.ajog.2021.05.045.

Yick Wo v. Hopkins, 118 U.S. 356 (1886).

Young, Iris Marion. "Pregnant Embodiment: Subjectivity and Alienation." *Journal of Medicine and Philosophy: A Forum for Bioethics and Philosophy of Medicine* 9, no.1 (1984): 45–62. https://doi.org/10.1093/jmp/9.1.45.

Zhao, Cindy, Phillip Dowzicky, Latesha Colbert, Sanford Roberts, and Rachel R. Kelz. "Race, Gender, and Language Concordance in the Care of Surgical Patients: A Systematic Review." *Surgery* 166, no. 5 (2019): 785–792. https://doi.org/10.1016/j.surg.2019.06.012.

Zuckerberg San Francisco General Hospital and Trauma Center. *FY 2021–2022 Annual Report*. Uploaded May 2024. https://www.zuckerbergsanfranciscogeneral.org/wp-content/uploads/2024/05/ZSFG-FY-Annual-Report-2021-2022.pdf.

Zuckerberg San Francisco General Hospital and Trauma Center. *FY 2022–2023 Annual Report*. 2023. https://www.sf.gov/sites/default/files/2023-10/05%20ZSFG%20FY%20Annual%20Report%202022-2023.pdf.

Zuckerberg San Francisco General Hospital and Trauma Center. "Home." Accessed August 17, 2024. https://www.zuckerbergsanfranciscogeneral.org/.

OTHER SOURCES

[name redacted]. "About [redacted] at [redacted]: Partners in Health" Accessed August 19, 2024. [url redacted].

[name redacted] Health. "Family Health Centers at [redacted]." [url redacted].

[name redacted] Health. "How [redacted] Became One of the Safest Hospitals in the Country." November 2, 2022. [url redacted].

[name redacted] Health. *In the Community 2023: Our Commitment to Nursing Excellence.* 2023. [url redacted].

[name redacted]. "Midwifery at [redacted]." Accessed August 8, 2024. [url redacted].

[name redacted]. "Our 340B Story." Accessed August 17, 2024. [url redacted].

[name redacted]. "Team Lily / Patient Information." [url redacted].

[name redacted]. "Training Sites." Accessed August 19, 2024. [url redacted].

[name redacted]. "The Value of an Integrated Healthcare Network." 2020. [url redacted].

Index

Adolescent pregnancy, 52
Advertising revenue, 126–127
Affirmative action programs, 206, 217–220
AFFIRM program, 183
Affordable housing, 37
African Americans. *See* Black people
African immigrants' babies, 90–91
Allostatic load, 101–102
Alpha Hospital, 1–4, 62–63, 76–77
American Indian/Alaska Native people, 97
"America's Black Mothers and Babies Are in a Life-or-Death Crisis," 119
Amniotomy, 176
Anderson, Dr., 148, 169
Andrews-Dyer, Helena, 117, 136
Annalise's story, 50–51
Annette's story, 11–13, 150–151, 165–170
Appointment booking, 77–78
Arbery, Ahmaud, 127

Babies, health outcomes of, 90–91, 99
Baldwin, James, 33
Bayview-Hunters Point area, 29–32, 35
BElovedBIRTH Black Centering, 183
Benjamin, Ruha, 113–114
Beyoncé, 119, 131
Biden, Joseph, 140
Bingham Ordinance of 1890, 27
Birth outcomes, 90–91, 99

Black Lives Matter movement, 120
Black maternal health crisis, 16, 117. *See also* Maternal mortality; Racial disparities in maternal mortality
articles about, 118–119
and doulas, 213–214
media coverage, 119–120, 123–125, 130–135, 137–139
mothers as political currency, 141
mothers as symbols, 135–141
mothers as victims, 123
news headlines, 117–118
as profit-making news, 127–128, 139, 141
Black Maternal Health Momnibus Act, 140
"Black Mothers Keep Dying after Giving Birth," 118
Black newborns, 204–205
Black people. *See also* Class-privileged Black people
commercially insured, 15, 67
culture, 92–96, 189–192
and educational advantage, 10
ER treatment, 103–104
and healthcare institutions, 13
and healthcare providers, 17
as homeowners, 32
and housing discrimination, 35
and illness-causing genes, 88–91
and implicit bias, 105–108

Black people (cont.)
  maternal morality rates, 6–7, 88, 139
  and medicalization of pregnancy, 156–157
  in medicine, 206–207
  as midwives, 166
  motherhood narratives, 121–123
  patient distrust, 110–114, 202, 215, 225
  police killings, 127–128, 131–132, 135, 140–141
  and poverty, 20–23, 96–97
  pregnancy outcomes, 100–102
  pregnancy-related death rates, 1, 7–8, 88
  and quality of care, 66
  in San Francisco, 19–20, 23–24, 29–31, 39
  and structural racism, 92
  and urban renewal, 33, 36–38
  weathering and stress, 100–102
Black providers, 151–164
  advocacy, 152–153
  and class-privileged Black patients, 147–149, 151–164
  and comfort, 151–153
  and implicit bias, 202
  midwifery, 166, 212
  and newborn care, 204–205
  and patient attitudes to medicine, 157–164, 167
  and patient expectations, 209–211
  and preventative screenings, 203–204
  and racial disparities in maternal mortality, 212–215
Black Wellbeing Clinic, 145, 172, 179, 181–183, 209, 211–212, 215–216
Bland, Sandra, 127
Bloody Sunday, 131
Bloody Thursday, 24–25
Body size, 165–166
Boling, Kelli, 118
Boone, Elaina and Talissa, 87
Breastfeeding, 213
Brighton Leary Foundation, 52

Brown, Michael, 127
Brown v. Board of Education, 109
Build Back Better Act, 140
Buttigieg, Pete, 140

Cable news channels, 129–130
Caesarian sections, 104
California
  Gold Rush, 26
  maternal mortality ratio, 139
  Medical Board of California, 222
  shipyards, 29–30
California Maternal Quality Care Collaborative (CMQCC), 139
Cal-WORKs, 57
Campbell, Colleen, 104
Canada, 7
Cardiac catheterization, 104
Cardiomyopathy, 89–90
Cardiovascular screenings, 204
Carson, Ben, 22
Castile, Philando, 127
Chalifour, Juliette, 63–64, 70–71
Charlotte's story, 216
Chauvin, Derek, 106, 119, 131–132
Chicago, 36
Childbirth, medicalization of, 154–156
Chinese immigrants, 26–28
Civil rights movement, 217, 221
Clarke, Marie, 60–61, 152, 181–182
Class-privileged Black people, 16–17, 46
  and Black providers, 147–149, 151–164
  choice of hospital, 47–48, 50, 66–67, 83
  healthcare strategies, 143–144
  navigating the system, 59
  performing privilege, 144–155
  and racial disadvantage, 22–23, 144, 147, 149–151, 169–170, 178
  and racial renunciation, 171–172, 178–180
  racism-associated stress, 101–102
  in San Francisco, 19–20, 39–43

wait times, 77, 79
white husbands, 150–151
CLAS standards, 187
CNN, 129–130
Cole, Haile Eshe, 121–122, 134
Cole Valley, 40
Commercial insurance, 49–50, 57
  Black people, 15, 67
  market orientation, 71–72
  and Medicaid, 68–69, 81
  and provider wages, 75, 77
  safety-net hospitals, 81
Consumerism, 170–171
Counterstereotypes, 185
COVID-19 pandemic, 92, 111, 140
CpG islands, 98
"Crack mother," 121–122
Crear-Perry, Joia, 7
Critical race theory, 221
Cultural competence training, 186–195, 225
  and cultural humility framework, 194
  and diversity within cultures, 191–192
  efficacy of, 194–195, 198
  and stereotypes, 189–191
  and structural competency framework, 198–201
  and structural racism, 188–189
Cultural explanations of health outcomes, 92–96, 188–191, 199
  culture concept, 94
  health behaviors, 95
  social disadvantages, 94–95
Cultural humility framework, 194

Daley, Richard J., 36
Davani, Sitara, 21, 58, 60–61, 67, 69–70, 75, 79
Davis, Dána-Ain, 7, 14, 212
Davis-Floyd, Robbie, 154–155
Delayed childbirth, 100–101
Democracy, 125–126

Dilation and curettage (D&C), 112–113
Diversity
  within cultures, 191–192
  genetic, 88–90, 95–96
Diversity, equity, and inclusion (DEI) initiatives, 196–198, 217–219, 221–222
Double-/triple-appointment booking, 77–78
Doula services, 139, 213–214
Dutch famine of 1944-1945, 99

East Hills campus, 51–53, 55, 72–73
Ebrahimji, Alisha, 131
Educational level, 8, 10
Eisenhower, Dwight D., 37
Ellington, Duke, 38
Elliott, Dr., 210–211
Eminent domain, 33
Employer-based health insurance, 6, 9
Endometriosis, 112
Epigenetics, 88, 97–100, 136–137, 224
Epigenome, 97–99
Evelyn's story, 40–43
Exhaustion, race-related, 43

Family Birth Center, 174–175, 178
Federal-Aid Highway Act of 1956, 37
Federally qualified health centers (FQHCs), 82
Feldman, Charles, 129
Feminist critique of medicalization, 156
Fillmore neighborhood, 30–35
Floyd, George, 106, 119, 127, 131–132, 141, 221
Food deserts, 94
Food insecurity, 99
Fortune's story, 112
Frakes, Michael, 204
Franklin Medical Center, 81–83
Fraser, Gertrude, 155

Garner, Eric, 127
Gaye, Marvin, 141

General, the. *See* Zuckerberg San Francisco General Hospital and Trauma Center ("the General")
Genes, 97–98
Genetic diversity, 88–90, 95–96
Genome, 97–98
Gentrification, 44
Georgia (midwife), 174–175
Geronimus, Arline, 100–102
Giselle's story, 113, 147–151, 169
Golden Health, 1–4, 7, 15, 17, 180
  AFFIRM program, 183
  Black Wellbeing Clinic, 145, 172, 179, 181–183, 209, 211–212, 215–216
  East Hills campus, 51–53, 55, 72–73
  and the General, 46, 50–51, 58–61, 63–64, 66–67, 69
  late arrivals/no-shows, 79
  L&D Department, 70
  and low-income/uninsured patients, 57, 60–61, 71, 79
  and Medicaid patients, 54–56, 58, 60, 79
  "on divert," 46–47
  patient insurance, 50
  patient satisfaction, 45, 75
  as public institution, 56
  racially concordant care, 212–213
  residency training, 64–65
  wait times, 76
  Women's Health Clinic (WHC), 77, 181
  Yerba Buena campus, 51–53, 55, 72–73
Gray, Freddie, 127
Group Prenatal Care (GPC), 183
Gruber, Jonathan, 204
Grutter v. Bollinger, 217–218, 220

Hansen, Helena, 187, 198–200
Harlem of the South, 37
Harlow's story, 157–162, 164–165, 167
Harris, Kamala, 140
Hartman, Saidiya, 130–132, 171
Harvey, David, 170

Healthcare. *See also* Healthcare segregation
  and poverty, 5–6
  private, 6
  as profit-making industry, 223–224
  quality of, 61–67
  and racial inequality, 224
  universal, 6–7
Healthcare segregation, 15, 48–55, 79–83
  causes, 50
  and class-privileged patients, 82–84
  between departments, 55
  within health systems, 51–54
  and low-income/uninsured patients, 83–84
  and Medicaid, 50, 81–83
  and Medi-Cal, 51–52, 54–55
  public vs. private hospitals, 57, 81–82
  and quality, 61–67
  and racially concordant care, 215–221
  and surplus revenue, 81
Health insurance, 6, 15. *See also* Commercial insurance
  the General's patients, 20–21, 49–50
  and hospital mergers, 53
  low-income patients, 59
Health outcomes. *See also* Maternal mortality
  cultural explanations of, 92–96, 188–191, 199
  doula-supported births, 213
  and environment, 98–100
  and implicit bias, 105–106, 184–186
  newborns, 90–91, 99, 204–205
  and parental genes, 99–100
  and racial discrimination, 43
  and racially concordant care, 203–205
  and structural competency, 198–201
Historically black colleges and universities (HBCUs), 66
Homecoming, 119, 131
Home Owners' Lending Corporation (HOLC), 32
Horror genre, 133–134

Hospital mergers, 53–54
Housing, affordable, 37
Housing Acts of 1949/1954, 32–33
Housing and Urban Development, Department of, 22
Housing policies, 32–35
Hunt, Francine, 181–182

Ifeoma's story, 157, 161–165
Iggi, Semret, 181–182
Implicit Association Test (IAT), 105
Implicit bias, 105–110, 215, 225
 and Black providers, 202
 and health outcomes, 105–106, 184–186
 and quality of care, 105–106
Income inequality, 42
Indigenous people, genocide of, 26
Individuation, patient, 185
Inequality, racial, 106–109, 224
 cultural explanation of, 96
 income, 42
 social/racial, 85
Infant mortality, 8
Insurance. *See* Health insurance
Irving, Shalon, 118
Isra's story, 210–211

James, Osamudia, 105, 186
Japanese immigrants, 28–30
Japanese internment, 28, 30
Jenna's story, 111–112, 143–144, 146–147, 151–153
Jim Crow South, 99–100
Jody's story, 172–173
Journalism, standard of, 124–125

Kuzawa, Christopher, 89, 91

Landrum, Simone, 133–134
Laundry ordinance of 1880, 27–28
Lazarus, Ellen, 71–72
Legacy media, 128–129

Lekas, Helen-Maria, 208, 213
Lewis, John, 132
Liaison Committee on Medical Education (LCME), 187
Lincoln Center, 36
Loren's story, 137–138
Los Angeles, 38
"Lost Mothers" series, 118
Loudon, Irvine, 154
Lowery, Wesley, 126
Low-income/uninsured patients, 59
 childbirth preferences, 156
 and the General, 57–58, 60–61
 and Golden Health, 57, 60–61, 71, 79
 and healthcare segregation, 83–84
 and H&H, 80
 and nonblack providers, 147
 no-shows, 77–78
 and poor people's hospitals, 84
 and quality of care, 62
 wait times, 76

"Mammy," 121–122
Martin, Trayvon, 127
Maternal CARE Act, 140
Maternal mortality. *See also* Black maternal health crisis; Racial disparities in maternal mortality
 high-black-serving hospitals, 103
 high-income nations, 7
 income and educational levels, 8, 97, 101
 media coverage, 120, 132–134
 political initiatives, 139–140
 and poverty, 97
 rates, 6–7, 88, 139
 and social class, 1–2, 8
 U.S. ratio, 139
 and white pleasure, 130–131
Matriarchs, Black, 121–122
McClain, Elijah, 127
McDaniel, Hattie, 38
McEwen, Bruce, 101–102

Meconium, 176
Media coverage, 119–120, 123–125, 130–134, 137–139
Media outlet income streams, 126–128
Medicaid, 48–49, 67–71
    and commercial insurance, 68–69, 81
    doula services, 139
    and Golden Health, 54–56, 58, 60, 79
    and healthcare segregation, 50, 81–83
    and hospital competition, 72
    and nonblack providers, 150
    patient race and class, 21
    postpartum care, 139
    and prenatal care, 5–6, 8–9
    and provider recruitment, 73, 77
    and racial disparities, 9
    reimbursement rates, 56, 68, 72–73, 77
    safety-net hospitals, 81
    wealthy people's hospitals, 81–82
Medi-Cal, 48–49
    Golden vs. the General, 58, 60–61, 69–71
    and healthcare segregation, 51–52, 54–55
    reimbursement coverage, 68
Medical schools, 80
Medicare, 48–49, 68
Mercy Medical Center, 52
Meredith's story, 145–147, 151, 169
Mergers, hospital, 53–54
Methylation, 98
Metzl, Jonathan, 187, 198–200
Miami, 37–38
Midwifery, 154–157, 165–167, 169, 174–175, 212
Milk, Harvey, 24
Minow, Martha, 124, 128
Molar pregnancy, 182
Morristown Flats, 51
Mowatt, Rasul, 132, 135
Moynihan, Daniel Patrick, 121–122
MSNBC, 130
Muwekma Ohlone, 26, 42

Nancy's story, 215–217
Nash, Jennifer, 119–120, 122, 135–136, 141, 213–214
Near West Side neighborhood, 36
"Negro removal," 38
Neoliberalism, 170–171
Newborns, 90–91, 99, 204–205
News industry, 126
Newspapers, 129
New York City, 36, 62–63, 79–83, 141–142
New York City Health and Hospitals (H&H), 80–81
New York City Health and Hospitals Corporation (HHC), 80–81
New York State, healthcare in, 5
Nichols, Tyre, 127
Nikki's story, 112–113
Noble, Safiya Umoja, 125, 130, 140
Nonprofit hospitals, 55–56

Obstetric practices, 154–156
Obstetric racism, 14, 212
Office of Minority Health, 187
Olivia, 173–180
Omega Hospital, 62–63
Overtown, 37–38

Patients
    attitudes to medicine, 157–164, 167
    distrust of providers, 110–114, 202, 215, 225
    experience of healthcare, 45, 67, 73–75
    patient individuation/perspective-taking, 185
    patient-provider confrontations, 2–3
    wait times, 2, 76–78
People of color. *See also* Black people
    and gene expression, 98
    illness-causing genes, 89
    patient distrust, 110
    and quality of care, 66, 103
    San Francisco hospitals, 49
    and urban renewal, 33, 36–37
Perspective-taking, 185

Police violence, 127–128, 131–132, 135, 140–141
Poverty
  and Black people, 20–23, 96–97
  and healthcare, 5–6
  rates, 22, 97
  in San Francisco, 23
Powell, Lewis F., Jr., 217–218
Preeclampsia, 119
Pregnancy
  medicalization of, 154–157, 162
  outcomes, 100–102
Pregnancy-related death. *See also* Maternal mortality
  and environment, 99–100
  income and educational levels, 8, 97
  rates, 1, 7–8
Prenatal care
  AFFIRM program, 183
  and Medicaid, 5–6, 8–9
  New York City program, 141–142
  scarcity of appointments, 59
  and stress, 98–99
Prenatal Care Assistance Program (PCAP), 76
Preventative screenings, 203–204
Print media, 129
Private hospitals, 80–81
Public housing, 35
Purnell, Derecka, 119

Quality of care, 61–67
  implicit bias, 105–106
  individual, 103–110
  and low-income/uninsured patients, 62
  and people of color, 66, 103
  racial disparities, 88, 102–110
  system, 102–103

Race. *See also* Racial disparities in maternal mortality
  and body size, 169
  and exclusionary zoning, 27
  and genetic diversity, 88–90, 95–96
  and healthcare outcomes, 13–14
  and maternal mortality, 1–2
  obstetric racism, 14, 212
  race-based affirmative action programs, 206, 217–220
  racial inequality, 42, 85, 96, 106–109, 224
  racial stereotypes, 185, 189–190
  racism-related stress, 43, 100–102, 136, 224
  racist housing policies, 32
  and social class, 9–10
  structural racism, 109, 188
  white experience of, 21
Racial discrimination
  and class privilege, 19
  and health outcomes, 43
  and racially concordant care, 220
  and stress, 43, 100–102, 136, 224
Racial disparities in maternal mortality, 1, 7–8, 16, 44, 96–115. *See also* Black maternal health crisis; Maternal mortality
  and Black providers, 212–215
  cultural competence training, 186–195
  and DEI programs, 196–197
  documentation of, 117
  epigenetics, 88, 97–100
  genes and culture, 92–96, 101, 115
  implicit bias, 105–110, 184–186
  media coverage, 119–120, 123–125
  patient distrust, 88, 110–114, 225
  poverty, 88, 96–97
  and profit motive, 224
  quality of care, 88, 102–110
  and racially concordant care, 184, 205, 212–215
  stress and weathering, 88, 100–102
  and structural racism, 188–189
Racial exclusion, 26–39
  Asians, 26–30
  Black people, 30–31, 38–39
  Chicago, 36
  Indigenous people, 26

Racial exclusion (cont.)
  intentional, 35
  Los Angeles, 38
  Miami, 37–38
  New York City, 36
  Washington, DC, 36
Racial identity
  awareness of, 21, 192
  essentializing, 208–211
  racial identity centrality, 208–209
  racial identity salience, 208–209
Racially concordant care, 17–18, 151, 182–184, 202–222
  AFFIRM program, 183
  aims, 202
  BElovedBIRTH Black Centering, 183
  Black Wellbeing Clinic, 145, 172, 179, 181–183
  critiques of, 207–221
  and essentializing identity, 208–211
  and healthcare segregation, 215–221
  and health outcomes, 203–205
  patient/provider communication, 202–203
  and race-based affirmative action, 219–220
  and racial disparities in maternal mortality, 184, 205, 212–215
  and reverse discrimination, 220
  and segregated spaces, 215–221
  universal, 206–207
Racial reckoning of 2020, 221–222
Racial renunciation, 17, 171–172, 178–180, 213
Racial segregation, 37, 102. *See also* Healthcare segregation
Racial stereotypes, 185, 189–191
Reagan, Ronald, 121
Regents of the University of California v. Bakke, 217
Reproducing Race: An Ethnography of Pregnancy as a Site of Racialization, 76–77
Reverse discrimination, 220

Rice, Tamir, 127
Rihanna, 181–182
Rita's story, 10–11
Roberts, Dorothy, 91
Roe v. Wade, 131
Rosenberg, Howard, 129
Rothstein, Richard, 29
Ruby's story, 193

Safety-net hospitals, 61–63, 76–77
  commercial insurance, 81
  Medicaid patients, 81
  private, 80–81
  and wealthy people's hospitals, 84
San Francisco, 14–15
  Bingham Ordinance of 1890, 27
  Black people in, 19–20, 23–24, 29–31, 39
  Chinatown, 34
  Chinese immigrants, 26–28
  inequality in, 25
  Japanese immigrants, 28–30
  laundry ordinance of 1880, 27–28
  poverty in, 23–25
  race and class in, 23–26
  racial exclusion, 26–30, 33–35, 38–39
  racial populations, 49–50
  racist housing policies, 32
  urban renewal, 33–35, 38
San Juan Hill neighborhood, 36
Santa Monica Freeway, 38
Scott, Walter, 127
Segregation, healthcare. *See* Healthcare segregation
Shange, Savannah, 24, 39
Shepherd, Stephane, 195
Slavery, abolition of, 171
Slum clearance, 32–33, 35–37
Social class. *See also* Class-privileged Black people
  and childbirth preferences, 156
  and inequality, 84–84

and infant mortality, 8
and maternal mortality, 1–2, 8
and race-based harm, 9–10
Social determinants of health (SDOH), 201
Social media, 124–125, 128–129
Sotomayor, Sonia, 185
Southwest DC, 36
Staff, hospital
   recruitment, 73–75
   shortages, 77
Starbucks incident, 106–107
Stellar, Eliot, 101–102
Stereotypes, racial, 185, 189–191
Sterling, Alton, 127
Stress, racism-related, 43, 100–102, 136, 224
Structural competency framework, 198–201
Structural racism, 109, 188–189
Students for Fair Admissions, Inc. v. Harvard (SFFA), 206–207, 220
Sugar Hill neighborhood, 38
Supplemental Nutrition Assistance Program (SNAP), 57
Sutherland, Tonia, 128
Sweet, Elizabeth, 89, 91
Synoptic Health, 52, 54
Syphilis, 110–111

Tal, Dr., 148–150, 169
Tax exemptions, 55–56
Taylor, Breonna, 127
Team Lily, 57
Thomas, Clarence, 220
Till, Emmett, 131–132
Till-Mobley, Mamie, 131
Trauma porn, 131
Truman, Harry, 32
Trump, Donald, 22, 198
Turner, Brianna, 58–60, 64–65
Tuskegee Experiment, 110–111, 113–114

United Kingdom, 7
United States
   birth outcomes, 90–91
   Black people in medicine, 206–207
   cardiovascular mortality, 204
   high-black-serving hospitals, 102–103
   hospital births, 154
   maternal mortality rates, 6–7, 139
   poverty rates, 22, 97
   pregnancy-related death rates, 1, 7–8
Universal healthcare, 6–7
Urban renewal, 32–36, 38, 44

Vaccines. *See* COVID-19 pandemic
Valerio, 51
Videos of police brutality, 131–132, 140–141
Villarosa, Linda, 119, 133–134
Volante, Helen, 145, 152–153, 181–182
Voting Rights Act of 1965, 132

Walker, Denetra, 118
Warren, Elizabeth, 140
Washington, DC, 36
Waters, Ethel, 38
Weathering, 100–101
Welfare queen, 121–122
Wells, Ida B., 131
White flight, 32
White immigrants' babies, 91
White newborns, 205
White people
   and black suffering, 130–134
   and diversity initiatives, 218–219
   pregnancy outcomes, 100–102
Williams, Serena, 119, 131
Women's Health Clinic (WHC), 77, 181

Yerba Buena campus, 51–53, 55, 72–73
Young, Iris, 155
Young Women's Clinic, 52–53, 55

Zoning, exclusionary, 27
Zuckerberg San Francisco General Hospital and Trauma Center ("the General"), 44–46, 182
  attitudes toward, 47–48, 65–67
  and commercial insurance, 57–58
  Family Birth Center, 174–175, 178
  and Golden Health, 46, 50–51, 58–61, 63–64, 66–67, 69
  and low-income/uninsured patients, 57–58, 60–61
  patient health insurance, 20–21, 49–50
  patient populations, 49–50
  patient satisfaction, 75
  as safety-net hospital, 61